Lecture Notes
Obstetrics and Gynaecology

Diana Hamilton-Fairley

MD, FRCOG
Consultant Obstetrician and Gynaecologist
Guy's and St Thomas's NHS Foundation Trust, London

Third Edition

WILEY-BLACKWELL

A John Wiley & Sons, Inc., Publication

This edition first published 2009, © 2009, 2004 by D. Hamilton-Fairley and © 1999 by Blackwell Science Ltd

Blackwell Publishing was acquired by John Wiley & Sons in February 2007. Blackwell's publishing program has been merged with Wiley's global Scientific, Technical and Medical business to form Wiley-Blackwell.

Registered office: John Wiley & Sons Ltd, The Atrium, Southern Gate, Chichester, West Sussex, PO19 8SQ, UK

Editorial offices: 9600 Garsington Road, Oxford, OX4 2DQ, UK
    The Atrium, Southern Gate, Chichester, West Sussex, PO19 8SQ, UK
    111 River Street, Hoboken, NJ 07030-5774, USA

For details of our global editorial offices, for customer services and for information about how to apply for permission to reuse the copyright material in this book please see our website at www.wiley.com/wiley-blackwell

The right of the author to be identified as the author of this work has been asserted in accordance with the Copyright, Designs and Patents Act 1988.

Library of Congress Cataloging-in-Publication Data

Hamilton-Fairley, Diana.
  Lecture notes. Obstetrics and gynaecology / Diana Hamilton-Fairley.—3rd ed.
     p. ; cm.
  Includes bibliographical references and index.
  ISBN 978-1-4051-7801-3 (pbk. : alk. paper)
  1. Obstetrics. 2. Gynecology. I. Title. II. Title: Obstetrics and gynaecology.
  [DNLM: 1. Obstetrics. 2. Gynecology. WQ 100 H217L 2008]
  RG526.C43 2008
  618–dc22
                                                2008023445

ISBN: 9781405178013

A catalogue record for this book is available from the British Library.

Set in 8/12 pt Stone Serif by SNP Best-set Typesetter Ltd., Hong Kong
Printed and bound in Singapore by Fabulous Printers Pte Ltd

1 2009

Contents

Preface

Welcome to the third edition of *Lecture Notes: Obstetrics and Gynaecology*, a book for medical, midwifery and nursing students as well as those in the early part of their professional careers, whether as midwives, general practitioners or specialists. The book aims to provide knowledge to understand, diagnose and treat the conditions that women may encounter throughout their lives, as well as the basic anatomy and physiology relevant to the subject.

This edition reflects the changes in practice that have taken place, including those more recently recommended in national guidelines in maternity from NICE and The Royal College of Obstetrics and Gynaecology. I have had the able assistance of two of our specialist trainees—Dr Inez von Rege and Dr Alexandra Tillett—in updating and correcting this edition. Their young minds have contributed some new spirit into the book and I hope that you will appreciate it as much as I do. Through them I have included an important section on the World Health Organization's Millennium Goals for maternity that demonstrate the stark contrasts that exist in maternity care across the world. Each edition causes me to realize that we are making progress in improving the health of women, through the increased use of simple medical regimens rather than surgery in gynaecology, and the emphasis on improved access to antenatal care with a wider range of services provided to care for the woman physically, psychologically and socially. This remains a luxury of the developed world, although increasing investment in simple health measures in the developing world will continue to reduce infant and maternal mortality and morbidity worldwide.

Feedback from the previous edition has led to an expansion of the sections on HIV and cardiac disease in pregnancy and the introduction of colour plates. I hope that these will enhance your ability to learn from this book. The sections on breast disease and genital infections have been updated and I am indebted to my colleagues once again for their contributions to the book.

Lecture Notes: Obstetrics and Gynaecology is now available in 64 different languages and I hope that those using it outside the UK will find it as useful in learning about this vital subject in health care although the content is largely based on the undergraduate and postgraduate curricula of British universities and training patterns. The health needs of women are similar throughout the world and providing the appropriate health care to them also leads to a healthier next generation of children.

I sincerely hope that this book helps you, the reader, understand, appreciate and learn about reproductive health care and that it may inspire some of you to decide to make the health care of women and their families your long-term career. If this book plays a part in either of these I shall be pleased.

Acknowledgements

I would like to thank Dr Wai Ching Loke, MRCP and Dr John White, FRCP, MD, Consultant in the genitourinary department of Guy's and St Thomas's Hospital for their revision of Chapter 6, Dr Sonji Clarke MRCOG for Chapter 11 and Mr Nicholas Beechey Newman, FRCS, MS, Senior Lecturer, Department of Endocrine Surgery, King's College Medical School, Guy's campus London, for his revision of Chapter 18. I would also like to thank my colleagues Dr Hilda Dunsmore, Mr Yacoub Khalaf MD, FRCOG, Mr Dattakumar Kunde MRCOG, Mr Toh-Lick Tan MRCOG and Alison Smith for providing the photographs and images used for the plates and within the text. I am as always indebted to the patience and detailed work of the editorial and publishing team of Blackwell Publishing.

List of abbreviations

AC abdominal circumference
AED antiepileptic drug
AF amniotic fluid
AFP α-fetoprotein
AIDS acquired immune deficiency syndrome
AIS androgen insensitivity syndrome
ALT alanine transaminase
APH antepartum haemorrhage
APS antiphospholipid syndrome
APTT activated partial thromboplastin time
ARM artificial rupture of the membranes
ASD atrial septal defect
AST aspartate transaminase
BMI body mass index
BPD biparietal diameter
BSO bilateral salpingo-oophorectomy
BV bacterial vaginosis
CAH congenital adrenal hyperplasia
CEA carcinoembryonic antigen
CEMACH Confidential Enquiry into Maternal and Child Health
CESDI Confidential Enquiry into Stillbirths and Deaths in Infancy
CIN cervical intraepithelial neoplasia
CMV cytomegalovirus
CNS central nervous system
CPD cephalopelvic disproportion
CRP C-reactive protein
CT computed tomography
CTG cardiotocograph
D&C dilatation and curettage
DCIS ductal carcinoma *in situ*
DIC disseminated intravascular coagulopathy
DOB date of birth
DUB dysfunctional uterine bleeding
DVT deep venous thrombosis
ECG electrocardiogram
ECV external cephalic version
EDD expected date of delivery
EFM electronic fetal monitoring

ELISA enzyme-linked immunoassay
FBC full blood count
FBS fetal blood sample
FFP fresh frozen plasma
FHR fetal heart rate
FL femur length
FNAC fine needle aspiration cytology
FNT fetal nuchal translucency
FPR false-positive rate
FSH follicle-stimulating hormone
GBS group B (β-haemolytic) streptococcal (infection)
GDM gestational diabetes mellitus
GH growth hormone
GIFT gamete intrafallopian tube transfer
GnRH gonadotrophin-releasing hormone
GFR glomerular filtration rate
GTN glyceryl trinitrate
GUM genitourinary medicine
HAART highly active antiretroviral therapy
HbA1c glycosylated haemoglobin
HC head circumference
hCG human chorionic gonadotrophin
HELLP haemolysis, elevated liver enzymes, low platelets
HIV human immunodeficiency virus 1
hPL human placental lactogen
HPV human papillomavirus
HRT hormone replacement therapy
HSV herpes simplex virus
ICSI intracytoplasmic sperm injection
IHD ischaemic heart disease
IPPV intermittent positive-pressure ventilation
IUCD intrauterine contraceptive device
IUD intrauterine death
IUGR intrauterine growth restriction
IUI *in utero* insemination
IUS intrauterine system
IVF *in vitro* fertilization
IVH intraventricular haemorrhage

IVU   intravenous urography
LBC   liquid-based cytology
LDH   lactate dehydrogenase
LDL   low-density lipoprotein
LFT   liver function test
LGV   lymphogranuloma venereum
LH   luteinizing hormone
LHRH   LH-releasing hormone
LLETZ   large loop excision of the transformation zone
LMW   low molecular weight
LMWH   low-molecular-weight heparin
LNMP   last normal menstrual period
LSCS   lower segment caesarean section
MCV   mean corpuscular volume
MCHb   mean corpuscular haemoglobin
MCHbC   mean corpuscular haemoglobin C
MMR   maternal mortality rate
MSU   midstream specimen of urine
MRI   magnetic resonance imaging
NAAT   nucleic acid amplification test
NICE   National Institute for Health and Clinical Excellence
NICU   neonatal intensive care unit
NNRTI   non-nucleoside analogue
NRTI   nucleoside analogue
NSAID   non-steroidal anti-inflammatory drug
NTD   neural tube defect
NtRTI   nucleotide analogue
OA   occipitoanterior
OC   oral contraceptive
OGTT   oral glucose tolerance test
OHSS   ovarian hyperstimulation syndrome
OP   occipitoposterior
OPCS   Office of Population Censuses and Surveys
OT   occipitotransverse
PA   pernicious anaemia
PAPP-A   pregnancy-associated plasma protein A
PI   protease inhibitor
PCOS   polycystic ovary syndrome
PCP   *Pneumocystis jiroveci* (formerly *carinii*) pneumonia
PCR   polymerase chain reaction
PET   pre-eclampsia toxaemia

PG   prostaglandin
PI   Pearl Index
PID   pelvic inflammatory disease
PIH   pregnancy-induced hypertension
PLP   prolonged latent phase
PMR/PNMR   perinatal mortality rate
POF   premature ovarian failure
POP   progesterone-only pill
PPH   postpartum haemorrhage
PPROM   preterm premature rupture of the membranes
PSA   prostate-specific antigen
PTT   partial thromboplastin time
RBC   red blood cell
RDS   respiratory distress syndrome
RMI   risk of malignancy index
RPR   rapid plasma reagin
SCC   squamous cell carcinoma
SCD   subacute combined degeneration
SCJ   squamocolumnar junction
SFH   symphysiofundal height
SGA   small for gestational age
SLE   systemic lupus erythematosus
STI   sexually transmitted infection
T_3 triiodothyronine
T_4 thyroxine
TAH   total abdominal hysterectomy
TB   tuberculosis
TED   thromboembolic deterrent
TENS   transcutaneous electrical nerve stimulation
TOP   termination of pregnancy
TPPA   *Treponema pallidum* particle agglutination
TSH   thyroid-stimulating hormone
TSI   thyroid-stimulating immunoglobulin
TV   *Trichomonas vaginalis*
UTI   urinary tract infection
VBAC   vaginal birth after caesarean section
VDRL   Venereal Disease Reference Laboratory
VIN   vulval intraepithelial neoplasia
VSD   ventricular septal defect
WCC   white cell count
WPC   woman police constable
WR   Wassermann reaction
ZIFT   zygote intrafallopian transfer

Chapter 1

Basic science

Female anatomy

A woman's body is less muscular than a man's body and therefore has a slighter skeleton to support the muscles. In the abdomen, the non-pelvic organs are similar and subject to the same diseases. Readers are therefore referred to books on general anatomy and this chapter is concerned with female pelvic anatomy. As much changes in pregnancy we introduce the pregnancy aspects in this chapter and Chapter 7.

Uterus (Box 1.1)

A hollow, muscle-walled organ in the pelvis communicating with each fallopian tube and, through its cervix, the vagina.
Pre-pregnancy: $7 \times 5 \times 3$ cm; weight, 40 g.
Full term: $30 \times 25 \times 20$ cm; weight, 1000 g.

Structure

The uterus is a muscle in three layers with vascular anastomoses between them:
1 Outer: thin, longitudinal, merging with ligaments

2 Middle: very thick, spiral muscle fibres with blood vessels between
3 Inner: thin, oblique with condensation at each cornu and at the upper and lower end of the cervical canal—the internal and external os.

Increase in size during pregnancy results mostly from hypertrophy of existing cells rather than an increase in number. Changes are stimulated by oestrogen and gradual stretch (maximum effective stretch about term).

The cavity of the uterus is lined by an epithelial layer (the endometrium), which undergoes changes in response to the steroids oestrogen and progesterone during the menstrual cycle in preparation for implantation of an embryo.

Blood supply (Fig. 1.1)

From the uterine and ovarian arteries, mostly the former. The uterine artery is a branch of the internal iliac artery. It runs in the lower edge of the broad ligament to the junction of the uterine body and cervix before running up the side of the uterus, giving off several branches into the myometrium. The ureter lies immediately beneath the uterine artery.

Cervix (Box 1.2)

Barrel-shaped canal at the bottom of the uterus (Fig. 1.2). Mostly connective tissue with muscle at

Lecture Notes: Obstetrics and Gynaecology, 3rd edition. By Diana Hamilton-Fairley. Published 2009 by Blackwell Publishing. ISBN: 978-1-4051-7801-3.

Box 1.1 Relations of the uterus

Peritoneum	The body and fundus are covered with peritoneum. In front, this is reflected to the upper surface of the bladder. Over the rest of the uterus, the attachment is dense and it cannot be stripped off the uterine muscle
Anterior	The uterovesical pouch and bladder
Lateral	The broad ligaments with their contents
Posterior	The pouch of Douglas
	The rectum

Box 1.2 Relations of the cervix above the attachment to the vagina

Anterior	Loose connective tissue
	Bladder
	Pubocervical ligaments
Lateral	The ureter 1 cm lateral to the cervix
	The uterine artery
	Uterine veins
	Parametrial lymph glands
	Nerve ganglia
	The transverse cervical ligament
Posterior	Peritoneum of the pouch of Douglas
	The uterosacral ligaments

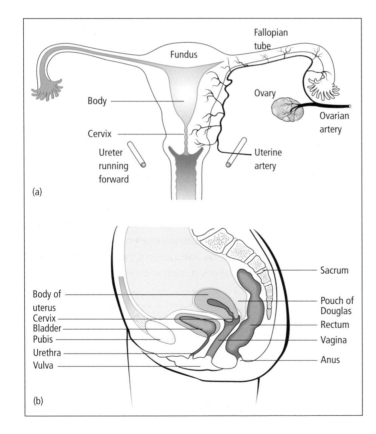

(a)

(b)

Figure 1.1 Relations of the uterus: (a) anteroposterior view; (b) lateral view. See also Box 1.1.

upper and lower ends (internal os and external os). In late pregnancy the ground substance of the connective tissue becomes less dense with a greater water content, and the cervix becomes softer clinically. The cervical canal is lined by columnar epithelium which undergoes squamous metaplasia at the external os. This is called the transformation zone and is the area where neoplasia can arise as the cells are constantly transforming from columnar to squamous epithelium. In the presence of high oestrogen levels (pregnancy, combined oral contraceptive pill) the transformation zone can be

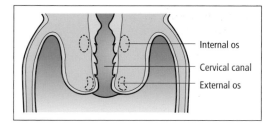

Figure 1.2 A longitudinal section of the cervix.

Internal os

Cervical canal

External os

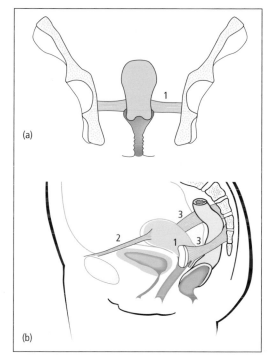

(a)

(b)

Figure 1.3 The ligamentous supports of the uterus: (a) frontal view; (b) lateral view. 1, transverse cervical ligament; 2, round ligaments; 3, uterosacral ligaments.

Box 1.3 Relations of the ovary

The ovary lies free in the peritoneal cavity

Anterior	The broad ligament
Posterior	The peritoneum of the posterior wall of the pelvis
	The common iliac artery and vein
	The internal iliac (hypogastric) artery
	The ureter
Lateral	Peritoneum over the obturator internus muscle
	The obturator vessels and nerve
	Further out, the acetabulum and hip joint
Above	The fallopian tube, which curls over the ovary
	Loops of bowel
On left	The pelvic colon and its mesentery
On right	The appendix if it dips into the pelvis

more difficult for sperm and bacteria to enter the uterus).

Ligaments

The uterus is supported by ligaments (Fig. 1.3). The principal supports of the uterus are the transverse cervical ligaments (cardinal ligaments), the uterosacral ligaments and the round ligament. The round ligament rises from the fundus of the uterus anterior to the fallopian tube and passes into the inguinal canal, ending in the labia majora. In pregnancy these ligaments are stretched and thickened. They soften because of the effect of progesterone and relaxin on collagen.

The broad ligament is made of two layers of peritoneum that run over the fallopian tubes anteriorly to the uterovesical reflection and posteriorly to the rectovaginal reflection.

Ovary (Box 1.3)

The ovaries have twin functions: steroid production and gametogenesis. They are a pair of organs on each side of the uterus, in close relation to the fallopian tubes. Each ovary is attached to the back of the broad ligament by a peritoneal fold, the mesovarium, which carries the blood supply, lymphatic drainage and nerve supply of the ovary. The

present on the outer surface of the cervix (an ectropion) whereas after the menopause it often retreats into the canal, making it more difficult to detect abnormal cells on a smear.

The cervix secretes fluid from glands present in the columnar epithelium. The nature of the secretion changes under the influence of oestrogen (making it thin and stretchy so that sperm can swim readily through it) and progesterone (more viscid and creamy coloured, making it

blood supply to the ovaries is principally from the ovarian arteries, which arise from the aorta just below the renal arteries. Medially the ovary is attached to the uterus by the infundibular/tubo-ovarian ligament.

The ovary is approximately 4 cm long, 3 cm wide and 2 cm thick and weighs about 10 g. A general view of the organs in the pelvis is shown in Fig. 1.1b.

Structure

The ovary has an outer cortex and inner medulla (Fig. 1.4) and consists of large numbers of primordial oocytes supported by a connective tissue stroma. It is covered by a single layer of cubical, germinal epithelium which is often missing in adult women. Beneath is the fibrous capsule of the ovary, the tunica albuginea, a protective layer derived from fibrous connective tissue.

The cortex of the ovary at menarche contains about 500 000 primordial oocytes which may become follicles—cysts about 0.1 mm in diameter. They have a single layer of granulosa cells that produce estradiol and specially differentiated theca cells that produce androgens.

The ovarian cycle is mediated through the hypothalamic pituitary axis (see p. 9). During each menstrual cycle many primordial follicles are recruited, but usually only one develops fully to become a mature graafian follicle and expels its oocyte. The granulosa cells multiply and secrete follicular fluid rich in oestrogen. The oocyte with its granulosa layer projects into the follicle (Fig. 1.4). The stroma cells outside the granulosa cell layer differentiate into:

- the theca interna (a weak androgen secretor)
- the theca externa (no hormone-secreting function).

Shortly before ovulation, meiosis is completed in the primary oocyte in response to the surge of luteinizing hormone (LH). The oocyte casts off the first polar body, resulting in the number of chromosomes in the remaining nucleus being reduced from 46 to 23. Thus the primary oocyte and the first polar body each contain the haploid number (23) of the chromosomes.

At this stage, the ripe follicle is about 20 mm in diameter. At ovulation it ruptures, releasing the oocyte usually into the fimbriated end of the fallopian tube.

The follicle in the ovary collapses, the granulosa cells become luteal cells whereas the theca interna forms the theca lutein cells. A corpus luteum develops and projects from the surface of the ovary. It can be recognized by the naked eye by its crinkled outline and yellow appearance. Its cells secrete oestrogen and progesterone. If the ovum is not

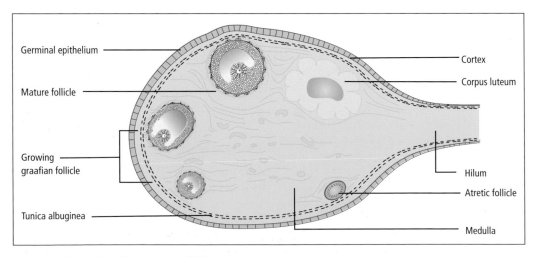

Figure 1.4 Maturation of the oocytes to follicles.

fertilized, the corpus luteum degenerates in about 10 days. A small amount of bleeding occurs into its cavity, the cells undergo hyaline degeneration and a corpus albicans is formed. If pregnancy does occur, the corpus luteum grows and may reach 3–5 cm in diameter. It persists for 80–120 days and then gradually degenerates.

The fallopian tube (Box 1.4)

The fallopian tube is the oviduct conveying sperm from the uterus to the point of fertilization and ova from the ovary to the uterine cavity. Fertilization usually takes place in the distal part of the tube. Plates 1 and 2 show the anatomy of the pelvis and the relationship between the ovary and tube visualized at laparoscopy.

The tube has four parts:

1 The intramural (cornual) part is 2 cm long and 1 mm in diameter.

2 The isthmus is thick walled, 3 cm long and 0.7 mm in diameter.

3 The ampulla is wide and thin walled, being about 5 cm long and 20 mm in diameter (Fig. 1.5).

4 The infundibulum is the lateral end of the tube. It is trumpet shaped and crowned with the fimbriae that surround the outer opening of the tube. The fimbriae stabilize the abdominal ostium over the ripening follicle in the ovary.

Structure

The tube has three coats:

1 An outer *serous* layer of peritoneum that covers the tube except in its intramural part and over a small area of its attachment to the broad ligament

2 A *muscle* layer with outer longitudinal and inner circular smooth muscles

3 The *mucosa* or endosalpinx that lines the tube and is thrown into numerous longitudinal folds or rugae. The rugae have a core of connective tissue covered with a tall columnar epithelium.

Three types of cell are found in the mucosa:

1 *Ciliated cells*, which beat a current usually in a medial direction

Box 1.4 **Relations of the fallopian tubes**	
Anterior	Top of the bladder
	Uterovesical peritoneal pouch
Superior	Coils of intestine
	On the right, caecum
	On the left, pelvic colon
Posterior	Ovary
	Pouch of Douglas and its contents
Lateral	Peritoneum over the obturator muscle
	Obturator vessels and nerve
Inferior	Structures in the broad ligament

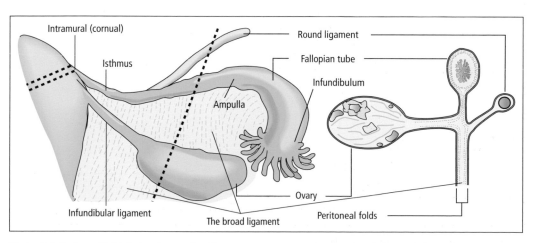

Figure 1.5 Peritoneal folds to two layers of peritoneum.

2 *Secretory cells*, which provide the secretion for the rapidly developing blastocyst, allowing exchange of oxygen, nutrients and metabolites

3 *Interciliary cells* with long narrow nuclei, squeezed between the other cells. There are rhythmic changes in the epithelium during the menstrual cycle; in the proliferative phase the cells increase in height and activity with increased secretions just after ovulation.

Vagina (Box 1.5)

The vagina is a fibromuscular canal extending from the vestibule of the vulva to the cervix, around which it is attached to form the fornices.

Structure

The anterior vaginal wall is about 10 cm long and the posterior wall 15 cm. It is capable of great distension, as in childbirth, after the prolonged hormonal stimulation of pregnancy. Normally, the anterior and posterior walls are in contact so the cavity is represented by an H-shaped slit.

Box 1.5 Relations of the vagina	
Anterior	The bladder and urethra
Posterior	Upper—the pouch of Douglas
	Lower—the rectum, separated by the recto-vaginal septum and perineal body
Lateral	The cardinal ligaments and the levator ani muscles

The walls have the following:
- An outer connective tissue layer to which the ligaments are attached—it contains blood vessels, lymphatics and nerves
- A muscular layer consisting of an outer longitudinal layer and an inner circular layer of variable thickness and function
- The epithelium of stratified squamous epithelium, which in women contains glycogen and is composed of three layers:
  — a basal layer
  — a functional layer
  — a cornified layer.

The epithelium undergoes cyclical changes during the menstrual cycle and characteristic changes during pregnancy. After the menopause it atrophies so that smears taken from postmenopausal women contain a high proportion of basal cells. There are no glandular cells in the vaginal epithelium and so the term 'vaginal mucosa' should not be used.

Vaginal fluid is composed of cervical secretion and transudation through the vaginal epithelium. The vagina allows colonization of lactobacilli which produce lactic acid from the glycogen in the epithelial cells.

Vulva

The vulva or external genitalia of the female includes the mons, labia major, clitoris, labia minor, vestibule, external urethra meatus, Bartholin's glands and hymen (Fig. 1.6).

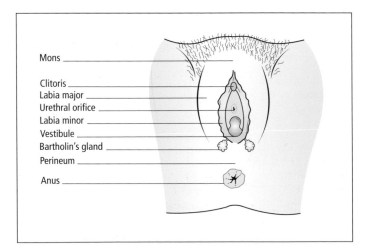

Mons

Clitoris
Labia major
Urethral orifice
Labia minor
Vestibule
Bartholin's gland
Perineum

Anus

Figure 1.6 The vulva.

The *mons* is a pad of fat that lies over the pubic symphysis. It is covered with skin in which hair grows profusely from puberty to the menopause.

The *labia major* are two folds of skin that enclose the vaginal opening. They are made up of fatty tissue that is very sensitive to oestrogen stimulation; the skin of the labia major is covered with hair after puberty.

The *clitoris* contains erectile tissue and is attached to the pubic arch by its crura. Folds of skin running forwards from the labia minor form the prepuce of the clitoris.

The *labia minor* are delicate folds of skin, containing fibrous tissue, numerous blood vessels and erectile tissue. The skin contains sebaceous glands, but no hair follicles, and epithelium that lines the vestibule and vagina.

The *vestibule* is the area between the labia minor into which opens the vagina, with the external meatus of the urethra in front and the ducts of Bartholin's glands behind.

The *external urethral meatus* is the opening of the urethra covered with squamous epithelium. Skene's ducts from the posterior urethral glands open on to the posterior margin of the meatus.

Bartholin's glands are a pair of glands, the ducts of which are lined by columnar epithelium. Each gland is the size of a pea and in structure the glands resemble salivary glands. The secretion is colourless and mucoid, and is produced mainly on sexual excitement.

The *hymen* is a circular or crescentic fold of squamous epithelium and connective tissue that partly closes the vaginal entrance in young women. Its shape and size vary. It is often ruptured or stretched by tampon insertion or intercourse; childbirth destroys it.

Perineum

The perineum is the area between the vaginal opening and the anus. The perineal body is a pyramidal mass of fibromuscular tissue into which the fibres of levator ani and the deep transverse perineal muscles are inserted. These are the muscles that are often torn or cut (episiotomy) during childbirth.

Bony pelvis

The false pelvis is to the true pelvis like a saucer on the top of a cup. The true pelvis is important in obstetrics; the false pelvis is not. Diameters of the true pelvis are shown in Fig. 1.7.

The longest axis of the pelvis changes through 90°, going from top to bottom. Hence the fetus passing through must rotate. There is a long curved posterior wall and a short anterior wall, so the fetus passing through takes a curved course (Fig. 1.8).

The three bones—two ilia and a sacrum—are held together at joints by ligaments (sacroiliac ligaments posteriorly and the symphysis anteriorly); these soften in pregnancy, allowing some laxity at these sites.

The coccyx is a fused group of the last vertebrae, hinged on the sacrum by a joint that easily allows bending back in childbirth.

Pelvic muscles

Lining lateral wall of pelvis
- Pyriformis
- Obturator internus.

Making pelvic diaphragm
- Levatores ani comprising:
  — pubococcygeus
  — iliococcygeus
  — ischiococcygeus.

Beneath pelvic diaphragm
- Anterior triangle:
  — deep perineal: compressor urethrae; deep transverse perinei
  — superficial perineal: ischiocavernosus; bulbocavernosus; superficial transverse perinei.
- Posterior triangle: sphincter ani.

Essentials of pelvic musculature

- The pyriformis muscles reduce the useful transverse diameter of upper and mid-cavities, thus thrusting the fetus forward.
- The pelvic diaphragm and its fascia are like a pair of cupped hands tilted slightly forward (Fig. 1.9).

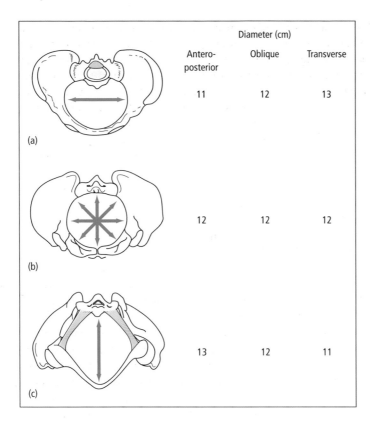

	Diameter (cm)		
	Antero-posterior	Oblique	Transverse
(a)	11	12	13
(b)	12	12	12
(c)	13	12	11

Figure 1.7 The bony pelvis: (a) inlet: longest diameter transverse, bean shaped; (b) midcavity: all diameters equal, circle; (c) outlet: longest diameter anteroposterior, diamond shaped.

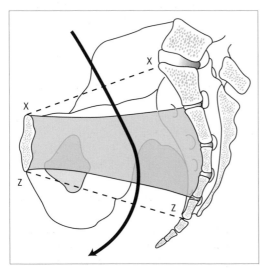

Figure 1.8 Side view of bony pelvis, showing the plane of the inlet (x–x), the zone of the midcavity (toned) and the plane of the outlet (z–z).

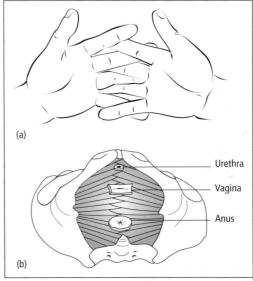

Urethra

Vagina

Anus

Figure 1.9 Interlocking hands (a) illustrate the lacing of the muscle fibres in the pelvic diaphragm (b).

Muscle fibres lace the one hand with the other, being especially thick around the three tubes which broach the diaphragm—the urethra, the vagina and the rectum. These muscle slings pull each of these forward making an extra sphincter.

Female physiology

The hypothalamic–pituitary–ovarian axis

The cyclical interaction of the hormones from the hypothalamus, anterior pituitary and the ovaries is shown in Fig. 1.10.

The ovarian cycle is determined by a complex series of biofeedback mechanisms that originate in the hypothalamus—a small area of the brain situated just above and anterior to the pituitary gland. The hypothalamus secretes a decapeptide called gonadotrophin-releasing hormone (GnRH) in a pulsatile fashion, which activates the production and secretion of follicle-stimulating hormone (FSH) and LH in the anterior pituitary. Its secretion is inhibited by high concentrations of oestrogen and progesterone.

Pituitary hormones

Follicle-stimulating hormone

FSH is a soluble glycoprotein. Production is activated by GnRH from the hypothalamus. FSH is produced in the anterior lobe of the pituitary gland and production is increased in the first half of the menstrual cycle, when oestrogen levels are low (positive feedback). This production is diminished by increasing oestrogen levels (negative feedback) (Fig. 1.11). FSH acts on the enzyme aromatase in the granulose cells surrounding the oocyte, converting testosterone (produced by the theca cells) into 17β-estradiol (E_2). This starts and maintains the recruitment of oocytes and their maturation.

Luteinizing hormone

LH is a soluble glycoprotein activated in the pituitary by GnRH. It acts on the theca cells at the start of the menstrual cycle to produce testosterone. As the follicle containing the oocyte grows under the influence of FSH, LH plays a role in choosing the dominant follicle and arresting the development of the other oocytes. As the oestrogen concentration rises, it reaches a level (800–1200 pmol/l) that causes LH to be released from the pituitary in a bolus at midcycle, initiating ovulation (rupture of the follicle and release of the oocyte) and completion of the first meiotic division. Ovulation takes place 36 hours after the LH surge. LH causes luteinization of the granulosa cells.

Ovary

There are seven million primordial oocytes in each ovary of the female fetus, which drops to two million at birth and is further reduced to half a million at puberty.

In each menstrual cycle over 400 primitive oocytes migrate to the surface of the ovaries under the influence of FSH. LH and FSH act in concert to select a single oocyte. When one follicle reaches approximately 20 mm in diameter, the oocyte is squeezed to the surface of the ovary (Fig. 1.12). The remaining follicles atrophy.

The process of ovulation is preceded by:
- the release of LH from the pituitary which initiates ovulation and completion of the first meiotic division
- a spurt of oestrogen from the tissues of the follicle.

The outward signs and changes associated with ovulation are:
- the cervical mucus becomes less viscid, becoming watery and increasing in amount
- in some women peritoneal pain is caused by irritation of released blood from the follicle (*mittelschmerz*)
- the body temperature may increase by about 0.6°C.

At ovulation the break in the follicle reseals and fluid builds up again to form a corpus luteal cyst. The large surge in LH causes a metabolic change in the granulosa cells so that they start to produce progesterone as well as oestrogen. This has a profound effect on the endometrium, which readies

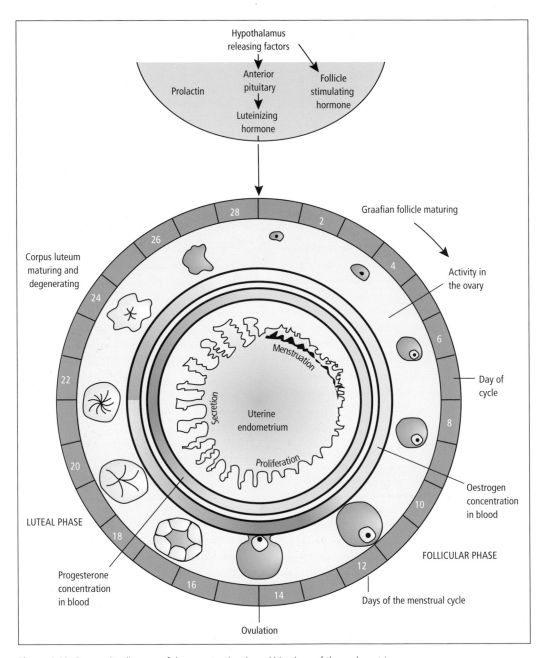

Figure 1.10 Composite diagram of the menstrual cycle and histology of the endometrium.

itself to accept an embryo 7–8 days after ovulation.

The oocytes that are unselected degenerate at a steady rate. At menopause there are no more follicles available for ovulation and so there is diminution of oestrogen production.

Fertilization

The fimbriated end of the fallopian tube, possibly excited by chemotaxis, closes to embrace the ovary like a hand holding a rugby football. The egg has virtually no transperitoneal passage.

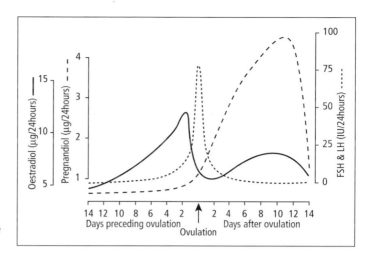

Figure 1.11 Hormone levels before and after ovulation.

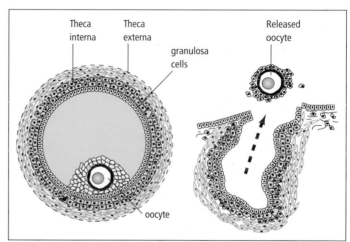

Figure 1.12 The follicle just before and just after the oocyte is released.

At the time of intercourse millions of sperms are deposited in the vagina. They travel in all directions, some through the cervix, where, in midcycle, the molecules of cervical mucus untangle their barbed-wire-like morphology to assume straight lines. A few sperm reach each fallopian tube where they swim countercurrent, the first arriving near the oocyte within 30 minutes of intercourse. One sperm only penetrates the zona pellucida by hyaluronidase activity; the tail is shed, the sperm's neck becomes the centrosome and the head is the male pronucleus containing half the genetic potential of the future fetus (Fig. 1.13).

Sperm penetration into the ovum initiates the second meiotic division of the ovum, with a reduction in chromosomes from 46 to 23 and the extrusion of a second polar body. The haploid nuclei of the oocyte and the sperm combine, restoring the diploid state of 46 chromosomes and fertilization is achieved.

Fertilization usually occurs at the ampullary end of the fallopian tube within 12–24 hours of oocyte production. The fertilized egg then travels along the tube propelled by:

- muscular peristalsis of the tube
- currents in the tube whipped by cilia.

During this period, nutrition and oxygenation are from the fluid secreted by the glandular cells of the fallopian tube lining. Arriving in the uterus 4–5 days later, the egg is in the cavity for 2–3 days and implants in the thick endometrium in the secretory phase on about day 22 of the cycle. The blastocyst starts to put out pseudopodia so that the surface area available for maternofetal exchange is increased. All transfer is by osmosis and diffusion at this stage.

Major ovarian hormones

Oestrogens

These are mostly produced by the maturing follicle. Levels gradually increase to a peak at the time of ovulation (Fig. 1.14).

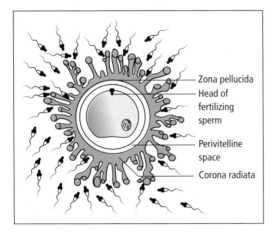

Figure 1.13 Several sperm surround the oocyte, but only one penetrates.

The recognized functions of oestrogens are to:
- stimulate growth of the vagina, uterus and oviducts in childhood
- increase the thickness of the vaginal wall and distal third of the urethra by increased stratification of the epithelium
- reduce vaginal pH by the action of Doderlein's bacillus on the glycogen to form lactic acid
- decrease viscosity of cervical mucus to facilitate sperm penetration
- facilitate the development of primordial follicles
- inhibit FSH secretion
- stimulate proliferation of the endometrium
- increase myometrial contractility
- stimulate growth of breasts with duct proliferation
- promote calcification of bone
- promote female fat distribution
- promote female hair distribution.

Oestrogen is metabolized by the liver and conjugated with glucuronic acid so that 65% is excreted in urine.

Progesterone

This hormone is produced by the corpus luteum in large amounts after ovulation and by the placenta in pregnancy. Its functions are to:

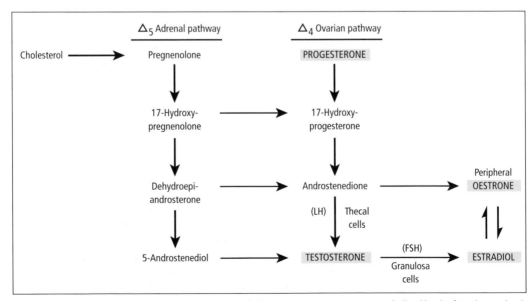

Figure 1.14 Pathways of oestrogen metabolism. Estradiol is a pregnancy oestrogen metabolized by the fetoplacental unit and does not appear here. FSH, follicle-stimulating hormone; LH, luteinizing hormone.

- induce endometrial secretory changes
- increase the growth of the myometrium in pregnancy
- decrease myometrial activity in pregnancy
- increase secretory activity in the uterine tubes
- decrease motility of the uterine tubes
- increase the glandular activity in the breasts.

Progesterones are metabolized in the liver; 80% becomes pregnanediol.

The endometrium during the menstrual cycle

The endometrium is the end organ of these changes responding to the changes in oestrogen and progesterone. Any disruption that occurs in the process of ovulation will cause a change in the pattern of bleeding experienced by the woman, which may lead to her seeking medical help.
- The production of oestrogen and later oestrogen and progesterone by the ovaries results in changes in the endometrium.
- The *endometrium* is the mucous membrane of the uterus, consisting of tubular glands with supporting stroma. There are numerous blood vessels that arise from the spiral arterioles, the terminal branches of the uterine arteries.
- The endometrium rests on the *uterine musculature*; its basal areas are so closely applied that they cannot be removed with a curette but can be reached at endometrial ablation.
- The *basal layer* comprises tubular glands that regenerate after menstruation.
- The *superficial compact layer* is covered with ciliated columnar epithelial cells, which extend down into the endometrial glands.

Changes in the menstrual cycle

At the end of menstruation, the endometrium enters a short resting phase, when it is thin, its glands are straight and the stroma compact and non-vascular. As oestrogen levels rise, the endometrium enters a proliferative phase with the endometrial glands becoming more tortuous, although the arterioles remain relatively straight; the stroma becomes cellular.

After ovulation, the corpus luteum is formed under the influence of LH; it secretes oestrogen and progesterone. In the luteal phase, the endometrium becomes secretory; it is thick, pale and glycogen appears in the glands, which in turn become full of secretions. The glands become more tortuous and the arterioles become more tightly coiled like springs.

If the ovum is fertilized
The endometrium grows to become the decidua of pregnancy. Stroma cells swell. Implantation occurs on the decidua, which provides nutrition for the rapidly developing blastocyst.

In the absence of fertilization
About 12–14 days after ovulation, there is an intense spasm of the endometrial arterioles leading to tissue hypoxia and death in the superficial layers. Fissuring of the endometrium follows with cleavage of the endometrium from its spongy layer. It is shed in small areas with accompanying bleeding—the menstrual loss. After this, regeneration occurs from the remaining basal layer and the cycle recommences.

The fallopian tubes

Their functions are to:
- convey a spermatozoon from the endometrial cavity to the ovum in the outer third of the fallopian tube
- transmit the fertilized oocyte into the endometrial cavity
- provide nutrients to the developing embryo on its 5-day passage.

Oestrogen increases the peristalsis of the tubes; at the time of ovulation there is a reversal of peristalsis to help the sperm travel more easily up the crypts between the folds of the mucus.

The oocyte is squeezed out of the follicle and sticks to the surface of the ovarian fimbria of the tube. The fimbria embraces the ovary and the oocyte moves directly into the fallopian tube with no transperitoneal journey. Fertilization is by a single sperm penetrating the zona pellucida.

Peristalsis of the muscle of the tube and the action of fine cilia move oviduct fluid and the passive ovum from the peritoneal end of the fallopian tube into the endometrial cavity, taking about 5 days.

During this passage, the fertilized ovum receives nutrition from secretions of the mucosa of the tube. Here gas exchange between the rapidly growing blastocyst and fallopian tube fluid also takes place. These tubal secretions are under the influence of oestrogen priming and increase greatly with progesterone. Mucopolysaccharide concentration and the calcium ions within the tubes also increase.

The vulva and vagina

The vagina is a tube lined by stratified squamous epithelium, which contains no mucous glands so there are no vaginal secretions. Any lubrication is a combination of secretions from the cervical canal mixed with secretions from vulval glands and a transudate from the vagina.

The labia minor are normally in apposition as are the fatter labia major in normal standing, sitting and lying down positions, only parted when the legs abduct.

Sexual activity

On sexual stimulation, there is a vascular engorgement of the labia major and minor and the clitoris. The sweat glands of the labia minor increase their secretions and at the same time mucus is secreted from Bartholin's glands and the endocervical glandular epithelium.

Abduction of the thighs opens the labia major and the voluntary musculature of the vagina and vulva helps to dilate the upper vagina while gripping the penis in the lower vagina.

The sexual response in women is usually slower than in men, but a plateau of response is more prolonged and it does not disappear so rapidly after orgasm as is often the case in men.

Part 1

The Woman

Chapter 2

The woman as a patient

Attitudes of women

Obstetricians and gynaecologists look after women who for the most part are not seriously ill. In obstetrics most are completely healthy and experiencing a normal physiological process in growing and delivering a new individual. In gynaecology women attend because they are having problems that are interfering with their daily lives but are rarely life threatening. The attitudes of women towards their medical attendants have changed in the last 50 years. The subservient doctor-knows-best approach has been modified among young and intelligent women who ask more questions. They are more informed about medical matters because of press articles and the television, radio and internet. They query the authority of the doctor more, not because they mistrust him or her but to ensure that they understand their condition.

In the 1960s there was a more aggressive approach by women asking for more recognition. This had its major opportunity with the onset of oral contraception, which for the first time put fertility squarely in the hands of women. Here too was a release from the doctor's benevolent paternalism.

Lecture Notes: Obstetrics and Gynaecology, 3rd edition. By Diana Hamilton-Fairley. Published 2009 by Blackwell Publishing. ISBN: 978-1-4051-7801-3.

About 70% of women prefer to be ·looked after by female doctors. This is understandable and, if staff ratios allow, this should be attended to.

Clinical approach

Doctors should remember the sensitive nature of gynaecological and obstetric problems, which are very personal to women. No woman wants to visit the gynaecologist but she does if she thinks that it would help. The attitude towards the obstetrician is mollified by the fact that women realize that there are two patients, and that problems may arise in pregnancy for both the mother and the fetus. In general, difficulties can be assuaged by allowing more time for such consultation. Many find it difficult to discuss the intimate sexual details of their lives with doctors, so tact and discretion are needed. Often, further more difficult personal details may come out while the examination is being performed or at the next visit.

When examining a female patient, all doctors should have a chaperone, who does not need to be present during the history but could be introduced at the time of the examination. The attitude of the doctor towards the woman is terribly important and can set the whole tone of the relationship. Friendly, but not affectionate, should be the tone of the doctor's behaviour.

Women's choice

The Patient's Charter issued by the Department of Health has raised expectations about women's choice of doctors. The general practitioners in a given area look after their population of men and women usually with complete confidence on both sides, but provision has been made for the rotation between practices of those who do not wish to accept the management and treatment protocols of a given practice.

When a woman has to be referred to hospital, she may request that she goes to a certain unit. This applies mostly in the big towns, because in rural areas there is usually only one district general hospital. There again the woman may request to see (or not see) any given consultant for her own reasons. In the outpatient department this can usually be arranged, but not at an emergency level where consultants work to a rota.

The presence of junior doctors or medical students at teaching hospitals is being highlighted at the moment. Naturally women want privacy, but, when it is explained to them that these are the doctors of the future, they usually understand and agree to them being present.

Ethics

Ethics is the science of morals but probably is better interpreted as the rules of conduct recognized in certain departments of human life. Those in the medical profession owe an ethical duty to do their best for those who seek their care. In latter years the subject has moved more towards developing evidence based medicine and working with agreed guidelines. In obstetrics and gynaecology there are particular areas of practice which may challenge the ethical and/or cultural beliefs of the doctor. These include the questions surrounding new technologies that enable previously infertile couples to conceive, and the rights of a woman to end a pregnancy within British Law (the Abortion Act of 1967 and its amendment in 1990). The doctor has a duty to provide women with access to such care by referral to a suitable practitioner/practice regardless of their own personal view. The doctor does retain the right not to provide such treatment and so can ask not to attend those clinics.

In an increasingly multicultural community such as that of the United Kingdom where there are people from many different cultures with different belief systems, rituals and cultural norms it is very important that the health care professionals and the systems they work within are sensitive to the individuals needs. They must however ensure that they are offering the best care that is available for that woman and her family.

Generally speaking, the ethics of medicine are covered by the General Medical Council, the British Medical Association and the Ethical Committees of the various Colleges including the Royal College of Obstetricians and Gynaecologists. Details proliferate but a central principle remains that you should do unto others as you would they should do unto you. Always imagine your mother or your daughter as the patient and how you would like them to be treated. This will generally lead to good ethical behaviour.

The pregnant woman

When a woman becomes pregnant she usually consults her family doctor first. There may be records going back many years and the doctor may know the woman from previous medical encounters. There is often already a rapport between the doctor and the woman. Although many of the items needed in the antenatal record for the history are already in the practice records, it is wise to keep a pro forma especially for each pregnancy with summaries of detailed notes held elsewhere.

A National Maternity Record has now been developed in the UK, which has three chapters that build into the record of the whole pregnancy—the antenatal, intrapartum and postnatal periods. With team obstetrics becoming common, midwives need to know of certain events in a woman's life. This raises the complication of the inclusion of events of a sensitive nature such as previous terminations of pregnancy or sexually transmitted infections. Practitioners must seek the permission of the woman as to how much of this goes into the woman's hand-held notes, but for obvious reasons this should be as complete as possible. If the woman wishes to keep confidential essential pieces of information that may affect the clinical management, marks such as an asterisk or euphemisms should be recorded in her notes that will alert your colleagues. For example, if a woman does not wish her HIV status to be recorded, it is acceptable to write that the woman should not have an instrumental delivery or breastfeed. This will clearly indicate to both midwives and doctors that she is HIV positive, but will not mean anything to a non-medically trained person who may see her notes.

If the woman attends an antenatal clinic where she is not known, one has to start from the beginning. The history, examination and investigation of the woman are taken at the booking clinic when she attends for the first time in pregnancy (see Chapter 9). Ideally, this should be at 8–10 weeks of gestation but more often in Britain it has slipped to 12–14 weeks, hence invalidating all the help that can be offered to the woman in the first trimester and passing the time when teratogenesis might have been avoided.

The gynaecological patient

Most women in their lives will consult a doctor about gynaecological symptoms. Initially this will be with a GP. If the condition warrants, the woman may be referred to a hospital gynaecologist. Whether specialist or GP, the same logical processes must be used to make a diagnosis and direct management. (The obstetric assessment is discussed in Chapter 9.)

The gynaecological assessment will be considered under three headings:
- History
- Examination
- Investigations.

History

This is best considered under systematic headings so that no important symptoms are omitted. It is often necessary to ask leading questions:
- The woman herself may not realize the significance of her symptoms

- She may be reluctant to mention symptoms connected with sexual troubles

The following is a useful pro forma.

Personal information
- Name, age, date of birth
- Married, single, widowed, divorced, separated
- Occupation past and present
- Hours and conditions of work
- Partner's occupation
- Type of housing/financial support.

Chief symptom
- Duration
- Periodicity
- Severity and description.

Any treatment of present complaint so far
All drugs taken recently must be noted, especially tranquillizers, oral contraceptives, hormones and antibiotics.

History of past major illness or operations
- All admissions to hospital/operations with approximate dates
- All illnesses requiring regular medication (eg asthma/hypertension)
- A written report obtained from another hospital may be helpful, especially with conditions such as infertility, to check what has been done.

Social history
- Home conditions (including nature and state of relationships with other people in the residence)
- Conditions of work
- Occupation
- Smoking habits
- Alcohol habits
- Drugs (cannabis, etc).

Family history
- Health of parents and siblings
- History of hereditary or familial disease.

Sexual history
- Dyspareunia
- Difficulty with coitus

- Use of contraception
- Sexually transmitted infections.

Obstetric history
- Number of pregnancies
- Dates
- Mode of termination of each, ie full-term birth, premature birth, stillbirth, miscarriage, ectopic pregnancy
- Abnormalities of:
  — pregnancy
  — labour
  — puerperium
- Birth weights of children and their sex (names are more personal)
- Their present state of health.

Menstruation
- Age at onset (menarche)
- Approximate duration of each menstrual bleed
- Interval from the first day of one to the first day of the next period
- Estimate of amount and character of loss
- Any recent change:
  — increase
  — decrease
  — clots or flooding
- Any pain associated with menstruation
- Date of last period
- Date of last cervical smear and the result.

Vaginal discharge
- Character of discharge:
  — mucoid
  — purulent
  — colour
  — quantity
  — bloodstained
- Discharge may be offensive or may cause:
  — soreness
  — irritation.

Micturition
- Frequency, day and night
- Pain on micturition
- Urge incontinence (micturition must occur on the urge)
- Stress incontinence (loss occurs on virtually any physical effort)

Bowels
- Regularity
- Use of purgatives
- Any history of piles, pain or difficulty on defecation
- Rectal bleeding.

Examination

The general appearance of the patient should be observed:
- Height
- Weight: calculate body mass index (BMI):

$$BMI = weight/height^2$$

(Normal range 19–25 kg/m^2)
- Does she look anxious or ill?

A systematic examination is made with special attention to the reproductive system.
- The lower eyelid mucous membrane should be inspected for anaemia.
- The breasts should be examined in women aged over 35 years (see Chapter 18).
- Other relevant symptoms, such as breathlessness or cough, call for examination of the heart and lungs.

Abdominal examination

The patient should be asked to empty her bladder before you examine her abdomen and pelvis. The abdomen should be exposed from the costal margin to the pubes and the patient should lie comfortably relaxed. A sheet or light blanket over the pubis is used to prevent unnecessary exposure.

Inspection
- Skin quality and fat or wasting
- Distension or any visible tumour
- Operation scars, especially a laparoscopy crescent at the umbilicus and/or lower abdomen, a curved low transverse scar for pelvic surgery (caesarean section or other open gynaecological procedure).

Palpation

This is done lightly at first to test for any localized tenderness or rigidity. Deep palpation is used to confirm the presence of a tumour or enlargement, especially of the uterus or ovaries. In the acute situation tenderness, guarding and rebound tenderness should be noted.

Percussion

If there is a central tumour it will be dull to percussion with hollow sounds from the flanks. Ascites may produce shifting dullness in the flanks and central resonance.

Auscultation

Although this will rarely help, it may give reassurance about intestinal activity, and bowel sounds may be heard. Fetal heart sounds may help make a diagnosis of pregnancy using a handheld Doppler machine after 12 weeks.

Pelvic examination

A chaperone should always be present when you perform a vaginal examination to act as an advocate for the woman and potentially to protect the doctor (male and female) from accusations of assault or inappropriate behaviour. You should offer a full explanation of the examination that you are about to perform. Verbal consent should be obtained from the woman in the presence of a chaperone. Before starting the examination, ensure that you have all the necessary equipment—speculum, swabs, spatulas/cytobrushes, slides—that you may require ready (Plate 3). If you are going to perform a cervical smear ensure that the slide is labelled in pencil (the fixative dissolves ink from biros and pens), or if using liquid-based cytology the pot is labelled with the patient's name, date of birth, hospital number/NHS number if she has one and the date of the examination before taking the smear.

The vagina

Vaginal examination can usually be satisfactorily performed by using the index finger alone. This causes less discomfort and muscle spasm. If the vagina is long or voluminous or your fingers are small, a second finger may be needed. The finger(s) should be inserted slowly up to the level of the cervix.

Assessment is by bimanual examination, the other hand being placed on the abdomen above the pubic symphysis. A three-dimensional image of the pelvis is built up from information obtained from both hands, not just the vaginal one (Fig. 2.1).

The vulva

The vulva is inspected for:
- swelling
- inflammation
- ulceration.

The urethra

The urethral orifice is inspected for:
- urethritis
- caruncle.

The patient is asked to cough or strain and any prolapse or stress incontinence of urine is noted.

Examination with a speculum

This is an essential part of the gynaecological examination. If it must be omitted because the vaginal entrance is too small or because of vaginismus, the examination is incomplete.

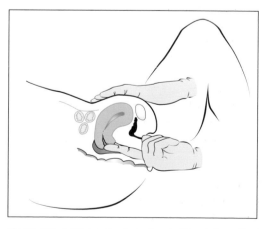

Figure 2.1 A bimanual examination gathers information about the pelvis with both hands.

The *bivalve speculum* (Cusco's) consists of two limbs jointed at the handle; it is made in various sizes and is useful for general cervical and upper vaginal examination (Fig. 2.2). It is also made in a disposable plastic form. Holding back the posterior wall with *Sim's speculum* gives a good view of the cervix and anterior vaginal wall (Fig. 2.3). The woman should be in the left lateral position (see p. 301).

When passing a speculum, it is important to remember that the vagina is directed upwards and backwards; warming a speculum under warm water makes it more comfortable.

The labia should be separated and Cusco's speculum lubricated with a small amount of aqueous jelly and gently inserted through the forchette. By maintaining gentle pressure the speculum will advance until the forward prong of the handle is reached. The two prongs should then be gently squeezed together to open the blades. The cervix should be visible at this point. If the uterus is very anteverted, it may take a few moments for the cervix to rotate between the blades. Moving the speculum to obtain a good view of the cervix should be done gently and slowly.

Sim's speculum is used to assess prolapse. The woman is placed in Sim's position. She is asked to lie on her left side with her superior shoulder falling forward so that she is semi-prone (see Fig 22.2). The lower leg should be naturally bent with the upper leg bent up towards her chest. The chaperone may help by holding the upper leg to part the labia. The speculum is lubricated beneath its lower surface and gently introduced along the posterior wall of the vagina. Any prolapse of the anterior wall will be seen bulging into the speculum. The cervix should be visible and its distance from the introitus noted. The patient should be asked to cough and any descent of the uterus or loss of urine noted. The speculum can then be gently rotated through 180° to view the posterior wall. The condition of the vagina should also be noted (well oestrogenized, atrophic, ulcerated).

Bimanual examination

When a cervical smear or a high vaginal swab is to be taken, it is best to pass the speculum before making a bimanual examination. This examination may be performed in the dorsal or left lateral position, a matter of personal preference among gynaecologists. In either case the patient should be spared unnecessary exposure by covering her with a sheet or light blanket. The gloved index finger may be lightly lubricated and is introduced gently into the vagina.

- The condition of the vaginal walls is noted
- The cervix is palpated for softening, tears or polyps—placing the finger behind the cervix and gently pushing upwards with the other hand palpating the abdomen just above the symphysis
- The uterus is palpated between the two hands noting:
  — size
  — consistency
  — shape

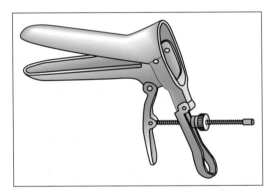

Figure 2.2 A bivalve or Cusco's speculum used to examine the cervix with the woman in the dorsal position.

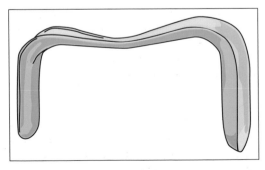

Figure 2.3 Sim's speculum used to hold back the posterior vaginal wall with the woman in the left lateral position.

— mobility
— tumours
— tenderness on pressure.

The finger in the vagina is now moved into the right lateral fornix; the hand on the abdomen follows to explore for any enlargement or tenderness of the tubes or ovaries. A similar examination is made of the left adnexa. The finger is passed to the posterior fornix to detect swelling in the pouch of Douglas.

If the woman complains of tenderness, the internal finger can move the uterus first to the left and then the right by pushing the cervix in the opposite direction. This is called testing for cervical excitation and, when present, often indicates tubal distension or an ovarian cyst.

Rectal examination

This can be valuable in certain aspects of gynaecology, but the patient may find it the most uncomfortable part of the whole examination. It permits bimanual examination of the uterus, tubes and ovaries if vaginal examination is impossible or undesirable. It may further be easier to feel a retroverted uterus or a swelling in the pouch of Douglas and allows an easier approach to the parametrium and uterosacral ligaments. The possibility of rectal disease must always be borne in mind.

Investigations

Blood

The haemoglobin level should always be measured before an operation, however minor. It should certainly be done in cases of excessive uterine bleeding (menorrhagia) and as a routine in early pregnancy. Blood disorders may be associated with a bleeding tendency so a platelet count, bleeding time and clotting time may also be done.

In black women, a sickle test should be done, and in women of Mediterranean or Middle Eastern origin there may be a thalassaemia trait that is diagnosed by electrophoresis.

Serological tests for syphilis, hepatitis and human immunodeficiency virus 1 (HIV-1) anti-bodies are done after counselling if there is any suspicion of any of these.

Blood urea and other tests for renal function should be done where indicated.

Human chorionic gonadotrophin (hCG) levels may be checked if a urinary pregnancy test is positive and a pregnancy cannot be seen on ultrasound. Other hormone levels in the blood may be measured in specific conditions. Their ranges are wide.

Urine

The urine should be tested as appropriate for:
• albumin
• sugar
• bacilluria by nitrite dipstick
• microscopy and culture.

Cytology

Exfoliative cytology in gynaecology examines cells desquamated from the epithelium of the genital tract. Material may be obtained by scraping the cervix with Ayre's wooden spatula, or a cytobrush. In the last few years liquid-based cytology has been introduced which uses a different spatula and specific methods for obtaining the specimen. In units where this is used (becoming universal within the UK) staff are specifically trained in how to take the sample. Cytology is principally used in the early detection of premalignant lesions of the cervix and is considered in Chapter 19.

Colposcopy

Colposcopy examines the cervix under magnification in the outpatient department. It is used together with cervical cytology so that biopsies can be accurately taken from suspicious areas and treatment performed (see Chapter 19).

Laparoscopy (Plate 1)

Visual examination of the pelvis and peritoneal cavity is invaluable when investigating pain or fertility potential. It is increasingly used for operations that used to be done as open abdominal procedures. The operating time is the same or longer than an open operation in some cases, but the reduction in postoperative pain and recovery time makes the benefit to the patient far outweigh the small loss in numbers of operations that can be done in a session.

Hysteroscopy

Endoscopy of the uterine cavity demands a fluid or gas under pressure to open up the cavity. Then the endometrium can be inspected and biopsied. Polyps and submucosal fibroids can be removed through the hysteroscope. Menorrhagia can be treated with instruments attached to the hysteroscope by removal or ablation of the endometrium.

Ultrasound

Abdominal or vaginal probes may be used. Transvaginal probes are preferred because the quality of the image is greatly improved. The uterine size is measured, and any fibroids or other abnormalities of the myometrium are noted and measured. The endometrial thickness is measured, and its consistency and shape are also noted. If there is any irregularity it can be further examined by introducing fluid into the cavity. Special fluids have been developed that can be seen travelling through the tubes so that tubal patency can be checked at the same time.

The ovarian morphology is noted and any ovarian cysts measured. These may be functional (part of the normal cyclical changes in the development and release of the oocyte) or pathological. Pathological cysts may have certain features that help to determine whether it is malignant—whether it has solid elements, its vascularity, the echogenicity of the fluid and its heterogeneity, its size and regularity of shape—or benign. The size of the tumour can be estimated accurately by measuring it in two planes: transverse and longitudinal (Fig. 2.4).

Ultrasound is used to monitor the progress of ovulation in assisted conception. A follicle can be found from day 10 of the cycle and its development monitored by a daily scan. When the follicle reaches 20 mm it is close to ovulation and is the best time for conception or the harvesting of oocytes. After ovulation the corpus luteum can be shown in the ovary.

Using ultrasound, a hydatidiform mole can be detected; the vesicles reflect echoes leaving a picture of a series of multiple semicircular reflections, rather like bubble foam/wrap. There is usually no fetus or fetal heartbeat.

In early pregnancy, an embryonic sac and/or yolk sac may be seen by five weeks with both embryonic tissue and heartbeat usually visible by 6 weeks. An early fetal death can be detected if a sac is present but no fetus. The scan should be repeated a week later and, if an empty sac is still found or a fetus but no heartbeat, a firm diagnosis made.

Ultrasound can be used in the diagnosis of ectopic pregnancy. Ultrasound may show a cystic area separate from the uterus, but free blood in the pouch of Douglas with an empty uterus and a positive pregnancy test raises high suspicion.

Doppler ultrasound examination can detect deep vein thromboses in the legs or pelvis.

Magnetic resonance imaging (MRI)

Pelvic tumours are seen easily; tumour invasion from the endometrium, the cervix or from the ovary can be seen on different cross-sections, enabling staging of these growths to be made without an invasive operation (Fig. 2.5). MRI is useful for delineating fibroids and adenomyosis. It is also used in pregnancy to image the fetus, particularly

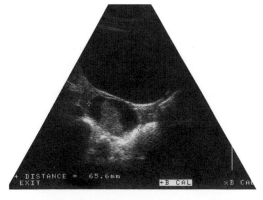

Figure 2.4 An ultrasound scan of an ovarian tumour.

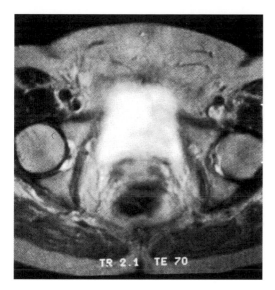

Figure 2.5 MRI of a pelvic tumour. (With acknowledgement to Dr Christine Heron, Radiological Department, St George's Hospital.)

if an intracerebral or skeletal abnormality or a tumour is suspected.

Computed tomography (CT)

These allow the visualization of many pelvic tumours to assess their position, size and consistency and any associated lymphadenopathy. It is increasingly used in conjunction with positron emission tomography (PET), which shows hotspots where malignant deposits may be present. CT is used to pinpoint the location of the hotspots.

X-rays

Straight films of the abdomen can show:
• gas and fluid levels in the obstructed intestine
• calcium in the urinary tract or dermoid ovarian tumour
• radio-opaque dye instillation shows the outline of the uterine cavity and spill seen from the fimbriated ends indicates patency of the tubes at fertility investigations.

Intravenous urography

The diagnosis of pelvic tumours and renal tract disease may be helped by intravenous urography. Before radical operations in the pelvis the course of the ureters can be checked. It may also be used to identify renal tract abnormalities associated with abnormalities of the genital tract.

Barium studies

A barium enema may be helpful in the diagnosis of rectal conditions. A barium meal with follow-through to the ileocaecal region may be useful in cases where symptoms are right sided.

Pelvic lymphangiography

By injecting radio-opaque contrast material into the lymphatics in the foot, the lymphatic drainage of the lower limb and pelvis is outlined. It is useful to detect secondaries in the lymph glands from malignant disease in the pelvis.

Ventilation/perfusion scan

This is used to detect a pulmonary embolism along with serum estimation of D-dimers. Sometimes a spiral CT scan of the chest may be used.

Part 2

The Young Woman

Chapter 3

Puberty and menstrual problems of young women

Puberty defines the period in a girl's life when she undergoes a series of physiological changes that lead to the achievement of sexual maturity and the ability to reproduce.

There are three phases of change:

1 *Adrenarche*: increased production of androgens by the adrenal glands which are converted centrally by the liver and ovaries and peripherally in the adipose tissue to oestrogens. This usually starts at the age of 8–10 years and leads to:
  - increased sebaceous gland activity
  - sweating
  - hair growth
  - pubic hair, which follows axillary hair.
2 *Sexual characteristics*:
  - Usually start at the age of 9–11 years.
  - Breast development usually precedes pubic hair growth and takes 5–6 years to reach Tanner's stage 5 (Fig. 3.1).
  - Pubic hair growth takes only 3 or 4 years and so is often complete before breast development.
  - Menarche usually coincides with breast development to Tanner's stage 3.
  - Average age of menarche in the UK is 12.9 years. It is earlier in countries nearer the equator.

3 *Growth*: the onset of puberty coincides with a rapid increase in growth velocity:
  - In girls growth gain is 25–28 cm and in boys 26–30 cm. Boys go through puberty later than girls and therefore start their growth spurt from a higher starting point, which accounts for their greater adult height.
  - The pituitary gland increases its frequency of pulsed growth hormone (GH) and luteinizing hormone (LH). The mechanism of this is unknown.
  - The greatest release of GH and LH is at night during sleep; this may account for the increased need for sleep in adolescents.
  - The increase in LH acts on the thecal cells of the ovary to increase androgen production. This starts the maturation of the oocytes in the ovary from the primordial phase to the antral phase, when they are ready to be recruited for final maturation and release. Once this begins the young girl starts her periods.
  - The onset of puberty is weight related; the average weight of a girl starting her periods is 45 kg. Anorexia in teenagers can arrest puberty if they become underweight for their age.

Germ cells

There are about seven million primordial oocytes or germ cells in each ovary of the female fetus at 15 weeks of intrauterine life. This drops to two million

Lecture Notes: Obstetrics and Gynaecology, 3rd edition. By Diana Hamilton-Fairley. Published 2009 by Blackwell Publishing. ISBN: 978-1-4051-7801-3.

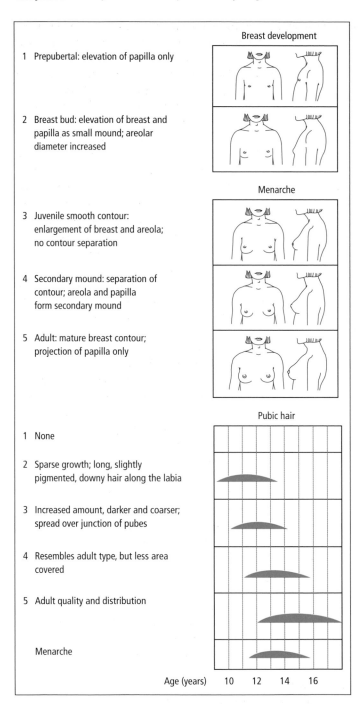

1 Prepubertal: elevation of papilla only

Breast development

2 Breast bud: elevation of breast and papilla as small mound; areolar diameter increased

3 Juvenile smooth contour: enlargement of breast and areola; no contour separation

Menarche

4 Secondary mound: separation of contour; areola and papilla form secondary mound

5 Adult: mature breast contour; projection of papilla only

Pubic hair

1 None

2 Sparse growth; long, slightly pigmented, downy hair along the labia

3 Increased amount, darker and coarser; spread over junction of pubes

4 Resembles adult type, but less area covered

5 Adult quality and distribution

Menarche

Age (years)   10   12   14   16

Figure 3.1 Tanner's classification of sexual maturity in girls. (After Tanner JM (1962) *Growth at Adolescence*. Oxford: Blackwell Scientific Publications.)

germ cells at birth and is further reduced to half a million at puberty.

About 400 will be recruited during each ovulation cycle during reproductive life; the rest degenerate at a steady rate. The stromal tissue of the ovary produces androgenic hormones which may be metabolized in peripheral fat to produce oestrogens.

Ovulation is controlled by the ovarian hormones and the gonadotrophins from the pituitary.

Menstrual cycle

Three structures are involved with the regulation of ovulation and menstruation:
1 The anterior pituitary gland
2 The ovary
3 The uterus.
These are all dealt with in Chapter 1, which considers the anatomy and physiology of these organs.

Amenorrhoea

Primary amenorrhoea

Definition: no periods experienced by the age of 16.

Investigations of this condition may be divided according to whether secondary sexual characteristics are present or not. If absent, girls should be investigated at the age of 16. If present, investigation can wait until the age of 18.

Causes of primary amenorrhoea

- Hypothalamic (absence of gonadotrophin-releasing hormone, GnRH) or hypogonadatrophic (no LH or follicle-stimulating hormone, FSH). This may be:
  — idiopathic
  — after radiotherapy of the brain
  — after surgery to the brain or pituitary, eg craniopharyngiomas in childhood
- Anorexia: excessive exercise (ballet dancers/gymnastics)
- Chromosomal
- Congenital.

Chromosomal causes

The normal human has 46 chromosomes, 44 autosomes and 2 sex chromosomes. The number is halved in both gametes—the oocyte and spermatozoon; when fertilization occurs the original number is restored in the resulting fertilized ovum (see Chapter 1).

In the normal female the sex chromosomes are XX, in the normal male XY. All oocytes carry the X chromosome, whereas about half the spermatozoa carry X and the others carry Y. Thus, the resulting offspring are either XX (female) or XY (male).

Sex chromosome abnormalities mainly arise from non-disjunction (Fig. 3.2). At the division of the primary oocyte while still sited in the ovary, the two chromosomes fail to separate, so that a primary oocyte is produced that may have two X chromosomes or none; conversely, the first polar body will contain the opposite—none or two. Fertilization by a spermatozoon, which may carry X or Y, can therefore result in abnormal patterns: XXX, XXY or XO. YO has not been described because this genetic combination is lethal.

The description is a simplification because more complex anomalies may occur, eg mosaics or individuals of mixed chromosomal patterns.

Turner syndrome
- Chromosome pattern XO
- Incidence about 3 in 10 000 full-term births
- Presents with primary amenorrhoea because there are either no ovaries or non-functioning streaks of tissue with no oogenesis
- Vagina and uterus present
- Poor breast development
- Little or no axillary and pubic hair
- Short stature (lack of growth hormone)
- Webbing of the neck (from lymphoedema)
- A wide carrying angle in the arms
- Coarctation of the aorta
- Congenital malformation of the kidneys may be found.
- Deafness
- Osteopenia
- Reduced intellectual capacity compared with siblings; occasionally this is severe
- Menopausal hormone profile.

Androgen insensitivity syndrome (AIS)
- Chromosomal pattern XY
- Due to lack of/abnormal androgen receptors (deletion on X chromosome)
- Active breast development (hepatic oestrogens)
- Absent or scanty axillary and pubic hair

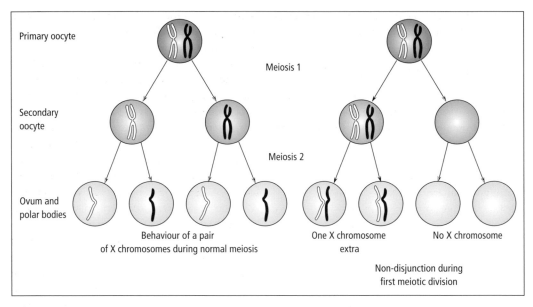

Figure 3.2 Non-disjunction during meiosis.

• Usually absent uterus with a very short vagina
• Gonads are testes or undifferentiated gonads and may be intra-abdominal or in the labia major
• Male serum androgen levels, raised LH and FSH resulting from failure of negative feedback from absent androgen receptor.

Congenital adrenal hyperplasia (CAH)
• Chromosomal pattern XX
• CAH is inherited as a mendelian recessive
• Female infants are often born with ambiguous genitalia from exposure to excess androgens in fetal life
• The clitoris is enlarged and the labia fused
• Vagina and uterus present
• Ovaries are usually polycystic in appearance and anovulatory
• Defective production of cortisol, most commonly as a result of 21-hydroxylase deficiency
• Leads to overproduction of corticotrophic hormone and enlargement of the adrenal cortex
• Increased adrenal androgen production
• Some of these babies are salt losers and become seriously ill in the first week of life

• Teenagers often develop severe hirsutism and acne.

Congenital causes
Menstruation not started by the age of 17 must be distinguished from cryptomenorrhoea—hidden loss caused by obstruction to menstrual flow. This is most often a result of a septum across the vagina just above the hymen at the embryological junction of the müllerian ducts and the urogenital sinus in the lower third of the vagina. It may be incomplete. A complete septum leads to cryptomenorrhoea (vagina filled with blood) and haematocolpos (uterus filled with blood). The lower part of the vagina may be a solid cord; haematocolpos and haematometra may form above this. On inspection of the vulva a bluish bulge is seen just inside the hymen. There may be cyclical attacks of abdominal pain and a mass may be palpable *per* abdomen, representing a large haematocolpos.

Treatment
Under anaesthesia, incise the septum and express the haematocolpos by suprapubic pressure. If

infection does not occur, subsequent menstruation and childbearing are normal.

Investigation of primary amenorrhoea

- A *history* is taken including a family history because AIS may affect other females in the family.
- *Physical examination*: the general examination should begin by recording the girl's height—if by 16 she is less than 147 cm there is a possibility of ovarian agenesis (Turner syndrome) or (pan)hypopituitarism. If there is a decrease in body weight, calculate body mass index (BMI = weight in kg)/height in m^2). A general examination checks the development of secondary sexual characteristics, hair patterns and density.
- A *pelvic examination* should be performed if the examiner really thinks that there is likely to be a positive finding. For most young women with primary amenorrhoea it will not be useful, particularly at first consultation. The vulva is inspected to see that the introitus is patent and there is no clitoromegaly; there may be cryptomenorrhoea, congenital absence of the vagina or a blind vagina as in AIS.
- *Investigation*: a full chromosome analysis should be performed to establish the karyotype, including any mosaicism and AIS.
- *Hormonal investigations* should include LH, FSH, estradiol and testosterone levels.
- *Ultrasound* will help determine the presence, state and size of the ovaries and any follicular activity. Uterine size can also be seen. It is rarely necessary to perform a laparoscopy to assess the pelvic organs.

Management

If the girl is normally developed, with normal breast development, normal uterus and vagina, and she has a normal female karyotype, the most likely diagnosis is delayed menarche. It is reasonable to await events; menstruation is not established in some individuals before age 18.

For those with a diagnosable pathological cause, the aim must be to restore normal function as far as possible and, although fertility may not be possible, enable the individual to lead as normal a sexual life as possible.

Cases of Turner syndrome should receive long-term treatment with cyclical hormones, oestrogen and progestogen (hormone replacement therapy, HRT). There is a small risk of uterine carcinoma.

In AIS, the gonads are testes that are often found inside the abdomen or inguinal canal. As these testes have a 25% risk of becoming malignant (teratoma or dysgerminoma), they should be removed soon after puberty and an artificial vagina may be constructed or dilators used to permit sexual intercourse. Treatment with oestrogen should also be given to augment breast development and prevent osteoporosis.

In cases of congenital absence of the vagina and uterus, the ovaries are usually normal. An artificial vagina may be constructed to permit sexual intercourse.

Abnormalities of pituitary secretion should be treated with oestrogen or progesterone until fertility is desired.

Secondary amenorrhoea

Definition: no periods for over 6 months, once having started.

Causes of secondary amenorrhoea

Physiological

Amenorrhoea occurs naturally in:
- pregnancy
- lactation
- after the menopause.

Pituitary

Total pituitary ablation or destruction by radiotherapy after puberty. Tumours may also destroy it. In Sheehan's syndrome, severe postpartum haemorrhage causes pituitary anoxia with failure of lactation, amenorrhoea and other manifestations of pituitary failure.

Hyperprolactinaemia may result from a definitive pituitary adenoma or scattered microadenoma causing galactorrhoea, visual disturbances and headaches. It may be a side effect of some drugs, particularly cimetidine and phenothiazine.

Anorexia nervosa may lead to pituitary damage and thus to permanent amenorrhoea and sterility. Periods may cease before weight loss becomes apparent.

Thyroid disease

All thyroid disorders that are symptomatic may be associated with amenorrhoea or excessive bleeding. Correction of the thyroid function may restore normal menstruation.

Ovary

Polycystic ovary syndrome (PCOS) is the most common cause of anovulation in young women, with one in five women having the morphological picture on ultrasonography and 1:20 affected by the symptoms of the syndrome. They have stromal hyperplasia of the ovaries, leading to an excess secretion of testosterone and the formation of multiple follicular cysts that fail or take variable amounts of time to mature; it is associated with amenorrhoea, oligomenorrhoea, hirsutism, acne and infertility, secondary to anovulation (Fig. 3.3). Women with PCOS are often hyperinsulinaemic. This predisposes them to obesity and late-onset (type 2) diabetes. Obesity increases the prevalence of anovulation and hirsutism. Anovulation and obesity both predispose women to endometrial hyperplasia/carcinoma because of the effects of unopposed oestrogen on the endometrium. Weight control and regular withdrawal bleeds are therefore essential.

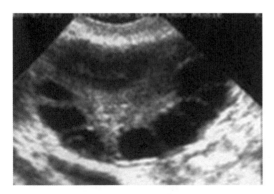

Figure 3.3 Ultrasound scan of a polycystic ovary.

These women are able to conceive spontaneously as most do ovulate, although irregularly. They should therefore receive the same advice about contraception as any other young woman because termination of pregnancy as a result of a mistaken diagnosis of infertility can be devastating both physically and psychologically. The women respond well to ovulation induction with anti-oestrogens or FSH if they fail to conceive but should try to keep their weight within the normal range to optimize the outcome of pregnancy. Hirsutism and acne are not curable but can be significantly improved through weight loss (if the woman is overweight or obese), the combined contraceptive pill, which reduces ovarian androgens and increases circulating sex hormone-binding globulin levels, or anti-androgens such as cyproterone acetate or spironolactone.

Spontaneous premature ovarian failure (POF) in the absence of disease causes premature menopause. The ovary ceases to respond to pituitary gonadotrophins, which are usually excreted in excessive amounts or may be normal. This follows a lack of oocytes or their autoimmune destruction in the ovary.

Castration by surgical removal of the ovaries or by exposure to irradiation leads to amenorrhoea.

Extensive destruction of the ovaries by infection or tumours is a rare cause.

Uterine

The endometrium can be destroyed by the following.

- Disease:
  — tuberculosis (TB)
  — severe postpartum infection
- Formal endometrial ablation (by laser or diathermy)
- Curettage usually after pregnancy, miscarriage or therapeutic abortion, particularly if there is any infection present (Asherman's syndrome).

General disease

Amenorrhoea may occur in any debilitating disease, eg pulmonary TB, not necessarily with involvement of the pelvic organs.

Terminal stages of diseases such as Addison's disease and uraemia caused by renal disease.

Starvation may lead to amenorrhoea, similar to that seen in anorexia nervosa.

Obesity can also cause amenorrhoea (most commonly associated with PCOS) and in grossly obese young women weight reduction may restore normal menstrual function.

Antipsychotic medication can increase the production of prolactin and induce anovulation.

History

- Family history
- Hot flushes
- Drugs such as reserpine, digoxin, phenothiazines and hormones, including oral contraceptives
- Change in body weight, ie obesity or sudden loss of weight
- Galactorrhoea
- Headache, visual disturbance (hemianopia).

Physical examination

- Height measurement
- Weight (calculate BMI)
- Blood pressure
- Breasts for evidence of pregnancy or milk secretion
- Pelvic examination to:
  — exclude pregnancy (a woman may still conceive in the course of a period of amenorrhoea)
  — assess the size and position of the uterus to exclude a pelvic tumour.

Investigations

- Pregnancy test
- Plasma hormone levels of FSH
- LH
- Estradiol
- Prolactin
- Testosterone
- Progesterone withdrawal test: give a progestogen for 5 days. If the woman bleeds afterwards, she has oestrogen in her circulation and a uterus.

Ultrasound assessment of:
- uterine size
- pregnancy
- ovarian size and morphology
- follicular function.

Computed tomography (CT) or magnetic resonance imaging (MRI) of pituitary area if has galactorrhoea/headaches/visual disturbance.

Examination under anaesthesia if congenital abnormality to:
- assess the pelvic organs
- perform a laparoscopy to inspect the pelvic organs and to take a biopsy of the ovaries.

The differential diagnosis of amenorrhoea is given in Box 3.1.

Box 3.1 Tests: differential diagnosis of primary and secondary amenorrhoea

	Chromosomes	FSH	LH	Estradiol	Testosterone	Prolactin	Progesterone withdrawal
Primary amenorrhoea							
Turner syndrome	XO	↑	↑	↓	=	=	Negative
Androgen insensitivity syndrome	XY	↑	↑	=/↓	↑	=	Negative
Hypogonadotrophic hypogonadism	XX	↓	↓	↓	=	=/↓	Negative
Secondary amenorrhoea							
Prolactinoma	XX	↓	↓	↓	=	↑	Negative
Polycystic ovary syndrome	XX	=	↑/=	=	↑	=	Positive
Premature ovarian failure	XX	↑	↑	↓	=	=	Negative

FSH, follicle-stimulating hormone; LH, luteinizing hormone.

Treatment

Treat the cause if one is discovered. If not, management will depend upon whether or not fertility is desired.

Women with low oestrogen levels should be treated with oestrogen and progesterone replacement (the oral contraceptive pill or HRT).

In *anorexia nervosa* the periods may cease before weight loss is evident; treatment should include efforts to restore weight to normal. In *gross obesity*, weight loss may result in normal menstruation.

Teenagers who over-exercise (ballet dancers and gymnasts) should be encouraged to reduce their training schedule.

In POCS, if the woman is obese, referral to a dietician is recommended to reduce weight. In some women metformin may help to restore ovulation in conjunction with a low-calorie diet. Regular progesterone therapy for 12 days every 3 months will give a regular withdrawal bleed or the oral contraceptive pill with cyproterone acetate (an antiandrogen) will give a regular period and improve hirsutism and acne.

A *premature menopause* is characterized by low oestrogen levels and high FSH. They should receive cyclical oestrogen and progesterone such as Cyclo-Progynova to prevent osteoporosis.

Where excess prolactin (>1000 µU/l) is secreted, perform CT/MRI of the pituitary fossa to exclude a tumour. In the absence of such a space-occupying lesion, microadenomas of the pituitary body are postulated. Treatment of amenorrhoea with prolactin excess is with bromocriptine or the longer-acting cabergoline (both are dopamine agonists) in perpetuity. Bromocriptine and cabergoline should be stopped if pregnancy occurs. Periods will return on treatment once prolactin levels return to normal.

Bleeding in infancy

Female infants may have vaginal bleeding during the first week of life. This is rarely significant and probably caused by withdrawal of maternally derived oestrogens that had crossed the placenta in pregnancy.

Precocious puberty is caused by premature maturation of the ovaries in most cases; very rarely there may be a granulosa cell tumour of the ovary. The breasts grow while pubic and axillary hair develops and endometrial bleeding occurs. Provided that a tumour of the ovary can be excluded, the child may be allowed to develop normally but the parents must be warned of the danger of pregnancy. They usually end up being short for their age because of the premature exposure of their bones to oestrogen, which makes bones fuse early. Early treatment with growth hormone may improve their final height.

The differential diagnosis includes:
- a mixed mesodermal tumour
- adenocarcinoma of the vagina; particularly at risk were adolescent girls whose mothers received stilbestrol during pregnancy, but this is now history.

Menorrhagia under 18 years

Adolescent bleeding of a sufficient amount to be considered as menorrhagia is usually dysfunctional, secondary to anovulation. There may be prolonged episodes of painless bleeding and the girl can become anaemic. Examination of the endometrium may show an anovulatory pattern or hyperplasia.

Treatment consists of eliminating any organic cause and correcting anaemia if present. Hormone treatment is usually successful using a progestogen such as norethisterone (15 mg daily) (see Chapter 16). When the treatment is stopped, withdrawal bleeding with shedding of the endometrium analogous with normal menstruation occurs. Treatment should be given cyclically for a further 3–6 months. An alternative is use of the oral contraceptive pill.

Chapter 4

Subfertility

Subfertility is defined as failure to conceive after 1 year of unprotected coitus at frequent intervals. A woman who has never conceived has primary subfertility, and a woman who has conceived before has secondary subfertility, even though this episode did not result in a live birth, eg miscarriage or ectopic pregnancy.

Causes of infertility (Table 4.1)

Both partners

- Mechanical difficulty in coitus with inadequate penetration, often associated with lack of ability in the male to maintain an erection.
- Periods of separation so that there is no intercourse at the most fertile time.

Male

- Impotence
- Premature ejaculation
- Azoospermia/oligospermia ($<20 \times 10^6$/ml)
- Poor sperm motility. (<50% progression)
- Less than 10% abnormal forms.

Lecture Notes: Obstetrics and Gynaecology, 3rd edition. By Diana Hamilton-Fairley. Published 2009 by Blackwell Publishing. ISBN: 978-1-4051-7801-3.

Female

- Fallopian tubes—infection may close or partly obstruct.
- Ovarian dysfunction (Table 4.2):
  — ovulation may not occur
  — ovulation is irregular with anovulatory cycles:
    — polycystic ovary syndrome (PCOS)
    — hyperprolactinaemia
    — perimenopausal
    — premature ovarian failure
- Intact hymen: a woman may complain of subfertility when her marriage has not been consummated
- Vagina: congenital malformation
- Uterus: congenital malformation or tuberculous endometritis.

Investigation of the infertile couple

History from the female

- Age, occupation, length of time with partner, use of contraception or avoidance of pregnancy, previous sexual activity.
- Previous pregnancies, including abortions, miscarriages, ectopic.
- Menstrual history: age at onset, cycle and duration of flow, dysmenorrhoea, ovulation pain, recent change in the cycle.

- Vaginal discharge: character, amount, whether associated with irritation or soreness.
- Previous illnesses, especially pelvic inflammatory disease (PID), diabetes, renal disease.
- Operations, especially in the abdomen or pelvis.
- Coitus frequency, difficulties, relation to fertile days.
- Previous investigation or treatment of infertility.

Examination of the female

- General examination: physical development, evidence of endocrine disorder.
- Abdominal examination: scars, tenderness, guarding, masses.
- Vaginal examination: state of introitus, presence/absence of vaginismus, size and mobility of the uterus, uterine enlargement, enlargement of the ovaries.

Table 4.1 Factors in infertility

Factor	Percentage
Ovulation disorder	30
Tubal factor	30
Male factor	30
Unexplained infertility	10

Table 4.2 Causes of anovulation

Cause	Percentage
Primary ovarian dysfunction	
Genetic, eg Turner syndrome	1
Autoimmune	
Secondary ovarian dysfunction	
Disorders of gonadotrophin regulation	
Hyperprolactinaemia	15
Functional	
Weight loss	10
Exercise	
Gonadotrophin deficiency	
Pituitary tumour	
Pituitary infarction	4
Pituitary ablation	
Polycystic ovary syndrome	70

History from the male

- Age, occupation, including absence from home, length of time with partner and duration of infertility.
- Sexual performance: frequency, ability to ejaculate in upper vagina.
- Previous relationships, fathering of any pregnancies.
- History of mumps with orchitis, injury to genitalia or operations for hernia or varicocoele, any recent debilitating illness.

Examination of the male

- General build and appearance
- Examination of genitalia, hypospadias
- Palpation of testicles, size, consistency. Relate size to standard models (Fig. 4.1).

Investigations

Seminal analysis (Table 4.3)

Best performed on a masturbation specimen, which should be examined within 2 hours of collection. It should not be from semen ejaculated at intercourse using a condom as most

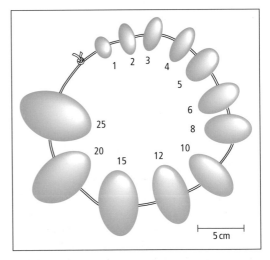

Figure 4.1 Models of testicular size to allow standardization of the examined testes size with an objective comparison (volume cm³).

Table 4.3 Normal seminal analysis

Volume (ml)	2–5
Liquefaction time	Within 30 min
Count (million/ml)	20–150
Motility	>50% progressive motility at 1.5 hours
Sperm morphology	>10% normal forms

modern sheaths are lubricated with spermicidal cream.

The motility of sperm is important; direct, straight moving sperms being the more likely to effect fertilization.

There should be at least 20 million sperms per millilitre. Fertility reduces progressively with numbers below this. Abnormal forms should not exceed 10%. Reliance should not be placed on a single sperm count.

In cases of severe oligospermia/azoospermia the cause should be sought. It may be caused by a chromosomal abnormality such as Klinefelter syndrome (XXY), or primary hypogonadism, when the level of gonadotrophic hormone will be high, or secondary hypogonadism, where gonadotrophic hormone will be low; in the latter there may be excess prolactin secretion, usually as a result of a pituitary tumour and possibly responsive to bromocriptine. Other causes of azoospermia may be related to congenital absence of the vasa deferentia or to obstruction in the epididymis.

Basal temperature charts

The woman may keep charts of her basal temperature for a period of 3 months. This is best taken first thing in the morning before leaving bed. In theory, the raised progesterone levels elevate the basal body temperature by 0.4–0.6°C within 12 hours of ovulation. The graphic chart produced bears some relation to ovulation when it is regular. However, the correlation of temperature to ovulation is less easily seen when ovulation is irregular. Other extraneous causes of temperature fluctuation (eg flu) intrude on this test as do unusual life rhythms (eg nurses on night duty). These charts are very difficult to use prospectively and have largely been abandoned.

Ovulation predictor tests

A daily test using a few drops of urine, which detects the LH (luteinizing hormone) surge by giving a colour change on a stick in the presence of a high LH. When it is positive the woman knows that she is going to ovulate within 36 hours. It is helpful in women with a regular cycle, but in women who have PCOS and an irregular cycle it is rarely helpful because they can have a raised LH in the follicular phase without a mature follicle or may take many weeks to produce an oocyte, making it almost impossible to time the test correctly.

Tests for tubal patency

Hysterosalpingography using a radio-opaque dye shows blockage of the tubes and indicates the site of the obstruction; it can also demonstrate abnormalities within the cavity such as polyps, submucosal fibroids or a congenital malformation of the cavity of the uterus (Figure 4.2). A new contrast medium containing microbubbles may be injected transcervically and its passage along the fallopian tube detected with ultrasound (HyCoSy; Plate 4).

Tubal patency may be tested under direct vision at laparoscopy. A solution of methylene blue is injected through a tightly fitting cannula in the cervical canal. The passage of the dye may be observed. When the tubes are normally patent, the dye pours out of the fimbriated end of the tube into the pouch of Douglas. Tubal obstruction may be recognized

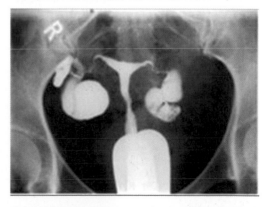

Figure 4.2 Hysterosalpingogram showing bilateral hydrosalpinges, normal cavity.

as can the presence of adhesions; a hydrosalpinx may be seen to fill with dye that does not spill. It may be possible to operate on the tubes at the same time by opening the fimbrial end in an attempt to improve fertility. The woman must be warned that she will have an increased risk of ectopic pregnancy if this is performed.

Hormone tests

Serum progesterone levels in the mid second half of the cycle (days 21–23 of a 28-day cycle) are 10 times as high as those of the rest of the cycle (30 ng/ml compared with 3–6 ng/ml) if ovulation has occurred. LH, follicle-stimulating hormone (FSH) and testosterone (if PCOS is suspected) should be taken between days 3 and 8 of the cycle.

Prolactin levels should be measured to exclude microadenomas of the pituitary gland; levels above 1000 μU/l are significant and should lead to magnetic resonance imaging (MRI) or computed tomography (CT) of the pituitary fossa.

Ultrasound

An ultrasound scan of the pelvis, especially with a vaginal probe, gives excellent views of the ovaries and uterus if pathology in either is suspected (eg PCOS—see Figure 3.3).

Treatment of subfertility

A couple seeking medical advice for subfertility are obviously anxious and concerned. They should always be offered help even if the period of subfertility is relatively short. In most couples, investigations should be done after 1 year of trying.

About 25–30% of women seeking advice for subfertility become pregnant during investigation and treatment. There are various lines of treatment that may prove successful depending on the condition found.

Correction of coital difficulties

An intact hymen should be removed or dilated. A longitudinal vaginal septum may have to be removed but usually they cause little difficulty unless menstrual blood becomes trapped behind them because they are blind ending. The woman should be taught to pass vaginal dilators and this helps to give her confidence. The use of a lubricant at coitus also helps.

Women who experience involuntary tightening of the vaginal walls, restricting the ability of the penis to penetrate, often have significant psychological reasons for this which may include previous sexual abuse or rape. These are obviously extremely sensitive issues and should be explored carefully. If you suspect that the woman is holding something back, ensure that you offer her an opportunity to discuss things with you on your own and when you have adequate time. She may agree to referral to a psychosexual counsellor. Although the counsellor may prefer to see the couple alone, it is perfectly usual for one or other to be seen first and the partner to be invited at a later time when the woman is ready.

In the male, the most common problems with fertility are premature ejaculation and inadequate erection. Both of these are discussed in Chapter 6.

Lesions of the uterine body

Removal of small uterine polypi (see pp. 233–6) at curettage is often successful. Myomectomy should be performed if the fibroids are blocking the fallopian tubes, intramural and > 5 cm in diameter or submucous (see Plate 9). Hysteroscopy is useful in identifying and treating intrauterine lesions. An intrauterine septum can also be resected, but may need to be done at the same time as performing a laparoscopy to reduce the risk of uterine perforation, by being able to visualize the external surface of the uterus.

Lesions of the tubes

Various operations may be undertaken to restore patency and function in cases where the tubes have been damaged by infection (most commonly with *Chlamydia* species).

- *Salpingostomy* where the fimbrial end is opened and held open by turning out a cuff (commonly done laparoscopically).
- *Tubal reimplantation* where the isthmus is blocked. The medial tubal end is freed and is reimplanted into the uterine cavity (rarely performed).
- *Salpingolysis* where peritubal adhesions are divided (usually at laparoscopy).
- *Reanastomosis* if the tube is blocked in midsegment; the obstructed area is resected and the open ends reanastomosed often using microsurgery.
- *Salpingectomy or sterilization at the cornu-isthmic junction*: removal or blockage of the tubes as close to the uterus as possible is now performed in an increasing number of women with damaged tubes undergoing in vitro fertilization (IVF) because it reduces the risk of an ectopic pregnancy after embryo transfer.

Results of many of these operations are disappointing because:
- *patency* can easily be restored but the tube may be too rigid to allow peristalsis
- *infection* may have caused the tube to be fixed to other organs by adhesions and so the fimbrial end cannot freely manoeuvre and thus harvest the oocytes
- after surgery there may be *too short a length of tube* so that passage of the fertilized oocyte is so rapid that the endometrium is not yet ready to receive it.

In consequence, the success rates of tuboplasty after infection range from 2% to 10%. The best results come after reanastomosis of sterilization procedures when most surgeons will report a 40–60% success rate, which can be improved to about 75% by the use of microsurgery. Despite these poor results there are some women who will be prepared to submit to such an operation even though the hope of a successful pregnancy is slight. For most women with tubal disease, IVF gives the best chance of a successful pregnancy (see p. 43).

Ovarian dysfunction (anovulation)

In cases of non-ovulation, further investigation is indicated (see Chapter 3). If there is a high level of prolactin on more than one occasion a CT scan should be done to exclude a pituitary tumour. Excess prolactin is treated with bromocriptine or cabergoline. As prolactin levels return to normal, menstruation restarts and normal fertility is restored.

Cases of primary or secondary ovarian failure show high levels of FSH and low levels of oestrogen. Induction of ovulation is impossible because there are no more oocytes, but the patient should be offered oestrogen replacement therapy.

Cases of ovulation failure with low FSH and LH levels may be treated by the use of gonadotrophins (FSH alone most commonly). Treatment with these must be monitored carefully with ultrasound to prevent multiple ovulation and thence multiple pregnancies, which carry significantly increased risks to the mother and fetuses compared with a singleton pregnancy. Ovarian hyperstimulation syndrome (OHSS) may develop after the release of excessive numbers of eggs and high oestrogen levels, which can cause coagulation disorders leading to a cerebral thrombosis/haemorrhage, and fluid–electrolyte imbalance that can be life threatening.

In practice, FSH is given regularly from about days 2–3 of the cycle. The dose is increased weekly, depending on the ultrasound examination of the ovary, which shows the number and size of follicles coming towards ovulation. When the response is satisfactory, an injection of human chorionic gonadotrophin (hCG) is given, which acts in a similar manner to the LH surge. Once a satisfactory dosage pattern has been established in one cycle, this can be repeated in other cycles in up to six treatment courses or until a pregnancy is achieved.

Cases of anovulation with PCOS may be treated with clomifene citrate (an antioestrogen) that makes the pituitary think that the oestrogen levels are low and therefore increases the production of FSH. One tablet is taken for 5 days starting during menstruation and mid-luteal progesterone levels on day 21 are measured to confirm ovulation. If facilities allow the woman should be scanned on day 10 to confirm the development of no more than two or three follicles (see Fig. 4.3 showing a single follicular cyst). If more than three are present the woman should be advised not to have intercourse to minimize the risk of higher-

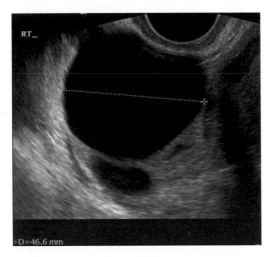

Figure 4.3 Ultrasound scan of follicular cyst.

order multiple pregnancies. Provided that ovulation occurs treatment should be repeated for 6 months or until the woman is pregnant. If the first dose is unsuccessful it is increased maximally to 150 mg daily. There is a rise of multiple follicular development from this hyperstimulation and therefore multiple pregnancies are more common (5–10%).

Treatment of male infertility

If it has been established that male factors are associated with infertility, treatment can proceed. This is best done in two phases:
- less invasive treatments
- more specific therapies.

Phase 1

The first phase should last about 3 months. Two specimens of semen should be examined to establish levels in the sperm count. Certain aspects of the man's way of life may need to be altered:
- over-exertion
- excessive smoking
- excess alcohol consumption
- poorly controlled diabetes
- hypertension
- being overweight.

If the scrotal temperature is raised, it is wise to wear boxer shorts to allow the testes to hang in a cooler atmosphere.

The timing of intercourse may need discussion so that, around the time of ovulation, the couple have intercourse. A few days of abstinence before this may boost the sperm count if there is a deficiency; otherwise timing is irrelevant.

Any varicocoele causing a raised temperature of the scrotum and the efferent ducts from the testes is managed by ligation. Three-quarters of men improve their sperm count after this if a varicocoele has been a feature.

Phase 2

Specific treatments will depend upon the results of investigations. A low sperm count with low FSH and testosterone level may indicate treatment with stimulating hormones (FSH—very rare).

In the absence of hormone deficiency, endocrine therapy is less easily justified. Hyperprolactinaemia is rare in males, but if it is present a dopamine agonist should be used.

Impaired fertility is sometimes associated with an increased incidence of chronic prostatitis. If present, long-term, low-dose antibiotic treatment may remove this potential cause (erythromycin 250 mg twice a day for a month).

Sperm washing has been described with variable results. Ejaculated sperm is washed in phosphate-buffered saline and resuspended for insemination into the uterus (intrauterine insemination, IUI). His partner is usually treated with clomiphene or FSH to increase the number of mature oocytes to two or three to increase the chance of conception. The risk of a multiple pregnancy is around 10% and OHSS 1%.

Generally speaking, this conservative management of male factors of infertility is disappointing and the success rate usually ranges between 20% and 40%. The introduction of assisted conception techniques has altered this considerably.

Assisted conception

Artificial fertilization methods have increased in use greatly in the last decade, with probably over

10 000 children in the world born as a result. Artificial fertilization has received considerable media coverage but should be considered as only one part of infertility management, particularly for those who cannot transmit sperms or eggs along the fallopian tubes as a result of damage or absence (Table 4.4) or abnormal sperm.

Patients selected for programmes are usually under 40 years of age and in a stable relationship. In most parts of the UK the NHS will fund couples under the age of 41 with normal gonadotrophin levels where neither partner has living children, although this varies. The National Institute for Health and Clinical Excellence (NICE) has recommended that the NHS should fund three cycles for each couple to increase the chance of success, but as yet adequate resources are not available for this.

Technique

For the process to take place, it is essential that oocytes be recovered. Most women now have ovarian cycles stimulated by gonadotrophins after treatment with a gonadotrophin-releasing hormone (GnRH) analogue to stop the woman's own hormone production; hCG is given to stimulate ovulation. This can be monitored by daily ultrasonography when follicle size can be measured; the follicle should measure about 20 mm in diameter for oocyte recovery.

Oocytes are aspirated through the posterior fornix of the vagina or bladder guided by ultrasound. Usually several (3–15) oocytes are recovered at the same procedure.

The oocytes are mixed on a warmed flat dish in special media with semen obtained from the husband by masturbation. Fertilization takes place in

Table 4.4 Indications for in vitro fertilization (IVF)

Cause of infertility	Percentage
Disease or absence of the tubes	50–70
Endometriosis	7–15
Sperm abnormalities or low count	5–20
Sperm antibodies	1–5
Idiopathic infertility	3–15
Failed donor insemination (DI)	1–5

vitro and under specially controlled conditions of temperature and atmospheric gases. The eggs are allowed to develop to the four- to eight-cell stage, and introduced to the woman's uterus through the cervix, using a fine cannula in as atraumatic a fashion as possible. A maximum of two or three fertilized ova are inserted 2 days after egg collection.

Luteal support with progesterone or hCG is given in the days after embryo replacement until 8–10 weeks of pregnancy or when menstruation begins if conception has not occurred.

More recently the embryo has been allowed to develop to the blastocyst stage before being transferred back to the uterus. This allows a single embryo to be transferred, reducing the risk of multiple pregnancies because its ability to implant is enhanced. The encouraging feature is that the conception rate and take-home baby rate is proving to be as high as or higher than multiple embryo transfer. This not only reduces the risks of pregnancy to the mother but also the number of premature deliveries and admission to special care baby units, reducing the cost to health systems of the outcomes of assisted conception.

Results

Conception rates at established IVF units are about 20–30% per cycle for all women. Success should be judged by a live birth and not just by the implantation of a fertilized egg—a biochemical pregnancy shown by a rise in hCG levels. The average take-home baby rate in the UK is 20%.

Gamete intrafallopian tube transfer

If the tubes are present and patent but conventional methods have failed, one may use gamete intrafallopian tube transfer (GIFT). The oocytes are recovered at laparoscopy under general anaesthesia. Prepared motile sperm from the male semen are then passed through the laparoscope into the fallopian tube and one or two of the oocytes are put into the same tube. The whole procedure takes about half an hour and there is no extracorporeal phase. Success rates are slightly lower than for IVF. It is no longer offered in the UK.

Zygote intrafallopian transfer

Zygote intrafallopian transfer (ZIFT) puts fertilized ova back into the fallopian tube 2 days after fertilization instead of replacement into the uterine cavity as in GIFT. This technique is no longer offered in the UK.

In utero insemination (IUI)

Washed semen are injected into the uterine cavity to meet an oocyte by travelling up the tube as happens naturally.

Direct injection of sperm into oocyte (intracytoplasmic sperm injection—ICSI)

Micromanipulation is performed at most UK centres, placing an individual sperm under the zona and into the oocyte. This has a similar success rate to IVF. Sperm may also be extracted from the epididymis or testis in cases of azoospermia.

Artificial insemination

In cases where the male is infertile, insemination with donor semen (donor insemination, DI) may be considered; this is best done by a doctor. Careful counselling of the couple about the implications is essential. Success rates are 15–40% per ovulation.

Donors

Facilities should be available for accumulating a sperm bank with samples from young donors, preferably of proven fertility. A sufficient variety of donors must allow the matching of height, hair colour and race by the doctor in charge of DI. Each donor's sample can only be used to help six couples.

Samples

Samples are produced by masturbation and are usually divided into tubes or straws of about 0.5 ml each, so that the average donor will produce enough to fill 6–10 tubes at any ejaculation. These are stored in liquid nitrogen under careful conditions and checked every 2 years.

DI and HIV

Until recently, fresh semen was used for DI; this was marginally better at achieving pregnancy than using frozen semen. One of the major fears of artificial insemination has become the theoretical risk of contamination from HIV. In consequence, all donor units now check their donors for HIV antibodies at the time that they produce their samples. The samples are then frozen and the donor is re-checked 3 months later in case he was incubating AIDS at the time that he produced the sample. If the second test is negative the sample can be used for insemination. The percentage of pregnancies achieved is 10–20%, less than with fresh semen.

Technique

The woman is positioned comfortably and a speculum inserted to expose the cervix. Insemination is usually performed into the cervical canal with recently defrosted semen; not more than 0.5 ml of semen is used because it would be painful to distend the canal with a greater volume than this.

Disclosure of donor

Changes in society have occurred that demand greater freedom of information. One of these is that a child from a pregnancy that started with DI may wish to know the identity of the donor. Recent legislation allowing children born by such techniques to trace their biological fathers when they reach the age of 18 has led to a significant reduction in the number of sperm donors.

Ovum donation

Women whose ovaries have never produced or have ceased to produce oocytes and have a uterus can use another woman's eggs to conceive. This is complex because it is more difficult to keep the donor anonymous because she will be attending the clinic at the same time as the recipient. In the UK the donor can be an altruistic volunteer, known to the woman, or a woman who is undergoing IVF herself at the time. She should be under the age of 35 and have completed her own family. In order to reduce the costs of a cycle, women who are prepared to donate their eggs share the costs with the recipient. All donors require counselling to discuss the various outcomes and make sure that they fully understand the situation. Recent legislation also means that any offspring can seek out their biological mothers from the age of 18.

The recipient has to take oestrogen followed by progesterone in order to prime her own uterus to receive the embryo, which will be fertilized with her partner's sperm.

In cases of intractable infertility, adoption may be considered (see below).

Preimplantation genetic diagnosis

Couples who carry genetic diseases that can prove lethal to their offspring can now undergo assisted conception techniques with IVF. After fertilization the embryo is allowed to develop to the eight-cell stage when a single cell is extracted and undergoes a test on its chromosomes. Until recently this was based on either the sex of the baby for X-linked disorders (Duchenne muscular dystrophy, haemophilia), where only female embryos would be replaced, or a lack of/excess of chromosome material for couples with robertsonian translocations or trisomies. More recently haplotyping (looking at the whole sequence) of the cell has been possible, matching the chromosomal abnormality in the carrier to those in the embryo so that only embryos that are carriers or free of the disease are replaced.

This requires considerable work-up of the couple and expertise in the genetics laboratory, so it is done only in very few centres worldwide. It has to be remembered that these couples conceive spontaneously and can therefore have normal children spontaneously without enormous technological support if they keep going long enough. It is a lottery and on some occasions all the embryos can be abnormal in the laboratory as well as in life.

Adoption

In cases of intractable infertility, adoption may be considered, although there is a great shortage of babies for adoption in the western world and increasingly couples are offered children who have been taken into care. Some couples travel overseas to adopt, which can be very protracted because of the bureaucracy involved.

Surrogate mothers

Increasingly, society is accepting the use of *surrogate parenthood*. If a woman has no uterus or has had it surgically removed, she still can make oocytes. Gametes, fertilized by her partner, can be cultured in the uterus of another woman, perhaps a relative such as a mother or a sister. This baby is genetically the same as the parents and only lodges for 38 weeks in the body of another.

In the UK, the baby is legally the child of the woman who bears him or her, ie the surrogate mother, and legal issues have arisen in the past when the surrogate mother changes her mind and wishes to keep the baby after birth.

Chapter 5

Pregnancy prevention

Contraception is the use of temporary techniques to prevent pregnancy while allowing intercourse to continue. The ideal contraceptive should be safe, harmless and not interfere with the sexual enjoyment of either party.

Distinguish between family planning and population control:

- *Family planning*, a personal matter demanding a low failure rate
- *Population control*, where the need for cheapness and ease of use may make a less exacting standard of efficacy acceptable.

The failure rate of any method of contraception is judged by the Pearl Index (PI): the number of women having regular intercourse who become pregnant within a year out of 100 couples using the method. See www.who.int/reproductive-health/family_planning/guidelines.htm

Contraception

Trends

Contraception has been available in the UK for several centuries, mostly in the form of barrier methods in the earlier days. In the 1960s, the hormonal method and intrauterine devices (IUDs) became

Lecture Notes: Obstetrics and Gynaecology, 3rd edition. By Diana Hamilton-Fairley. Published 2009 by Blackwell Publishing. ISBN: 978-1-4051-7801-3.

popular. In the 1970s, free family planning was available from the National Health Service. This led to an increase in availability and uptake of all methods in all groups of age, sex or marital status. In the 1970s doubts were raised about the risks of hormonal contraception, which, by the 1980s, had been resolved somewhat, only to be followed by the fears of HIV, which led to wider use of condoms for safer sex. At the same time, the long-lasting IUDs came on the market and offered less intrusion on sexual life. In the mid-1990s long-lasting injectables also became more widely used. Table 5.1 shows the World Health Organization (WHO) data in 2002 of various usages in different regions. The WHO no longer collects these data in this form so no update is available. The usage of condoms has increased in countries such as Botswana where the government have taken the threat of AIDS very seriously and provided condoms free of charge in an attempt to reduce the spread. Unfortunately this is not universal.

Sterilization, a permanent method, has also increased in popularity since the late 1970s, so that about a quarter of couples choose this as their method.

Family planning services

Family planning services in the UK are based in the community and run by doctors and nurses who are specifically trained in family planning. Many run with a no appointment needed system; others have

Table 5.1 Worldwide usage of contraceptives by percentage

	Oral contraceptives	Intrauterine device	Condom	Other methods	Sterilization	
					Male	Female
More developed regions	17.3	7.6	15.0	2.7	7.0	10.4
Less developed regions	5.9	16.3	3	3.9	3.6	22
World	7.8	14.9	5	3.6	4.1	20.1

Data from the World Health Organization, 2001.

appointment times. They often offer cervical screening and increasingly sexual health screens (see Chapter 6). School nurses are able to provide contraceptive advice and addresses of suitable clinics. Sexual health and contraceptive advice are also provided in schools through the Public Health and Life Style syllabus. Despite this women continue to have unwanted pregnancies and the UK has the highest rate of teenage pregnancy in Europe.

Access to contraception advice and its methods may be affected by a number of factors:
• Consultations are rarely free
• Clinics are seldom open access or rooted in the community
• A lack of adequately trained personnel
• Lack of awareness of methods or availability by women
• Cultural issues surrounding the acceptability of contraception
• Women having little control over their own lives and bodies because of attitudes within couples and/or the family.

It is therefore very important for health services to strive to provide high-quality services, for educational materials to be available for all women. and to break down the myths and taboos that may surround contraception so that women can make informed choices.

Counselling

Family planning and birth control need discussion of more than just the mechanics of the methods. They are part of reproductive life linked with emotional and sexual life. There is sometimes embarrassment surrounding family planning and so this matter may not be discussed openly. It is for profes-

Box 5.1 Checklist of contraceptive counselling

When discussing any methods of contraception consider:
• suitability
• side effects
• risks
• benefits
• how it works
• after-sales service
• professional care needed

sionals to try to help break these barriers by discussing the matter in a clear and simple fashion. There are many factors that medically influence the choice of contraception offered to women. Over the years many myths have been promulgated about the various methods and who can or cannot use them (suitability).

The influence of peer comments is probably even greater than that of professionals. If a woman has met someone who had a bad time on the pill, this will be remembered more than advice given by the family planner. When counselling, the professionals should listen as much as they should advise. There are not enough data available on the use of methods to be absolute. The failure rate is not the only thing that influences people. When counselling, the items in Box 5.1 should all be included. The provision of contraception is one of the most intimate areas of an individual's life and requires high skills in communication and information giving.

In 2004 the WHO published a guideline on the medical eligibility criteria for contraceptive use. Associated with this is a wheel for easily determining whether a woman can use the method (Table 5.2).

Table 5.2 Medical eligibility criteria for contraceptive use

Criteria	COCP/ combination inject	Progestogen- only pills	Depo- progesterone	Implants	Copper IUD
Age					
Menarche to <18	1	1	2	1	2
>40	2	1	1 or 2	1	1
Parity—nulliparous	1	1	1	1	2
Breastfeeding					
Up to 6 weeks	4	3	3	3	48 h–4 weeks
6 weeks to 6 months	3	1	1	1	1
Sepsis—puerperal/post-abortion	1	1	1	1	4
Cancers:					
Breast cancer (current)	4	4	4	4	1
Cervical cancer (pre-treatment)	2	1	2	2	4
CIN (see Chapter 19)	2	1	2	2	1
Vaginal bleeding (unexplained)	2	2	3	3	4
PID					
Now	1	1	1	1	4
Past	1	1	1	1	1 or 2
STI					
Gonorrhoea/chlamydia infection	1	1	1	1	4
Other STIs	1	1	1	1	2
Increased risk of STIs	1	1	1	1	2 or 3
HIV infection	1	1	1	1	2
Smoking					
<35	2	1	1	1	1
>35	3	1	1	1	1
Hypertension					
Moderate	3	1	2	1	1
Severe	4	2	3	2	1
Deep vein thrombosis—past	4	2	2	2	1
Current	4	3	3	3	1
Major surgery/prolonged immobility	4	2	2	2	1
Cardiovascular disease	4	2	3	2	1
Headaches					
No migraine	1	1	1	1	1
Migraine	4	2	2	2	1
Diabetes	2	2	2	2	1
Liver diseases	4	3	3	3	1
Drug interactions					
Rifampicin	2	3	2	3	1
Some anticonvulsants	2	3	2	3	1
ARV therapy	2	2	2	2	2
Obesity	2	1	1	1	1
Uterine fibroids	1	1	1	1	1

ARV, antiretroviral; PID, pelvic inflammatory disease; STI, sexually transmitted infection.

For each perceived risk factor listed in Table 5.2 a score of 1–4 has been awarded for each method of contraception:

1 Use the method in any circumstance
2 Generally use the method
3 Use of the method is not generally recommended unless more appropriate methods are not available or acceptable
4 Method not to be used.

The use of contraception is influenced by many factors other than just the regulation of reproduction, including:

• cultural background
• religion
• partnership status
• personal health
• personal habits.

Methods used by the female

Hormonal

• The pill—combined oral contraceptive (oestrogen and progestogen)
• The emergency pill: high-dose progestogen
• The mini-pill: progestogen-only pills
• Injectable hormones: combined or progestogen only (Depo)
• Implantable hormones: progestogens
• Transdermal progestogen or combined.

Intrauterine contraceptive devices (IUCDs)

• Copper-bearing devices
• Progestogen-bearing devices.

Barriers

• Diaphragm or Dutch cap
• Cervical cap
• Vault pessary
• Vaginal sheath.

Chemical spermicides

• Soluble pessaries.
• Creams, foams and jellies.

• Medicated sponges.
• Douching.

Hormones: oral contraceptives (OCs)

Combined pill

The pill is used by about a third of women in the UK who use contraception. There is a wide range of oral contraceptives. Most are a mixture of oestrogen and a progestogen taken for all of the 21 days of the packet. The most common oestrogen used is ethinylestradiol combined with one of the following:

• Norethisterone
• Levonorgestrol
• Desogestrel
• Drospirenone
• Gestodene.

The pill:

• inhibits ovulation by interfering with gonadotrophin-releasing hormones
• modifies the endometrium, preventing implantation
• makes the cervical secretion more viscid and less permeable to spermatozoa
• The progestogen norelgestromin is combined with ethinylestradiol in a transdermal patch.

Advantages

• The pill is the most effective method of reversible birth control provided that the instructions are followed and it is taken regularly.
• The method is not related to the act of intercourse.
• Women who suffer from dysmenorrhoea or heavy periods often find their periods less painful and the flow diminished.
• Menstruation occurs at regular intervals of 4 weeks.
• Haemoglobin levels are maintained so that anaemia is less common.
• Acne and hirsutism may improve.

Metabolic effects

In different women there may be as much as a 10-fold variation in tissue levels of the hormones and therefore of their effects because of:

- difference in absorption
- difference in liver metabolism of steroids
- difference in fat layers of body as fat absorbs steroids avidly.

Glucose tolerance may be impaired. There may be an increase in:

- low-density lipoproteins (LDLs)
- cholesterol
- serum iron
- serum copper
- circulating blood coagulation factors VII and IX
- fibrinogen.

Side effects

- There may be fluid retention and weight gain.
- Break-through bleeding may occur in the first cycle and later if the amount of oestrogen is too low.
- Thromboembolism may occur, mainly with high oestrogen dosage and a very small increased risk in users of desogestrel/gestodene preparations.
- Skin pigmentation such as the chloasma of pregnancy may develop.
- Migraine may be aggravated.
- Depression occurs in a few.
- There is a little evidence that the pill is carcinogenic to the cervix or the breast. Much of this relates to the higher-dose oestrogens and progestogens used in oral contraceptives 40 years ago.
- There is a lower incidence of cancer of the ovary (by 40%) and endometrium (by 50%).

Contraindications

- The most serious hazards are:
  — thromboembolism
  — coronary thrombosis
  — cerebrovascular accident.
- The pill should be avoided in women:
  — with a history or family history of thrombophlebitis, severe heart disease or cerebrovascular accidents
  — aged over 40 if they are obese and smoke heavily
  — with liver damage including recent infective hepatitis or glandular fever
  — with a history of breast cancer
  — with excess weight, more than 50% of ideal

  — with moderate hypertension
  — with true sickle cell disease—genotype SS or SC (but not sickle trait, genotype AS).

Women taking the pill who undergo surgery face an increased risk of thrombosis and embolism during the postoperative period. The pill should ideally be stopped 4 weeks before elective surgery and immediately in the case of illness or accidents leading to long immobilization.

Drug interactions

Certain drugs may interfere with the absorption, metabolism or efficacy of oral contraceptives:

- Phenytoin
- Barbiturates
- Anti-tuberculous drugs (eg rifampicin)
- Antibiotics (eg griseofulvin and tetracycline).

The dose of hypoglycaemic agents may need increasing whereas the effect of corticosteroids may be enhanced. Women who have epilepsy may need double the normal OC dose to inhibit breakthrough bleeding and achieve maximum safety if they are on sodium valproate or clonazepam.

Prescribing the pill

A careful *history* should be taken with reference to conditions such as heavy smoking that may increase the risk of the pill.

Examination should include a record of blood pressure and body weight. The breasts, heart and abdomen should be examined. A pelvic examination should be made to exclude pelvic pathology.

The choice of oral contraception often depends on the doctor's preference; the list of available pills is extensive. In general:

- 20 µg pills are best kept for very slim women
- 50 µg pills are only used as emergency contraception or for women with epilepsy.

Watch for interacting drugs that are also being taken. The choice lies between a 30 or 35 µg pill to be taken either continuously or as one of the biphasic or triphasic pills.

The first pill is taken on the first day of menstruation. Successors are either taken for 21 days with 7 pill-free days during which a withdrawal bleed occurs or continuously depending on the brand.

Good instructions come with each packet and should be read.

There may be some side effects, such as early morning nausea, breast tenderness and slight bleeding during the first cycle. The *tricyclic regimen* suits some women; here a 35 µg pill with varying doses of progestogen is given for 21 days, then 7 pill-free days when bleeding should occur. This may help sufferers from migraine or epilepsy.

The combined pill should not be given during lactation, the progestogen-only pill being preferred then. The pill may be started on the second day after a miscarriage or termination of pregnancy.

The method should be carefully explained and discussed. The woman is advised to report adverse effects immediately. Regular examination with tests for blood pressure, glycosuria and excessive weight gain is essential.

Forgotten pills

If a pill is missed, advise the woman to take the missed one as soon as she realizes. The most critical time is at the beginning of the packet (starting late) or at the end because either will prolong the pill-free interval and may allow ovulation to occur. If it is within 24 hours of the usual time, contraception is probably secure. If longer than this, the pill may not work. Additional contraception (ie condom) or abstinence is advised for 7 days. If the missed OC is within the last 7 days of the pack, go straight into the next cycle's pack—there will probably be no period but the contraceptive effect will be maintained. If the missed pill is within the first 7 days of a pack, the couple should be advised to use additional barrier contraception for at least 2 weeks. Emergency contraception should be used if unprotected intercourse has taken place since finishing the last packet.

Combined transdermal patch

The patch should be applied to a dry and hairless part of the body away from a joint. The day of application is days 1, 8 and 15 (weekly), and the patch should be removed on day 21. The next patch should be reapplied on day 28. It is recommended that a different site be used each month to prevent dermatitis.

If the patch becomes detached mid-week for less than 24 hours and is reapplied or replaced, no added contraception is needed, but if for more than 24 hours then extra contraception should be used for 7 days. The time of attaching the new patch should be considered a new day 1 and that patch should be retained until the new day 22. If there is a delay in starting the patch, the same rules apply as for the combined pill. If the patch is not changed on day 8 or 15, a 48-hour rule comes into play: <48 hours continue the cycle as if it had been changed correctly; >48 hours then a new cycle should be started as described above and additional contraception used for 7 days. If the patch is not removed on day 22 the next cycle should start on the original day 28 with no loss of contraceptive effect.

Emergency pill (postcoital contraception/ the morning-after pill)

High-dose levonorgestrel alone is now the recommended emergency contraceptive. Treatment should be given within 72 hours of a single incident of unprotected intercourse. The earlier it is taken, the more likely it is to be effective. Hormonal treatments are not as effective as the insertion of an IUD but the latter requires attendance at a clinic and a trained professional, and is not ideal for younger women who are not in stable relationships. The 'morning-after pill' is now available without prescription at any pharmacy in the UK to all women over the age of 16, but they have to pay for it.

The doctor, nurse or pharmacist giving out the morning after pill must inform the woman that:

- the next period can be early or be late
- the woman should have a pregnancy test if she does not menstruate
- she should use barrier methods of contraception until the next period
- she should attend a clinic promptly if she experiences any abdominal pain or her period is very light or strangely timed because she may have an ectopic pregnancy.

The main side effects are nausea and vomiting.

Oestrogen and progestogen are no longer used in the UK. An alternative, which is being evaluated and may be more effective, is the antiprogesterone mifepristone.

Progestogen-only pill

Progestogens are used for oral contraception; they probably act not by inhibiting ovulation but by their effect on the cervical mucus and the endometrium. They also reduce tubal motility so increasing the risk of ectopic pregnancy.

The progestogen-only pill is taken continuously at the same time of day from the first day of menstruation. If the pill is delayed more than 3 hours, additional precautions or abstinence is needed until the pill has been taken continuously for 14 days.

There is a failure rate of 1–4/100 women-years. There may be irregular bleeding or amenorrhoea and the risk of thrombosis is less than that for the combined pill. They are useful in older women and in women with serious medical disorders, e.g. sickle cell disease.

Injectable contraceptives

Those most commonly used consist of a progestogen given either by intramuscular injection or as subcutaneous implants. They are not the first choice for contraception but are widely used in less developed countries and in the UK for women when other methods are unacceptable or contraindicated.

Depo-medroxyprogesterone acetate (Depo-Provera) is given in a dose of 150 mg repeated every 12 weeks or 90 days. Norethisterone enanthate (Noristerat) is given in doses of 200 mg every 8 weeks.

Side effects include weight gain, irregular bleeding and amenorrhoea.

Implantable contraceptives

A progestogen called etonorgestrol is available for subdermal implantation (Implanon). It consists of several rods that can be removed if needed or replaced after 3 years. If a woman is not using hormonal contraception, it should be implanted in the first 5 days of the cycle to give immediate effective contraception. If she is using hormonal contraception, is post partum or after a second trimester abortion then it should be done between day 21

and day 28 after delivery. After a first trimester abortion it should be inserted immediately after the procedure/abortion is complete.

Intrauterine devices

IUDs have existed for centuries. In the past devices were made solely of plastic and they have been superseded in British practice by devices incorporating copper; some also have a silver core or extra copper on the horizontal arms. One of these is shown in Fig. 5.1.

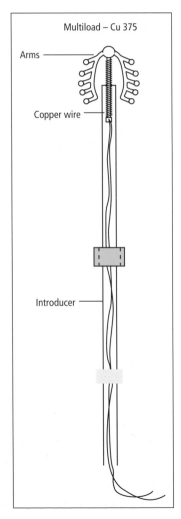

Figure 5.1 One type of intrauterine contraceptive device in current use.

- Copper devices (copper inhibits sperm motility):
  - Multiload
  - Cu 250
  - Cu 250 short—copper wire on stem
  - Cu 375
  - Gyne T 380 (copper wire or stem and arms).
- Copper devices with silver core: Nova-T.

Advantages

An IUD gives permanent protection and requires no attention at the time of intercourse. Provided that there are no complications, a device can remain in the uterus for up to 5 years; in the last decade of reproductive life, this time may be extended as potential fertility is less.

Disadvantages

A skilled doctor or nurse is required to insert an IUD. When first inserted there may be pain and bleeding. The menstrual flow may be increased and the periods prolonged for a few months. There is risk of a flare-up of pre-existing tubal infection.

Complications

- The device may pass unnoticed, especially during menstruation.
- Pelvic infection may occur.
- Increased risk of rejection in nulliparous women.
- Perforation of the uterus may occur with the coil moving into the peritoneal cavity. This is usually at the time of insertion, particularly with an acutely anteflexed or retroflexed uterus. If it occurs with a copper device it should be removed, by either laparoscopy or laparotomy.
- There is no evidence that IUDs are carcinogenic.
- The thread may disappear. The continued presence of the device can be checked by ultrasound. Removal is usually easy in the outpatient department.
- Although the rate of intrauterine pregnancy is reduced, that of ectopics is not. Hence, there is a relative increase in ectopic pregnancy after IUD insertion.

Progestogen devices

Mirena (levonorgestrel 20 μg/day)—called an intrauterine system (IUS) because its profile is very different from the copper IUDs. It has the same effects on cervical mucus and the endometrium as the progestogen-only pill but very little progestogen is released into the systemic circulation, so the side effects of breast tenderness and bloating are minimized.

- It reduces menstrual flow and often dysmenorrhoea.
- It has a lower incidence of pelvic inflammatory disease (PID).

It is particularly useful in older women who have heavy periods. Its Pearl Index is very low and similar to that of sterilization. Periods and fertility return to normal within a few weeks of removal.

Contraindications

An IUD should not be inserted in the presence of:
- pelvic infection
- large or submucosal uterine fibroids
- genital malignancy
- abnormal bleeding, except Mirena
- menorrhagia.

Method of insertion

The device is supplied in a sterile pack with full instructions for insertion. This should be done with aseptic and antiseptic precautions (Fig. 5.2):

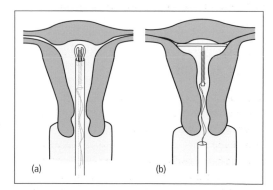

(a)   (b)

Figure 5.2 Method of insertion: (a) the T-shaped intrauterine device (IUD) is straightened inside a plastic tube and inserted through the cervix. (b) When pushed from the hollow tube it resumes its old shape.

- The best time is at the end of menstruation.
- The cervix is exposed and may be steadied with a single-toothed forceps.
- A uterine sound measures cavity length.
- The device is loaded into the introducer and inserted to touch the fundus.
- The introducer is withdrawn and the nylon threads cut, leaving 1.5–2.0 cm in the upper vagina.
- The woman should be taught to identify the threads.

A vasovagal attack may occur at the time of insertion, after cervical stimulation. This usually responds on stopping the insertion and lowering the woman's head. Formal resuscitation is very rarely needed, but facilities should be available at the family planning clinic for the rare occasion.

Postcoital contraception
An IUD may be used for postcoital contraception to prevent implantation if inserted within 5 days of unprotected intercourse. The woman must be seen again to ensure that menstruation has occurred. This is an emergency measure, but if normal menstruation occurs the device may be left as permanent contraception.

Pregnancy
The pregnancy rate with copper devices is reported as 1.4/100 women-years. Should pregnancy occur the possibility of ectopic pregnancy must be excluded:
- If the tail of the device is visible the device should be removed by pulling gently on the thread.
- If the tail of the device is not found the position of the device must be checked by ultrasound.
- The device may be left in the uterus throughout pregnancy.

Barrier contraception
The most effective is the *vaginal diaphragm* or Dutch cap, which consists of a watch spring or coiled spring edged with a dome of latex. They are made in various sizes and for maximum safety must be used with a spermicidal jelly or cream:
- The correct size must be selected before examination (Fig. 5.3).

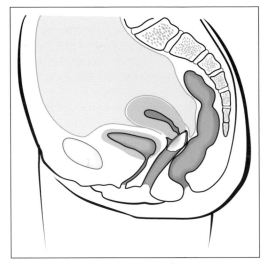

Figure 5.3 The diaphragm fits snugly to the walls of the vagina occluding the cervix from the rest of the vagina.

- The woman should be taught how to insert and remove it.
- Always use it with a spermicide.
- Leave it in for 8 hours after intercourse.
- A check of the fit and, if needs refitting, after 6 months and after childbirth.

If there is prolapse or a retroverted uterus, an alternative is the *cervical cap* made of rubber or plastic. This is harder to get in place and easier to displace at intercourse.

The *vaginal sheath* is like a plastic bag that lines the vagina. It retains its place by a spring ring in the fornices. The woman can insert it at leisure. It has mixed popularity among women and their partners.

Chemical contraceptives
These are mainly spermicides. They may be bought over the counter and do not need professional advice. Creams, gels, soluble pessaries and foaming preparations exist. The failure rate is relatively high if used alone.

A disposable plastic sponge impregnated with spermicide (Nonoxinol-9) can be placed high in the vagina. It is less effective than the diaphragm with a pregnancy rate of about 9/100 women-years.

Douching

Douching immediately after intercourse with warm water or a weak solution of vinegar (one teaspoon to a pint) is a time-honoured but ineffective method. It does not affect those sperm that have already passed up the cervical canal.

Methods used by the male

The sheath

The sheath or condom is one of the most common methods of contraception. It requires no medical intervention and can be bought in many non-medical places. For maximum safety the woman should insert a chemical contraceptive (spermicide) in case the sheath bursts or slips off. Another advantage is that it reduces the spread of sexually transmitted infections, including HIV.

Coitus interruptus

This is the oldest and a widely practised method: the male withdraws before ejaculation. It is not always reliable because human beings are frail. It may prevent complete satisfaction to both partners. In *coitus reservatus* the man enters the vagina but does not ejaculate. This is even more unreliable, for who wants to stop?

The male contraceptive in injectable or tablet form continues to be researched and is coming closer to reality. As yet there are none on the market commercially.

Methods used by both partners

The safe period or natural family planning

In theory ovulation occurs at a predictable time in each menstrual cycle, so there are days when a woman can expect to be infertile. These can be calculated in various ways:

- The calendar method based on working out the fertile period from previous cycles (Fig. 5.4).
- The basal temperature method depends on the rise of basal temperature that follows ovulation. Intercourse is stopped for 3 days before and after ovulation.

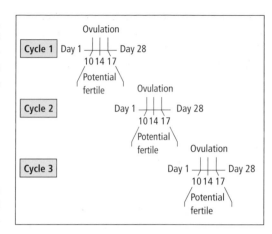

Figure 5.4 The fertile time to avoid when using the calendar method of contraception.

- Teaching the woman to note the changes in cervical mucus that occur at ovulation and mark the peak of fertility. Instead of sticky glue-like mucus, it becomes thin and runny. Motivation is important as is adequate instruction.
- Ovulation predictor tests, but these are expensive.

The disadvantage of the safe period is that it is not really safe and has a high failure rate. Very few women have absolutely metronomic cycles and this is made worse if menstruation is irregular, after childbirth or abortion, or in women approaching the menopause.

Contraception for the under 16s.

In British Law, a person under the age of 16 requires a parent or guardian to give consent for them to undergo any surgical, medical or dental procedure. In 1985 a legal case was brought by Mrs Victoria Gillick that challenged the right of doctors to prescribe contraception to minors under the age of 16 without informing their parents. Subsequently in 2001 the Department of Health produced advice for the medical profession to enable them to establish whether the child had sufficient understanding and intelligence to enable him or her to understand fully what is proposed, known as 'Gillick' or 'Fraser' competence. Competence according to the Department of Health, is not a simple attribute that a child either possesses or does not possess.

The rules state that each child must be assessed as an individual, their competence to consent is not age specific and concerns their capacity to make a decision and thus their competence should be judged in the same way as for an adult. The GMC has produced two documents of relevance in this area in 2008 '0–18 years guidance for all doctors—paragraphs 22–41' and 'Consent: patients and doctors making decisions together— paragraphs 54–56.'

Good practice is to encourage the young person to confide in their families and involve them in the decision. If the child insists that their confidentiality should be respected then the doctor has a duty to do so unless there are grounds to suggest that the child may suffer significant harm as a result. Consideration must be given to factors such as whether the child is in an appropriate relationship (with a boy of her own age or one who is much older which may be abusive/considered statutory rape in law), and the risk to her of an unwanted pregnancy.

Sterilization

Sterilization is an operation aimed at the permanent occlusion of tubes carrying the gametes.

Counselling for sterilization

Sterilization is an important step in the life of any man or woman. It should be considered as irrevocable because, although reversal is possible for both men and women, success cannot be guaranteed even in the most expert hands. Counselling is important and consent must be given in writing. The consent of the spouse is no longer necessary legally, but it is desirable that the couple should be seen together and the full implications of the procedure explained.

A girl under 16 cannot consent to sterilization, nor can her parents insist on it. The same applies to individuals who do not have mental capacity to understand the meaning and consequences of the operation. At present such operations can be performed only with the consent of a High Court judge. An advocate for the patient is usually involved to ensure that his or her best interests are upheld in an objective and fair manner.

Female sterilization

The most practical place to block the female genital tract is at the fallopian tubes. These are deep inside the peritoneal cavity, so their approach is a bigger procedure than operating on the male. The use of the laparoscope has reduced much of the need for large incisions in most cases, but it is still an intraperitoneal operation requiring a general anaesthetic and the availability of full surgical skills.

Laparoscopic sterilization

This operation is performed through a small incision but is potentially just as hazardous as a larger operation (Plate 5). It should be performed only by those who are skilled in general gynaecological surgery, because the abdomen may have to be opened at any time to deal with complications. These are, however, uncommon and usually the laparoscopic sterilization can be done as a day case. The women should be advised to avoid unprotected intercourse for at least a week before the procedure. IUDs should be left in situ until the next period. The progestogen-only pill and combined pill can be stopped at the end of the current packet.

The tube is then blocked by one of three methods:

1 A *mechanical clip* (Hulka-Clemens, Filshie) may be applied to each tube. This may be a spring-loaded clip or a plastic one with a grip (Fig. 5.5).

2 A *Silastic ring* (Falope ring) may be applied to the medial narrow part of each tube through the laparoscope (Fig. 5.6). A knuckle of tube is drawn up and over it is slipped a Silastic ring, which constricts the neck of the knuckle. This causes necrosis of the tube at the bound point, which then fibroses, blocking the lumen, and then pulls apart leaving the tube with a gap.

3 *Unipolar or bipolar diathermy* used to cauterize the fallopian tube in two places about 1 cm apart in

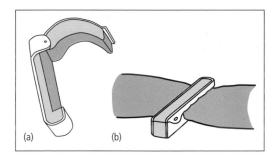

Figure 5.5 Clip sterilization: (a) a Filshie clip and (b) its method of application (Plate 5).

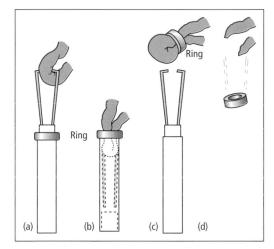

Figure 5.6 A Silastic ring and its method of application: (a) the springy forceps grasp the tube; (b) retracting the forceps draws the tube through the plastic ring; (c) passing the forceps back releases the tube and the tube is constricted at its neck by the ring; (d) the loop becomes hypoxic, dies and the ends separate when the ring drops off.

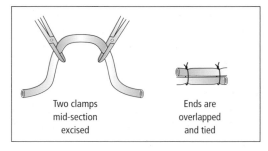

Two clamps
mid-section
excised

Ends are
overlapped
and tied

Figure 5.7 Division and overlapping of tubes at mini-laparotomy.

the isthmus area. There is a risk of heat damage. For this reason, it is less commonly used in the western world.

Photographs are usually taken to show that the correct structure has been occluded, the ring or clip has been correctly applied across the whole tube and the clips are securely tightened. This has become important when the sterilization fails.

Failure rates of laparoscopic sterilizations are about 2–3/1000 operations.

Laparotomy sterilization

This is virtually never done these days except at the same time as a caesarean section. The operation of formal surgical division is commonly performed these days while doing an elective caesarean section when the abdomen is open. The failure rate is about 2–4/1000 operations.

More rarely the Irving method, where each tube is divided and separated and the medial end implanted in a tunnel in the wall of the uterus, is used. The simplest operation was described by Pomeroy but is very rarely performed.

A lesser abdominal operation (Mini-Lap) can be performed by an experienced surgeon. A 5 cm transverse suprapubic incision is extended to the rectus sheath and the surgeon then separates the rectus muscles. This allows a bivalve speculum to be introduced through the incision into the peritoneal cavity. Through this, each fallopian tube in turn can be sought, drawn up and operated upon. It is divided and the two ends overlapped so that the ends are separated. This operation is often done in developing countries where laparoscopy is not readily available. The failure rate for this operation is about 1–2/1000 operations (Fig. 5.7).

Other methods

Transuterine methods of sterilization without anaesthesia are attempted using a hysteroscope and placing occlusive devices into the cornu of the tube. These have the advantage of being more readily reversible. None of these methods has yet been shown to produce reliable results.

Causes of failure

Despite these operations, a woman may still get pregnant in 2–3/1000 cases in the UK:

• The woman may already have a fertilized oocyte in the proximal tube or even the uterus at the time of the operation. Hence try to operate in the first 2 weeks of the cycle.

• All women undergoing sterilization should have a pregnancy test before the procedure.

• The occluding clip or ring may be correctly placed but spring off or break after the operator has left the abdomen. Unless a good knuckle of tube is brought through the Silastic ring, it may not be pinching it securely. The clip may re-open under pressure of the tissues, although this is less common with the beaked Filshie clip. Very rarely sterilization clips have broken. Thus they have no occlusive effect on the fallopian tube and have been removed subsequently from the abdomen in pieces.

• Although the tube is blocked by the clip and the short length of fibrosis that it causes, the two ends of the tube may not separate. A small fistula can form between the contiguous ends, bypassing the occluding device or burrowing through the short length of fibrous tissue. This would allow sperm to pass up readily although fertilized eggs might pass down less commonly; in consequence an ectopic pregnancy may result.

• The occluding device may be put on the wrong structure. Laparoscopic sterilization should be done only when the surgeon has good vision. Occasionally, however, with less than perfect sight, a clip is put on the round ligament just in front of the fallopian tube.

A hysterosalpingogram is occasionally performed 16 weeks after the operation to ensure tubal blockage. It is unwise to do it before as the pressure of the injected dye may disrupt healing tissues and produce a fistula between the blocked parts of the tube.

Male sterilization

Blockage is performed by division of each vas deferens in the groin, a lesser surgical operation than for the female, and done under local anaesthesia (Fig. 5.8). Unguarded intercourse should await two

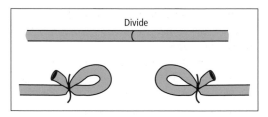

Figure 5.8 Male sterilization: divided ends of the vas deferens are turned back and ligated to ensure that the open ends are not just separated but point in opposite directions.

semen specimens showing no sperm, often as long as 16 weeks after the surgery.

Complications are few:

• Haematoma of the scrotum
• Infection
• Failure of blockage
• Long-term generation of sperm antibodies and non-specific antibodies in later life.

Termination of pregnancy

Pregnancy may be terminated by intervention with instruments or drugs. If done incorrectly, there is a high risk of trauma and death of the mother. It is illegal in some societies, but many sovereign states have now passed laws that allow a termination to be performed by doctors under certain constraints.

Religious and cultural factors dictate whether termination is allowed in a country. Generally, termination of pregnancy (TOP) is unacceptable to the Roman Catholic church, to Moslems and to some other major world religions. In actuality, women seek termination of unwanted pregnancies worldwide, irrespective of the official religion or laws of a country.

In some countries, TOP is used as a part of the contraceptive programme; in communist eastern Europe, up to a third of women used termination as their primary means of contraception. In most of the western world this is not so, because it is appreciated that TOP has many more complications than the more conventional methods of contraception.

Four factors have recently rendered TOP safer in western society.

1 Better training of doctors in the subject

2 Safer general anaesthesia or wider use of local anaesthetic agents

3 Asepsis and antisepsis have reduced infection:
— screening for chlamydia infection and gonorrhoea before the procedure
— use of prophylactic antibiotics

4 Liberalization of abortion laws encourage early medical advice.

Position in the UK

Major changes in TOP were associated with the 1967 Abortion Act (which does not apply in Northern Ireland) and the subsequent 1991 amendment. Before then, a few TOPs had been carried out under an *obiter dictum* or case law, which said that a physician may recommend a pregnancy be terminated if he thought that the continuation of pregnancy would harm the mother's physical or mental health. Since the 1967 Abortion Act, the position has been codified into statute law. This was modified in 1991 so that now there are five indications that must be certified in advance by two doctors who should have seen and examined the woman. These are reproduced in Box 5.2, taken from the Abortion Act Certificate A.

In addition, in an emergency, one doctor alone may recommend TOP to save the woman's life or health. This indication is very rarely used.

In England and Wales, the various indications are used in the proportions (2006) in Table 5.3.

Assessment of the data by age is shown in Fig. 5.9, along with the proportion of births reported in these age groups. There is a shift to younger women in the distribution of terminations.

Ninety per cent of TOPs in Britain take place before week 12 of pregnancy and only 2.5% are performed after week 20 even though the law at present allows this up to completed week 24. A legal TOP must be notified by the operating surgeon to the appropriate Department of Health in England, Scotland or Wales within 7 days.

Methods

Any woman presenting with a request for a TOP should be assessed carefully. Her GP may know the

Box 5.2 Extracts from the Abortion Act Certificate A 1991

A The continuance of the pregnancy would involve risk to the life of the pregnant woman greater than if the pregnancy were terminated

B The termination is necessary to prevent grave permanent injury to the physical or mental health of the pregnant woman

C The pregnancy has NOT exceeded its 24th week and that the continuance of the pregnancy would involve risk, greater than if the pregnancy were terminated, of injury to the physical or mental health of the pregnant woman

D The pregnancy has NOT exceeded its 24th week and that the continuance of the pregnancy would involve risk, greater than if the pregnancy were terminated, of injury to the physical or mental health of any existing child(ren) of the family of the pregnant woman

E There is a substantial risk that if the child were born it would suffer from such physical or mental abnormalities as to be seriously handicapped

Table 5.3 Various indications for termination of pregnancy

Category	Percentage
A	0
B	1
C	94 (from 85 in 1995)
D	4
E	1
Emergency	<0.01

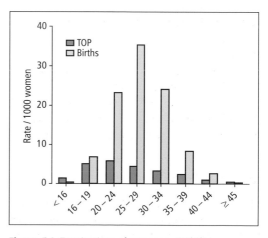

Figure 5.9 Terminations of pregnancy (TOP) by age compared with births.

circumstances of the family well, but the hospital doctor will not. The alternative to abortion is continuation of the pregnancy and its sequelae must be considered:

- adoption
- placing child with foster parents
- the mother's parents taking the child.

Often none of these is acceptable and the woman wishes to go on with the abortion. The GP usually sends her on to a gynaecologist for a second opinion and action, having signed the first half of the Abortion Act Certificate A.

In the hospital, if in agreement with the GP, the specialist signs the second part. Time should be allowed for the woman to reconsider; if she wishes to go ahead she is checked for fitness for operation under anaesthesia and tested for *Chlamydia*. The future method of contraception is discussed to avoid a repeat unwanted pregnancy. Many women are day-case admissions, especially those seen in the earlier weeks of gestation (before 14 weeks). A TOP must be performed in an NHS hospital or clinic specifically licensed for the purpose.

Early abortion

Surgical termination

For pregnancies up to 12 weeks' gestation, TOP is often by a vacuum aspiration of the uterine cavity. A hollow plastic catheter is passed through the cervix, which has been gently dilated, usually after prostaglandin ripening. A vacuum suction then removes the uterine contents and a gentle curettage ensures that the uterus is empty. This technique has few complications and a high success rate.

Medical termination

The use of antiprogesterone steroids such as mifepristone has spread from Europe to the UK, but is not used widely in the USA because of the views of their politicians. An increasing number of women at less than 9 weeks' gestation elect for this day-case TOP, which is very effective in producing total abortions in 96% of cases—a figure comparable with the success rate of aspiration TOP. Women opt for this because it avoids anaesthesia and surgery; they consider it more natural and it gives them control.

Used in the outpatient department, a single oral dose of mifepristone is given, followed 36–48 hours later by 200–600 µg oral misoprostol or a 0.5 mg gemeprost vaginal pessary. Although the measured blood loss in both medical and surgical methods is the same, women report a longer period of blood loss after medical TOP.

Mifepristone is also most useful at 16–18 weeks' gestation when 200 mg is given 24 hours before prostaglandins ($PGE_{2\alpha}$) and works swiftly.

Mifepristone can also be injected into ectopic gestational sacs in ectopic pregnancy (see Chapter 8) and can be used for postcoital emergency contraception.

Complications of early TOP

- *Haemorrhage*: separation of the sac and forming placenta causes blood loss. Syntometrine is often needed intravenously to help the myometrium clamp down.
- *Perforation*: if the uterus is perforated, laparoscopy with examination and repair of the uterus may be required.
- *Infection*: TOP is an invasive procedure, passing instruments through the potentially septic area of the vagina into the sterile area of the uterus. The operator cleans the upper vagina with antiseptic before starting and antibiotics may be given before the operation if vaginal infection is suspected. If infection occurs, particularly with *Chlamydia*, it must be treated promptly with antibiotics or a tubal infection may follow leading to future infertility.
- *Incomplete termination*: this leads to retention of products of conception. Bleeding occurs and re-evacuation of the uterus is necessary.
- *Psychological complications*: many women have a natural grief reaction after early TOP; if the abortion was voluntary, that reaction passes in a few weeks or months. Should the woman have been coerced into termination, the reaction can continue for much longer; up to 25% of women in this latter group may require psychotherapy.

Future pregnancies

Early TOP usually has no effect on future pregnancies. If the cervix is properly dilated (usually not more than 8 mm), there should be no cervical incompetence after early TOP; this is more commonly found after 10–12 mm dilatation, particularly if no prostaglandin was given preoperatively to ripen the cervix.

Mid-trimester abortion

After 14 weeks of gestation, pregnancy termination becomes more difficult. In the UK it is most commonly performed for fetal abnormality beyond 18 weeks.

Morcellation and extraction

In the hands of an expert and experienced gynaecologist, under anaesthesia the cervix can be dilated to well beyond 10 mm. Crushing instruments are introduced into the uterus to break up the fetus which is then extracted piecemeal. This is an unpleasant and potentially hazardous way to abort, but in expert hands it does mean that the whole procedure is over in a few minutes with the mother asleep and unaware of the abortion. She often goes home later the same day.

Prostaglandins

The uterus can be made to contract by giving prostaglandins ($PGE_{2\alpha}$) *per vaginam*, orally, intra-amniotically, extra-amniotically or intravenously. Usually the woman is given the antiprogesterone mifepristone 48 hours before the prostaglandins as it has been shown to shorten the time to delivery. In most cases the progestogen misoprostol given vaginally or orally is effective.

A mini-labour follows and delivery usually takes place in 10–20 hours. This is painful and so should be well covered with analgesia, even an epidural. Evacuation of the placenta is needed in some cases.

Hysterotomy

If prostaglandins are not available, pregnancies after about 14 weeks require a surgical termination and a mini-caesarean section is performed. There is no lower segment and so the uterine incision has to be vertical. This is rarely done anywhere in the world now.

Complications

• *Bleeding*: this is uncommon after prostaglandin TOP, because the uterus has been contracting

through the mini-labour. However, the placenta is often retained in terminations between 14 and 22 weeks of pregnancy and requires removal under general anaesthesia. Bleeding is not a major problem after hysterotomy because it is a surgical procedure at which haemostasis is achieved at the time of the operation.

• *Infection*: infection is not common after mid-trimester abortion procedures and should be prevented as it is in any labour or surgical operation by good asepsis and antisepsis.

• *Psychological problems*: these are more common after mid-trimester abortion. The woman has been pregnant for a longer period and the fetus is more developed. This is an area of great sensitivity that the attendants must be very careful in handling. Some people wish to bury the fetus with a religious service; these natural reactions should be assisted.

• *Future pregnancies*: after mid-trimester TOP, the cervix has been dilated and cervical incompetence can follow.

A vertical hysterotomy scar on the uterus might cause a problem, because it is more liable to rupture in a subsequent pregnancy than a lower segment transverse incision.

Later terminations

Until 1991, TOP was permitted in England, Wales and Scotland only before 28 weeks, the time of presumed viability in law. With modern neonatal developments, the law has reduced this to 24 weeks. Clauses C and D limit terminations to below 24 weeks, but the other clauses (risk of death, grave permanent injury to the mother or fetal abnormalities) are not time limited. Sometimes ultrasound may show a fetal abnormality only at 26–28 weeks or cordocentesis done for karyotyping studies may give results as late as 28–29 weeks.

Late termination is difficult to accept for the woman and for all who have to care for the woman, but it is a logical extension of the law's previous position with more up-to-date diagnostic tests on the fetus. Such terminations are usually done with mifepristone and prostaglandins.

Chapter 6

Benign diseases, genital tract infections and sexual problems

Introduction

This chapter addresses benign conditions and infections affecting the lower genital tract. In reading the chapter, it is useful to remember that many infectious conditions may be sexually transmitted and therefore it is essential to consider this possibility in all women who are, or have recently been, sexually active. It is important to have knowledge of these diseases, which are among the most widespread infectious diseases in the UK and many other parts of the world. Some sexually transmitted infections (STIs) have significant long-term sequelae including infertility, ectopic pregnancy and chronic pelvic pain, as well as the possibility of mother-to-child transmission during pregnancy or at delivery and post partum (if breastfeeding).For example, HIV shares the same route of transmission as STIs and STIs facilitate sexual transmission of HIV. In the presence of HIV and STI co-infection, cervicovaginal HIV RNA shedding is increased. This increases the risk of chorioamnionitis and preterm labour, which in turn are linked to an increased risk of mother-to-child transmission of HIV.

The increase in the reported incidence of STIs in the UK and other countries reflects a number of

factors, including worsening of access to over-burdened sexual health services, a more liberal attitude to sexual intercourse, the younger age of starting sexual activity, a lack of political will to deal with STI-related issues, and less than ideal sex education in some schools and homes (Table 6.1).

In addition, the introduction of more sensitive DNA amplification-based diagnostic tests has resulted in more diagnoses of some conditions, eg infection with *Chlamydia trachomatis*. The UK has a well-established network of genitourinary medicine (GUM) clinics that provide primary care access to patients at risk of STIs. These clinics provide quarterly statistical returns on their workload—a statutory requirement in the UK (KC60). In addition, these clinics have health advisers who oversee partner notification (contact tracing) of all patients diagnosed with important STIs. They also possess expertise in risk assessment for HIV infection and provide pre- and post-test counselling for those at high risk of HIV infection.

In an attempt to deal with the alarming increase in STI diagnoses and the increasing waiting times in GUM clinics, the British government released a National Strategy for Sexual Health and HIV in 2001, which aims to increase the amount of STI testing and treatment undertaken in general practice and community reproductive and sexual health (family planning) services. Any health-care worker who takes on the responsibility of treating an STI (presumed or confirmed) must ensure that sexual part-

Lecture Notes: Obstetrics and Gynaecology, 3rd edition. By Diana Hamilton-Fairley. Published 2009 by Blackwell Publishing. ISBN: 978-1-4051-7801-3.

Table 6.1 Number of new diagnoses of sexually transmitted infections in the UK in 2006

		Percentage change	
	Numbers in 2006	2005–2006	1997–2006
Chlamydia infection	113 585	4	166
Genital warts	83 745	3	22
Genital herpes	21 698	9	31
Gonorrhoea	19 007	−1	46
Syphilis	2 766	−1	1607

Data from the Health Protection Agency.

ners are treated as well. There is little or no point in treating the index case when they will simply be re-infected by an untreated partner. Even if they are no longer at risk of reacquiring the STI from a previous partner, it is important from the public health perspective that sexual contacts are treated.

Taking a sexual history

History of presenting condition

Describe the current symptoms and establish their duration and nature.

- For vaginal discharge, try to establish if the discharge is different from normal and, if so, how has it changed? What is it about the discharge that bothers the patient?
- Details of the onset, eg postcoital, post-antibiotics, premenstrual.
- The volume—does it soil underwear or require sanitary towels to be used?
- The colour and consistency:
  — white, thick and lumpy, 'cottage cheese'— suggestive of **candidiasis**
  — yellow, green and frothy—classically **trichomoniasis** although variation is seen
  — stringy, clear, mucoid—likely to be cervical in origin.
- Bacterial vaginosis and trichomoniasis are common causes of offensive discharge, often described as a 'fishy' odour.
- Extreme odour is often associated with anaerobic bacterial activity caused by retained foreign bodies and carcinoma.
- Remember that cervical infection may manifest only as vaginal discharge.

- Vulval soreness is suggestive of secondary bacterial infection, herpes genitalis or dermatitis.
- Dysuria, frequency and urgency are symptoms commonly seen with cystitis/urinary tract infection (UTI) in women but STIs such as chlamydia infection, gonorrhoea, trichomoniasis and herpes genitalis commonly give rise to dysuria or other urethral symptoms.
- Intermenstrual and postcoital bleeding may be seen in women with cervicitis.
- Deep dyspareunia and pelvic pain may alert the practitioner to salpingitis or pelvic inflammatory disease (PID).
- Superficial dyspareunia can be caused by a wide range of conditions including STIs (eg herpes), non-STI infections (eg candidiasis), genital dermatoses or vulvar pain syndromes.
- Genital lumps and bumps: women display a wide range of normal anatomical variants in the vulvovaginal region that may cause concern if noticed recently by the patient. Nevertheless, STIs such as genital warts and molluscum contagiosum are common causes of new lumps.
- Cuts, sores or ulcers may be presenting symptoms of STIs (eg herpes, syphilis, lymphogranuloma venereum [LGV] and chancroid), non-STI infections (eg candidiasis) and genital dermatoses (eg eczema). Painful inflammatory ulcers may be seen with severe aphthosis, Behcet's syndrome and Crohn's disease.
- Inguinal lymphadenopathy is an important symptom because it usually indicates a significant infection (eg herpes, syphilis, LGV and chancroid) or other morbidity in the anogenital region or lower limb (eg metastatic vulval/vaginal/anal cancer). Common conditions such as candidiasis,

bacterial vaginosis, cystitis, warts and Chlamydia do not usually cause lymphadenopathy so other pathology should be sought.

Sexual contact history

• Cover sexual contacts for the past 3 months (6 months if acute hepatitis B and 2 years if secondary syphilis are likely)
• Sexual orientation of patient
• Gender of partner(s) and whether regular or non-regular partner
• Country of origin of partner(s)
• Type of sexual intercourse: vaginal, oral, anal, fingers, sex toys
• Use of condoms and other contraceptive methods. Self-reported condom use is not always predictive of risk of infection.

Past history of STIs

• Past infections with warts and herpes may recur spontaneously.
• Document fully any previous treatments for positive treponemal serology along with previous syphilis test results.
• Document previous HIV test results (with year).

Recent antibiotic and drug history

• Relevant for gonorrhoea as resistance is common.
• Antibiotics may trigger some conditions such as candidiasis and genital fixed drug eruptions.
• Oral contraception may influence symptoms such as discharge and bleeding.
• Document allergies.

Hepatitis B immunization

Hepatitis B immunization is recommended for those using intravenous drugs, sex workers, and those who are sexual or household contacts of hepatitis B carriers.

HIV risk assessment

• Necessary only for period since 3 months before last negative HIV test. This 'window period' is being reduced with the use of newer HIV antibody/antigen assays and such tests should reliably detect evidence of infection after 4–6 weeks since sexual exposure.
• Number of recent sexual partners with whom patient has had unprotected vaginal or anal sex.
• Has the patient had unprotected sex with men *in or from* countries with high HIV prevalence, eg sub-Saharan Africa, Caribbean, south-east Asia, Latin America, some Eastern bloc states?
• Injecting drug use with sharing of needles.
• Blood transfusion at a time when blood supplies were not checked for HIV antibodies or in a less developed country.

Benign conditions

The vulva and vagina

Pruritus vulvae

Pruritus vulvae is a common symptom—an itch or irritation of the vulva sufficient to lead to scratching.

Causes
• Irritating vaginal discharges of *Trichomonas vaginalis* or vulvovaginal candidiasis. As many infections are common to the vulva and vagina, these are considered collectively in later sections.
• Parasitic infestations such as scabies and pubic 'crab' lice. More likely to manifest as pubic or perineal itching.
• Superficial mycoses such as tinea can affect the feet, the groin and the vulva.
• Sensitivity to drugs or chemicals can lead to an irritant or contact dermatitis. Chronic itching and scratching may lead to lichen simplex in the affected vulval skin, with erythema, lichenification and fissuring. Sensitizing agents include:
   — soap and disinfectants
   — detergents used for washing underwear
   — contraceptives made of latex
   — commercial spermicides
   — ointments containing benzocaine and amethocaine.

- Iron deficiency anaemia, also associated with glossitis.
- Gross vitamin deficiencies, A and B group, especially in elderly women.
- Glycosuria from any cause, but principally diabetes. Glycosuria probably causes irritation because it exacerbates vulvovaginal candidiasis. Dipstick urinalysis and further blood testing for impaired glucose tolerance should be performed.
- Degenerative conditions of the vulva occur mainly in postmenopausal women and are associated with irritation and soreness. There are two main varieties: squamous cell hyperplasia and lichen sclerosus:

Squamous cell hyperplasia *(formerly known as vulval dystrophy)* is an important but uncommon condition specific to the vulva. It presents as a thickening and hypertrophy of the vulval skin, often spreading into the groin and around the anus. The hypertrophic keratin layer causes white patches (called leukoplakia). It may be precancerous and tends to recur in time after surgical excision of the vulva. Diagnosis is by biopsy; this shows thickening and increase in depth of the keratin layer, while the basal papillae are hypertrophied and dip deeply into the dermis.

- Lichen sclerosus is a condition usually seen in postmenopausal women and pre-pubertal girls. It differs from squamous cell hyperplasia in that it does not usually spread beyond the skin of the vulva, perineum and perianal areas. Biopsy shows a general thinning of all the skin layers; the keratin layer is deficient and the basal papillae are flattened. There is hyaline change in the dermis, which is infiltrated with lymphocytes.

True pruritus must be distinguished from soreness of the vulva, also a common symptom, and is often caused by herpes genitalis, vaginitis, oestrogen deficiency states and postmenopausal atrophy.

Investigations

These should include the following:
- A careful history, including the use of any substance that might lead to contact allergy
- Examination to determine characteristics and limits of physical signs
- Microbiological examination of vaginal secretions and scrapings from the skin
- A full blood count, urinalysis and fasting blood glucose if relevant; exclude thyroid dysfunction if lichen sclerosus is present
- Biopsy of the skin of the vulva is important to confirm uncertain diagnoses and to exclude both premalignant and malignant conditions.

Treatment

Women may delay seeking advice for vulval symptoms and often self-medicate with topical and oral preparations, especially antifungal treatments; this may obscure the diagnosis and exacerbate the symptoms.

No treatment should be prescribed without a full vulvovaginal examination and relevant investigations. Empirical treatment based on symptomatology alone may result in serious pathology, such as an early carcinoma, being overlooked. With full investigation, the cause can be found in most cases and the help of a dermatologist may be useful in difficult cases. The treatment for many women is to address the underlying cause, eg diabetes or anaemia.

Fungal infections should be treated with imidazole drugs and intravaginal applications (creams or pessaries) should be supplemented with antifungal creams for vulvitis. General advice should be provided about the avoidance of vulval irritants including soaps and douches; simple emollients such as aqueous cream are suitable for use as soap substitutes.

Squamous cell hyperplasia and lichen sclerosus should be treated with potent topical steroids. In cases which do not improve, vulval dermatologist advice should be sought. Surgery may be indicated for the treatment of coexistent VIN/SCC (vulval intraepithelial neoplasia/squamous cell carcinoma) or fusion, although disease tends to recur around the scar.

Non-STI conditions of the vulva

- Folliculitis around the pubic and perineal region has become commonplace in an era when many women deploy various methods of depilation.

Topical antibiotics will usually clear infection but ingrown hairs can be problematic for some and alternative hair removal methods may be needed to avoid recurrences.

- Infections, boils and carbuncles may affect the vulva, especially in women with glycosuria and diabetes.
- Hidradenitis suppurativa may present in the vulval, perineal and perianal areas, and can be difficult to treat.
- Swellings of Bartholin's glands: cysts of Bartholin's duct, bartholinitis and Bartholin's abscesses are common. They present as swellings in the fourchette. An acute abscess is painful and tender like a boil; an abscess may rupture spontaneously, but tends to recur. Treatment of both cysts and abscesses is best managed by marsupialization, which permits adequate drainage and in many cases the function of the gland is retained. The pus in an abscess should always be cultured and a search made for gonococci and *C. trachomatis* in the urethra and cervix, because some Bartholin's abscesses result from these STIs.
- Vaginal and uterine causes: a patient complaining of a lump in the vulva may be suffering from:
  — uterine prolapse
  — a large polyp
  — inversion of the uterus
  — a vaginal cyst.

The urethra

Urethral caruncle occurs mostly in postmenopausal women. It presents as a bright-red swelling at the posterior margin of the urethral meatus. Most urethral caruncles are asymptomatic; however, some may be painful and tender, often associated with dysuria and dyspareunia. Occasionally bleeding or blood on the undergarments may occur. Some lesions may mimic urethral carcinoma. Conservative treatment with Sitz baths (small tub that fits over the toilet) and topical oestrogens may suffice. Surgical therapy may be required for larger symptomatic lesions or if the diagnosis is uncertain.

Prolapse of the urethra, which may be acute or chronic, involves the whole circumference of the urethra and not just the posterior margin of the meatus. It may give similar symptoms to a caruncle. Medical therapy includes local measures such as Sitz baths and topical antibiotic, steroid or oestrogen creams. If symptoms are severe or persistent, the prolapsed urethra should be excised and repaired.

The vagina and cervix

Infections of the vagina may or may not be STIs, whereas infections of the cervix are usually caused by STI pathogens, especially *Neisseria gonorrhoeae* and *C. trachomatis*.

Natural protection of the genital tract is provided by:
- squamous epithelium thickened by oestrogens
- low pH (about 4–4.5) from lactic acid derived from intraepithelial glycogen breakdown by lactobacilli (Doderlein's bacilli)
- mucus from the cervix, Bartholin's gland and Skene's glands, rich in bactericidal lysozymes.

This protection can be diminished in a number of ways:
- Pre-pubertal and postmenopausal women have lower oestrogen levels resulting in a thinner epithelium, a higher pH and less mucus production.
- Antibiotics can alter the balance of commensal flora in some women, although this effect is not consistent
- Chemical douches that wash away the natural protective secretions.
- Ulcerative STIs that breach the protective mucosa.
- Vaginal microbicides.
- Foreign bodies in the vagina such as retained pessaries or tampons.
- Cervical instrumentation and menstruation can remove the protective discharge from the endocervical cavity.

During pregnancy:
- Immunocompetence is diminished, eg decreased number of T-helper cells and decreased lymphocyte responses to certain antigens.
- Vaginal pH increases, influencing vaginal flora.
- Cervical secretions become viscous, forming a cervical mucus plug.

Examination

Inspect the vulva for:
- reddening
- oedema
- excoriation from scratching
- fissuring
- ulceration: multiple shallow tender ulcers ± vesicles are typical of herpes simplex virus (HSV) infection; syphilitic chancres tend to be indurated and may be non-tender
- Inspect the external urethral meatus for prolapse or caruncle.

Vaginal examination to check for:
- Patchy mucosal reddening may be associated with trichomoniasis.
- White plaques and vaginitis are associated with candidiasis.

Examine the cervix and urethra for:
- reddening
- punctate haemorrhages on the cervix seen in trichomoniasis ('strawberry cervix')
- mucopurulent cervical discharge
- contact bleeding

Palpate the urethra for thickening tenderness and purulent discharge. Check that Bartholin's glands are not enlarged or tender.

All women with pelvic pain should undergo a bimanual pelvic examination. Palpate for cervical motion tenderness, adnexal tenderness, and any midline, adnexal or retrovaginal masses.

Palpate the inguinal lymph nodes for swelling and/or tenderness. Lymphadenopathy is an important sign NOT usually associated with conditions such as candidiasis, bacterial vaginosis (BV), trichomoniasis or cervicitis.

Investigations

- Swabs should be taken from the cervical canal and lower urethra for *Neisseria gonorrhoeae*, posterior fornix for BV, *Candida* spp. and *Trichomonas vaginalis*, and any overt lesions on the walls of the lower genital tract.
- Microscopy of a Gram-stained vaginal smear can be performed for BV and candida infection and microscopy of a saline wet mount can enable detection of *T. vaginalis* (sensitivity depends on the experience of the microscopist but is usually no greater than 60%).
- Nucleic acid amplification tests for *C. trachomatis* should be used, sampling the endocervix (or self-taken vulval/vaginal swab). First catch urine is often used to screen women but is a suboptimal specimen.
- If ulcers are seen, swabs for HSV polymerase chain reaction or PCR (type-specific HSV PCR if available), and if appropriate, dark-ground microscopy for detection of *Treponema pallidum* can be performed in addition to syphilis serology.

Treatment

The principles of therapy for STIs are to:
- avoid and manage complications and long-term sequelae
- notify and adequately treat sexual partners concurrently to avoid re-infection
- test for other STIs
- educate patients on STI transmission and safe sex.

Foreign bodies in the vagina

This usually presents with a foul discharge caused by overgrowth of anaerobic organisms around/within the foreign body. This is most common in:
- children: beads or toys, etc
- developmentally delayed: beads or coins, etc
- women in custody: the vagina may be used to hide objects (eg drugs), which might then be forgotten.

Treatment requires the removal of the foreign material. A stat dose of metronidazole may help to restore vaginal flora although no clinical trials support this practice.

Toxic shock syndrome

Caused by staphylococci.

Symptoms
Shivering, diarrhoea, erythematous rash and fainting. Occurs mostly on second and third days at the peak of menstrual flow.

Physical signs
- Hypotension.
- Fever, tenderness of vagina and cervix.

Treatment
- Removal of tampon
- Intravenous fluid resuscitation
- Systemic antibiotics.

Microbiology and therapy of common genital tract infections

Bacterial vaginosis

This condition is caused by an imbalance in the vaginal microflora, although the exact mechanisms that result in this change remain uncertain. There is a decrease in the number of acid-producing lactobacilli and an increase in other vaginal organisms, including *Gardnerella vaginalis*, *Mycoplasma* spp., *Mobiluncus* spp. and other anaerobes. It appears to be more common in certain ethnic groups, eg African–Caribbean individuals, and also in those who are sexually active. Some studies report a higher rate in lesbian women and a high rate of concordance between lesbian couples.

BV has been linked to an increased risk of pregnancy complications including post-abortion infections, late miscarriages, preterm labour and delivery, preterm rupture of membranes and postpartum endometritis. However, there is conflicting evidence about the value of screening or treatment of BV in pregnancy to improve pregnancy outcomes.

Symptoms and signs

Typically there is a non-purulent, homogeneous vaginal discharge, often with an offensive fish-like smell. Patients sometimes present complaining solely of the odour. The symptoms may be more noticeable perimenstrually, and the smell may be exacerbated after unprotected sexual intercourse as a result of the alkalinity of semen releasing more of the volatile amines.

Investigations

The diagnosis of BV should be made by Gram staining of a specimen taken from the lateral wall of the vagina. It is no longer recommended to culture for *Gardnerella vaginalis* because this organism is a normal commensal in the vagina of many asymptomatic women. Features consistent with BV include a reduction in numbers (or absence) of Gram-positive lactobacilli, the presence of mixed Gram-variable bacteria consistent with an increase in anaerobes and *Mobiluncus* spp., and the presence of more than 20% 'clue cells'. Clue cells are vaginal epithelial cells with an adherent mixture of small Gram-negative and -positive organisms that obscure their normal microscopic appearance (Fig. 6.1).

Alternatively, clinical (Amsel's) criteria can be used. Three of the four following criteria need to be present:
1 Presence of homogeneous discharge
2 Presence of clue cells on wet film
3 An increased vaginal pH (>4.5)
4 Release of a fishy odour on addition of alkali (usually 10% KOH).

Treatment

Asymptomatic women do not require treatment, although some may report beneficial change to their vaginal discharge. Treatment should be offered to women undergoing termination of preg-

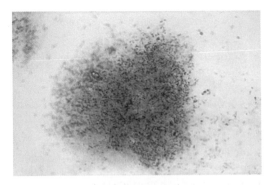

Figure 6.1 Gram-stained slide showing 'clue cell' in bacterial vaginosis. (With acknowledgement to Professor Catherine Ison, Sexually Transmitted Bacteria Reference Laboratory, London.)

nancy or other gynaecological surgery regardless of symptoms because this can reduce postoperative infections.

Appropriate regimens include:
- Metronidazole 2 g single dose orally
- Metronidazole 400 mg twice a day orally for 5 days
- Intravaginal metronidazole 0.75% gel once at night for 5 nights
- Intravaginal clindamycin 2% cream at night for 7 nights
- Clindamycin 300 mg twice daily orally for 5 days
- Tinidazole 2 g single dose orally
- In pregnant women the 5-day oral courses of metronidazole or clindamycin should be used.

There is no indication to treat the male partner because this is not an STI.

Vulvovaginal candidiasis (thrush)

This is caused by a commensal dimorphic fungus that exists in both yeast and mycelial forms. It thrives in sugar-rich environment and symptomatic overgrowth occurs in up to 75% of women at some stage. It occurs more commonly in:
- pregnancy
- diabetes mellitus
- oral contraceptive or oestrogen therapy
- in some women after exposure to broad-spectrum antibiotics.

Symptoms and signs

- Vulval itching or soreness
- Superficial dyspareunia
- A change in vaginal discharge, reported variously, including thick 'cottage cheese' and watery 'milky' types
- Vulval stinging on urination

Clinical findings vary from minimal change to severe inflammation:
- Erythema of the vulva and vagina
- Fissuring and excoriation
- White curdy discharge: there may be adherent white plaques

- Candidal overgrowth may be asymptomatic and found incidentally on speculum examination or cervical cytology
- Men in contact with candidiasis may develop a blotchy red rash on their glans penis or foreskin.

Treatment

- Topical antifungal creams to the vulva are soothing but it is also important to treat intravaginally with a pessary or cream. These are available over the counter without prescription.
- A number of suitable imidazole agents are available with equivalent efficacy, eg clotrimazole 500 mg pessary as a single dose with 5–7 days of topical 1% clotrimazole cream to the vulva twice daily.
- Oral fluconazole 150 mg as a single dose or itraconazole 200 mg twice daily for 1 day may be used with similar efficacy when topical therapy is not suitable. (Avoid oral azoles in pregnancy and breastfeeding.)
- Male *Candida*-associated balanitis responds well to a combination of 1% hydrocortisone and an antifungal, eg Canesten HC or Daktacort, given twice a day for 5–7 days.
- In pregnancy, asymptomatic carriage and symptomatic recurrences are more common. As this is not usually sexually transmitted, there is no proven benefit from treatment of the male partner.

Sexually transmitted infections

Trichomoniasis

The causative organism is a flagellated protozoan, *Trichomonas vaginalis* (TV). In women it causes a vaginal infection, and is usually also found in the urethra. This organism is transmitted sexually; the male is transiently colonized from the infectious reservoir in the female vagina. This occurs because the adhesion proteins of this organism are expressed preferentially in acid pH, typically found in the vagina, whereas the male urethral pH is approximately 7.4. In addition, trichomonads are repeatedly washed out of the urethra when men micturate. The organisms can colonize the sub-preputial sac, the prostate and the paraurethral glands (male equivalent of Skene's glands).

Symptoms and signs

Trichomoniasis in women is asymptomatic in 10–50% of cases. Symptoms include an irritating vaginal discharge with inflammation of the vulva, vagina and ectocervix. The cervical appearance may manifest as a 'strawberry cervix', also termed 'colpitis macularis'. The vaginal discharge may be greenish-yellow, frothy and offensive with a fish-like smell. Up to 15% of infected women have no visible signs. Men typically have no symptoms but, when present, the symptoms include urethral discomfort, dysuria and occasional urethral discharge.

Investigations

The diagnosis may be made within the clinic by the use of a saline wet mount in which a drop of vaginal fluid from the posterior fornix is placed in a drop of saline on which a coverslip is floated. The trichomonads have a characteristic motility as a result of their five flagella. Culture is more sensitive and regarded as the current gold standard. Nucleic acid amplification tests with sensitivities and specificities approaching 100% are currently in development, but still unavailable in many clinical settings. It is important to screen for other common STIs in TV-infected women.

Treatment and follow-up

Trichomoniasis is an STI, so sexual partner(s) *must* be treated with antimicrobials to reduce the re-infection rate:
• Metronidazole 2 g single dose orally (avoid in pregnancy or breastfeeding) or 400 mg twice daily for 5 days.
• Tinidazole 2 g single dose orally.
• Various complicated regimens exist for metronidazole-resistant trichomoniasis and referral to an STI specialist is recommended.

• Partner notification (contact tracing) should be initiated at diagnosis.
• Patients should return for a test of cure at least 7 days after they finish antibiotics.
• Trichomoniasis in pregnancy is linked to preterm labour and preterm rupture of membranes. However, there is no evidence that treatment improves pregnancy outcomes. It is not recommended to screen for TV in asymptomatic pregnant women.
• Neonatal infection with TV is infrequent but vaginitis and UTIs have been described.

Chlamydial infection

Chlamydia trachomatis is the most common bacterial STI in the UK and the predominant organism responsible for PID and ectopic pregnancy. Between 5% and 10% of sexually active women under 24 and men aged 20–24 in the UK are infected. There has been a recent increase in chlamydia cases in men and women in the UK (Fig. 6.2) and a national screening programme for chlamydial infection is being rolled out. *Chlamydia* is a potent mediator of chronic inflammation and can cause fine adhesions in the pelvis surrounding the tubes and ovaries. Untreated chlamydial infection has been reported to result in PID in 10–40% of infections and tends to present with relatively mild symptoms, although more recent studies suggest lower complication rates. PID is an important cause of tubal factor infertility, ectopic pregnancy and chronic pelvic pain. There may be inflammation with adhesions between the liver capsule and diaphragm from perihepatitis (Fitz-Hugh–Curtis syndrome—Plate 6). Other complications include epididymo-orchitis in men, seronegative reactive arthritis and Reiter's syndrome, neonatal and adult conjunctivitis and neonatal pneumonia. In pregnancy, chlamydial infection has been associated with chorioamnionitis and preterm delivery.

Symptoms and signs

Up to 70% of women and 50% of men may be asymptomatic. Male partners may complain of either dysuria or a urethral discharge, usually cloudy

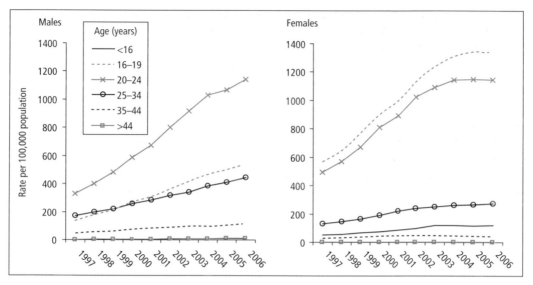

Figure 6.2 New diagnoses of genital chlamydia infection by sex and age in the UK (1997–2006). (Data from the Health Protection Agency.)

or mucopurulent in nature, and may occasionally present with epididymo-orchitis. If symptoms/signs are present in women, they may include any of the following: vaginal discharge, dysuria, postcoital or intermenstrual bleeding, mucopurulent cervical discharge, cervicitis, deep dyspareunia, pelvic pain, cervical excitation and other signs of PID.

Infection of the pharynx and conjunctiva may be present without genital infection but are rare.

Investigations

• *C. trachomatis* is difficult to culture and this technique requires a specialist laboratory.
• Nucleic acid amplification tests (NAATs), which have increased sensitivity over other diagnostic methods, are the tests of choice (eg Strand Displacement Amplification (SDA), PCR, Transcription Medicated Amplification (TMA)).
• NAATs for *C. trachomatis* can be performed on swabs from the endocervix as well as non-invasive specimens such as first void urine or vulvovaginal swabs, although the sensitivity in urine is less than from the endocervix and vulva/vagina as a result of the reduced organism load in female urine. These tests will detect both dead and viable DNA but will not provide data on antimicrobial susceptibility.

Hence, testing within 6 weeks of treatment completion is not recommended due to the potential for persistent chlamydial DNA.
• Enzyme-linked immunoassay (ELISA) techniques are less sensitive and should be replaced in British laboratories by NAATs.
• Fluorescent labelled within the clinic; this technique is labour intensive and not suitable for screening.
• It is important to screen for other common STIs in *Chlamydia*-infected women.

Treatment and follow-up

• *Chlamydia* is an STI, so sexual partner(s) *must* be treated. Patients are advised to abstain from sex for 7 days after they and their partners have been treated. Suitable regimens include:

— azithromycin 1 g single dose orally (not licensed for use in pregnancy although available data indicate that it is safe and is recommended by the World Health Organization; the *British National Formulary* advises use when no alternatives but most GUM clinics use this treatment)
— doxycycline 100 mg twice daily for 7 days (contraindicated in pregnancy)

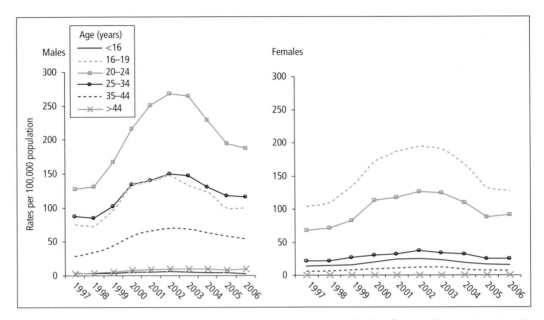

Figure 6.3 New diagnoses of gonorrhoea by sex and age in the UK (1997–2006). (Data from Health Protection Agency)

— erythromycin 500 mg four times daily for 7 days or 500 mg twice daily for 14 days; can be used in pregnancy but both regimens are associated with significant side effects and lower efficacy.

• Longer regimens of a minimum 2 weeks are recommended for treatment of PID and epididymo-orchitis.

• Tests of cure are not necessary with the above regimens, although they are recommended with erythromycin-containing regimens. It is also recommended in pregnancy when cure rates seem to be lower. If using NAATs, non-viable organisms may be detected up to 6 weeks after treatment. Re-screening infected women at 3–6 months seems to be a better strategy because re-infection or treatment failure is likely to be detected at this time.

• Partner notification (contact tracing) should be initiated at diagnosis. Re-infection is common. Only up to 50% of sexual partners will test positive for *Chlamydia*.

Gonorrhoea

This STI is caused by *Neisseria gonorrhoeae*, a Gram–negative diplococcus that is often visualised within neutrophils in Gram-stained genital specimens. There has been a recent increase in gonorrhoea cases in men and women in the UK (Fig. 6.3).

Symptoms and signs

Primary sites of infection in women include the endocervix, urethra, oropharynx, anorectum and Bartholin's glands. In men, the urethra, oropharynx and anorectum are the sites of primary infection. The conjunctivae can also be infected, especially in neonates.

Up to 50% of infected women are asymptomatic. When symptomatic they may present with vaginal discharge (50%), lower abdominal pain (<25%), dysuria (12%), deep dyspareunia, intermenstrual or postcoital bleeding, or signs of ascending infection suggestive of PID. The last occurs in about 10% of cases although the rate is lower in pregnancy. Endocervical mucopurulent discharge can be present but is not a sensitive sign of infection.

Men with urethral gonorrhoea usually have evidence of a purulent urethral discharge and/or dysuria (90%). Complications such as epidydimitis and prostatitis occur rarely (<1%).

A sore throat is unusual with oropharyngeal infection, which usually clears spontaneously within 3 months. Proctitis symptoms including anorectal discharge (12%), discomfort, bleeding and tenesmus may occur with anorectal infection, although most anorectal infections are asymptomatic. Disseminated gonococcal infection is well recognized (<1% of infections). Haematogenous spread of *N. gonorrhoeae* can lead to a pustular rash, tenosynovitis, arthritis/arthralgia and fever with occasional serious sequelae such as endocarditis and meningitis.

Investigations

A swab from the endocervical canal will be culture positive in 80–90% of infected women:
- There will be an increased diagnostic yield if the female urethra and anal canal are also cultured. About 2% of female genital gonorrhoea is detected only if the anal canal is sampled in addition to the urethra and endocervix; it is thought that most cases of anorectal colonization result from self-inoculation via spread of vaginal discharge rather than through unprotected anal sex.
- The organism is extremely fastidious and so the swabs should either be inoculated directly onto appropriate culture medium (as happens in some GUM clinics) or be sent to the laboratory as soon as possible. Stuart's transport medium may increase the yield if a delay is envisaged in the transport process.
- Once cultured, the gonococci can be further analysed for antimicrobial susceptibility.
- NAATs are now available for the diagnosis of gonorrhoea in women using non-invasive specimens such as urine or vulval swabs in addition to the endocervix. The sensitivity of these tests is higher than for culture. These tests will detect both dead and live organisms but will not provide data on antimicrobial susceptibility. Whenever possible, when NAATs return a positive result, cultures should be taken from the patient before treatment in order to ascertain antimicrobial sensitivity. Specificities of NAATs for *N. gonorrhoeae* are <100% and so false positives occur, particularly in low prevalence populations. It is important to convey the possibility of a false-positive result to the patient, in whom a diagnosis of an STI may have a devastating effect.
- It is important to screen for other common STIs.

Treatment and follow-up

- The following regimens remain highly efficacious:
  — ceftriaxone 250 mg i.m. single dose
  — cefixime 400 mg p.o. single dose
  — spectinomycin 2 g i.m single dose.

These regimens are safe to use in pregnant and breastfeeding women. Longer courses are recommended for the treatment of upper genital tract complications and disseminated disease.
- No documented treatment failures with ceftriaxone treatment have yet been reported. The prevalence of microbial resistance is rising mainly in the homosexual population. Surveillance data from 2006 have shown increased resistance to penicillin (9.5%) and ciprofloxacin (26.5%) in *N. gonorrhoeae* strains acquired in the UK, which has required a change in first-line antibiotics used for treatment. Treatment should be guided by local antibiotic sensitivities with the aim of efficacy in a minimum of 95% of cases locally. Where local penicillin and ciprofloxacin resistance rates are lower than 5% or where a strain is shown to be sensitive, the following regimens can be used:
  — amoxicillin 2 g oral with Probenecid 1 g oral, both as a single dose (less effective in pharyngeal and rectal infections)
  — ciprofloxacin 500 mg oral single dose.
  Concomitant chlamydia infection is frequent (up to 40% in women) and thus epidemiological treatment of *Chlamydia* should be considered when treating for gonorrhoea, unless it is known that *Chlamydia* is absent.
- When treating pharyngeal infection, single dose treatment with amoxicillin and spectinomycin is not adequate.
- Patients should return for a test of cure at least 3 days after the completion of antibiotic treatment.
- Partner notification (contact tracing) should be initiated at diagnosis.

Herpes simplex infection

Genital herpes is caused by HSV types 1 and 2, which enter the host through mucocutaneous surfaces. These viruses are able to establish latency and subsequent reactivation may give rise to repeated episodes of the disease. Herpes genitalis is the most common ulcerative STI in the UK. The rise in new diagnoses is steepest in women, especially in the 16–24 age groups (Fig. 6.4). In primary HSV, ie infection in those who have never been infected in the oral or genital areas by either strain of the virus, the causative agent is equally likely to be HSV-1 or -2. The natural history of HSV-1 genital herpes is more favourable, with fewer, less symptomatic reactivations and less viral shedding.

Symptoms and signs

The first episode is often characterized by extensive genital ulceration together with local regional lymphadenopathy and systemic symptoms. The ulceration may last up to 3 weeks if untreated, and first episodes are more severe in vulval and perianal locations compared with penile infection. The typical lesions present initially as vesicles that burst to leave a superficial tender ulcer with an erythematous halo and a greyish-white exudate. Complica-

tions include dissemination to distant sites (eg finger, thighs), meningitis, sacral radiculomyelopathy, and urinary difficulties or retention. Recurrent infections are shorter and less severe than primary infections, often lasting only 3–5 days. Factors involved in reactivation include local trauma, menstruation and stress, although this varies between individuals. HSV-2 infections recur much more commonly than HSV-1 ones. Prodromal neuralgia-type pain radiating down the thigh or buttocks is common.

Up to 80% of HSV-2-seropositive people are unaware of their HSV infection. Most are asymptomatic and others have their recurrent symptoms attributed to other causes, eg recurrent thrush.

Investigations

- Culture of HSV is performed using a swab of vesicular fluid (best) or from the ulcer base, which is sent to the laboratory in viral transport medium. This technique is widely available in the UK but is slow and labour intensive, and requires optimal sample storage and transport.
- NAATs for HSV such as PCR are superseding culture and appear to be the most sensitive diagnostic test for genital ulcers.

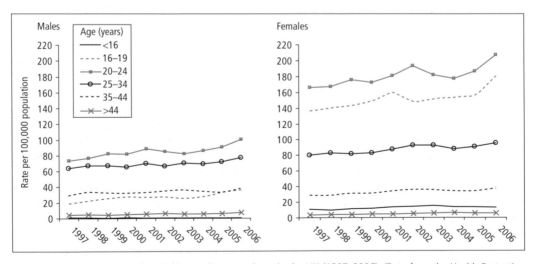

Figure 6.4 New diagnoses of genital herpes by sex and age in the UK (1997–2006). (Data from the Health Protection Agency.)

- Typing the HSV strain (1 or 2) from a first episode lesion allows for a more informed discussion on transmission and prognosis.
- Serology is not very helpful in individual diagnosis. It has a role in the management of a first episode of HSV in a pregnant woman to determine if it is a primary episode, as well as in counselling partners of patients with known HSV-2 recurrent genital lesions. The positive predictive value of serological tests in asymptomatic individuals is determined by the prevalence of HSV in that population. Testing of anonymized sera from individuals aged 16–64 years seeking health care through the NHS in 1991 and 2000 showed that HSV-2 seroprevalence across England was 9.7%.

Treatment

- Primary episodes should be treated with the following:
  — aciclovir 200 mg five times daily for 5 days (double dose in HIV-positive patients)
  — aciclovir 400 mg three times daily for 5 days
  — valaciclovir 500 mg twice daily for 5 days
  — famciclovir 250 mg three times daily for 5 days.
  Consider extending treatment to 10 days if new lesions appear after the initial 5-day course.
- Recurrent episodes are self-limiting and generally do not need treatment. General advice includes saline baths and analgesia. Patients who have frequent episodes with well-recognized prodromal symptoms may be given episodic antiviral treatment, which should be initiated in the first 24–48 hours of the attack.
- After a first episode, the frequency of recurrent episodes decreases year by year in most infected individuals. For frequent recurrent disease (eg more than six episodes per year) or for those with severe symptoms or psychosexual sequelae, consider suppressive antiviral therapy with aciclovir 400 mg twice a day for 6 months initially, and continue as long as required with trials off therapy every 6–12 months. If breakthrough recurrences occur on standard treatment, the daily dosage should be increased or alternative regimens (valac-

iclovir or famciclovir) tried, although these are much more expensive and generally no more efficacious.
- Condom use has limited efficacy in preventing HSV transmission, and is more effective for prevention in women than in men. Infectiousness is greater during a symptomatic episode, although asymptomatic shedding of the virus occurs quite often and so the chance of transmission on symptom-free days still exists. Evidence suggests that daily suppressive treatment with valaciclovir reduces the risk of HSV acquisition by the HSV-negative partner in HSV-discordant couples. The value of partner notification (contact tracing) for first episode HSV is debatable because symptoms may occur for the first time many years after initial infection.

Herpes in pregnancy

The management of herpes in pregnancy requires good communication among the obstetric team, GUM clinicians, paediatric team and patient to avoid unnecessary or unsafe procedures and anxiety. Neonatal infection is very rare in the UK and is mostly acquired during delivery. Risk factors for neonatal herpes acquisition include first episode genital herpes, premature rupture of membranes for more than 4 hours, invasive monitoring, preterm delivery before 38 weeks' gestation and maternal age <21 years. Herpes neonatorum has a high mortality rate (up to 50%) in those who develop encephalitis, but it is rare. A third of those surviving will have some residual neurological damage.

It is important to establish the stage of the maternal HSV infection to allow appropriate management, although this may not always be easy. HSV serology may be useful if samples taken at the episode and 6 weeks later show development of antibodies, indicating a primary infection. In practice the results can take a few weeks and this limits its use.

First and second trimester acquisition
- First episode genital herpes has been associated with first trimester miscarriage but has not been

linked with developmental abnormality if the pregnancy continues.

• Manage the episode as in non-pregnant women. Although aciclovir is not licensed for use in pregnancy, there is substantial clinical experience supporting its safety.

• Vaginal delivery should be anticipated.

• Consider daily suppressive aciclovir from 36 weeks in order to reduce the likelihood of HSV lesions at term.

Third trimester acquisition

• It takes about 6 weeks for the pregnant woman to develop antibodies in response to HSV infection, and transplacental transfer of HSV-specific antibodies protects against neonatal HSV. Although the evidence for caesarean section to prevent neonatal HSV is limited in this situation, it should be offered to all women presenting with first-episode genital herpes lesions at the time of delivery, or within 6 weeks of the expected date of delivery or onset of labour. However, caesarean section may not be of benefit in reducing transmission for women presenting with ruptured membranes for >4 hours.

• If vaginal delivery is unavoidable or where the mother opts for a vaginal birth, prolonged rupture of membranes and invasive procedures should be avoided. Intravenous aciclovir given intrapartum to the mother and subsequently to the neonate may be considered. The paediatricians should be informed of the HSV risk to the neonate.

Recurrent genital herpes in pregnancy

• Women should be reassured that recurrences during pregnancy are no more severe than when non-pregnant and pose no threat to the pregnancy or neonate. The risk of transmission to the newborn is low even if lesions are present during labour. Transplacental transfer of maternal antibodies provides protection at the time of delivery.

• The benefits of obtaining specimens for culture at delivery to identify women who are shedding HSV asymptomatically are unproven.

• The use of suppressive treatment with aciclovir from 36 weeks reduces HSV recurrences and caesarean section deliveries for HSV and may also be cost-

effective. An aciclovir dose of 400 mg three times daily should be considered because of the altered pharmacokinetics of the drug in late pregnancy.

• Women who have never had genital HSV and who have partners known to have HSV should be advised to avoid sex in the third trimester and during symptomatic recurrences. This should include oral sex if the partner has orolabial herpes.

Genital warts

Genital warts, also known as condylomata acuminata, are caused by various genotypes of the human papillomaviruses (HPVs). Infection with the low-risk types account for >90% of warts whereas high-risk HPV types (eg 16 and 18) are associated with malignant potential or intraepithelial neoplasia, but are not usually associated with exophytic warts. Genital warts are transmitted sexually although inoculation from extragenital sites (eg hands) has been reported. It is the second most frequently diagnosed STI in the UK. Routine HPV immunization of girls aged 12–13 is to be introduced in the UK in 2008 and aims to prevent infection with the two most common oncogenic HPV types (HPV-16 and -18) responsible for most cervical cancers. It may also prevent genital warts caused by low-risk genotypes (usually type 6 and 11) depending on the vaccine used.

Symptoms and signs

In most cases HPV infection is subclinical. When present, warts do not usually cause discomfort apart from some irritation; in the perianal area bleeding may occur. In women, genital warts typically occur on the vulva at the vaginal introitus, posterior fourchette, on the labia, around the clitoris, and in the perineal and perianal regions. In men, warts usually occur at the frenulum, around the coronal sulcus, on the inner aspect of the prepuce, on the penile shaft, within the meatus and at the perianal margin. Proctoscopy may reveal internal warts as far as the squamocolumnar junction between the anal canal and the rectum. Perianal lesions occur in both sexes. Warts feel hard to the touch and are often raised with an irregular surface. Patients can be quite distressed by warts despite their benign nature, especially when chronic and not responding to treatments. Warts are more difficult to treat when patients have cell-mediated immune deficiency, eg in people with diabetes, immunosuppressed transplant recipients or HIV-positive patients.

Investigations

• The diagnosis is a clinical one. If required, confirmation can be obtained histologically.
• It is important to screen for other common STIs.

Treatment

• Treatment is cosmetic and is aimed at eliminating or reducing the size of the warts. It does not eliminate the virus as it remains latent within the basal skin cells. The following may be used:
— cryotherapy: treatment should be applied until a 'halo' of freezing has been established a few millimetres around the treated lesion; a freeze–thaw–freeze technique should be used and lesions held frozen for 10–30 seconds, depending upon their size
— self-application of podophyllotoxin may be undertaken whereby the solution or cream is applied to the warts twice daily for 3 days followed by a 4-day break; this cycle may be repeated three more times before the patient is reviewed by a clinician; it should be avoided in pregnancy
— imiquimod topical therapy 3 nights a week for 4 weeks, followed by clinical review; not licensed for use in pregnancy
— trichloroacetic acid (caustic agent to be handled with care)
— electrocautery
— surgery (curettage, scissor excision).
• Warts tend to recur in pregnancy when they can enlarge with gestation and be difficult to treat. Treatment modalities are also limited. Caesarean section is only very rarely indicated when warts are potentially large enough to obstruct labour. There is also the small risk of perinatal transmission, resulting in infant or childhood laryngeal papillomatosis.

General advice

• Warts may recur within the first year after therapy in up to one-third of cases.
• Condoms should be used with new sexual partners although protection may be limited because the virus has a 'field effect' and can be shed from a wide area of genital skin and mucosa.
• Long-term partners are likely to be already infected with the same HPV genotypes as the patient, so instructions on condom use may not be helpful in this situation.
• It is important to ensure that cervical smears are being undertaken in line with the recommendations for national screening programmes (see Chapter 19).
• There is evidence that smoking is linked to diminished response to treatment.
• Girls aged 12–14 should be encouraged to have the immunization against HPV-16 and -19.

Syphilis

This disease, caused by *Treponema pallidum*, was a major cause of morbidity and mortality in the pre-antibiotic era. It remains an important disease in resource-poor settings and has recently re-emerged as an important STI in homosexual or bisexual men, many of whom are HIV positive. There continue to be outbreaks of syphilis among women in the USA and, more recently, this has occurred in the UK. There are epidemiological links to crack cocaine use, social deprivation and ethnic minorities in these cases. Many women arrive in the UK from parts of the world with high syphilis prevalence. Sexual contact in these regions or with partners from these regions may result in symptomatic or latent syphilis infection.

Syphilis in pregnancy

Congenital syphilis may occur in infants born to those women who are infected and book late for their antenatal care, or in whom infection is acquired after their initial booking blood tests have been performed. The outcome for the fetus varies depending on the gestational stage at which infection is acquired. All pregnant women should be screened for syphilis at the initial antenatal visit. In pregnant women with untreated early syphilis, 70–100% of infants will be infected. Stillbirths are seen in up to a third of cases. Vertical transmission has been reported in women with untreated syphilis of many years' duration. All pregnant women with positive treponemal serology should be evaluated for clinical evidence of syphilis and treated as for syphilis, even when non-venereal treponematoses are suspected to be the cause of their underlying seroreactivity. Ideally treatment should be initiated before a confirmatory second serology is available, to prevent neonatal complications if the patient defaults follow-up.

Women who had documented treatment for syphilis in the past do not need re-treatment during current or subsequent pregnancies if there is no clinical evidence of syphilis and the non-specific serology (Venereal Disease Reference Laboratory [VDRL] or rapid plasma reagin [RPR] titre) is negative or serofast in low titre compared with the patient's previous results. Re-infection still needs to be excluded by checking recent sexual partners, and babies should also be followed up by a paediatrician to exclude congenital syphilis.

Symptoms and signs

Syphilis can present in the primary stage (9–90 days), secondary stage (6 weeks to 6 months) or tertiary stage, which includes gummatous lesions, neurosyphilis and cardiovascular syphilis (10–40 years). Alternatively, latent syphilis may be detected in patients during opportunistic serological screening at GUM or antenatal clinics. Patients are usually only infectious during the first 2 years of the infection, ie primary, secondary or early latent stages, which are the focus of this chapter. Tertiary syphilis is rarely seen in the UK, even in women from high prevalence regions.

The primary stage usually manifests as an ulcer at the site of inoculation, often associated with rubbery regional lymphadenopathy. Characteristically the ulcer is painless and indurated with a serous exudate, although ulcers in women tend to have more subtle clinical appearances and may be tender, especially if secondary bacterial infection ensues. In women, the ulcer is usually on the vulva but may be intravaginal, on the cervix, or in the perineal or perianal regions. In men, the ulcer may be in the coronal sulcus, on the penile shaft or on the glans penis. Homosexual and bisexual men may present with primary lesions at the anal margin, or on the tonsils, lips or nipples. Women who practise fellatio or receptive anal sex may also experience primary lesions at these sites.

Secondary syphilis typically manifests with a widespread maculopapular rash, which may affect the palms and soles, as well as with generalised lymphadenopathy, mouth ulcers and alopecia. Condylomata lata may occur in moist areas where they mimic anogenital warts, so treponemal serology should be performed to exclude syphilis in these cases.

Investigations

In centres equipped with a dark-ground microscope, examination may be made of lesional material placed in a drop of saline under a floating coverslip. Suitable material includes ulcer exudate, samples from open skin lesions and condylomata lata, as well as sterile aspiration of lymph nodes. Pathogenic *Treponema* spp. have a characteristic appearance and motility, although an experienced microscopist is needed to achieve high sensitivity. NAATs are becoming available in the UK that should allow for sensitive detection of *T. pallidum*-associated lesions.

Serology remains the mainstay of diagnosis but is unable to distinguish between the different pathogenic treponemes, which include *Treponema pertenue* (yaws) and *T. carateum* (pinta). In the primary stage, treponemal serology is generally positive in 70–80% of cases but should be positive in 100% of secondary and early latent disease. It is important to repeat negative serology at 3 months in patients with genital ulceration to ensure that syphilis has been excluded. Most laboratories now screen with a *Treponema*-specific ELISA method detecting IgG, and confirm this with the *T. pallidum* particle agglutination (TPPA) test. Syphilis IgM assays are also available and appear to improve the sensitivity of diagnosis of early primary lesions. Activity of the treponemal disease is estimated with non-treponemal tests, which detect anticardiolipin antibodies, such as the RPR or VDRL test. Measurement of activity is useful because it provides a marker with which to monitor the therapeutic response as evidenced by a fall in RPR/VDRL titre. Once infected with syphilis, the specific treponemal tests generally remain positive, so the only way to detect a subsequent re-infection is by testing with the RPR or VDRL. A 2-titre rise or fall in the RPR/VDRL is usually the minimum significant change considered to be clinically relevant in this somewhat subjective assay.

It is important to screen for other common STIs.

Treatment and follow-up for early syphilis

This includes primary, secondary and early latent syphilis (<2 years' duration):
- Benzathine penicillin 2.4 MU i.m. as a single dose; two doses are recommended in pregnancy (days 1 and 8).
- Procaine benzylpenicillin 750 mg i.m. daily for 10 days.
- Doxycycline 100 mg twice daily for 2 weeks.
- Azithromycin 2 g orally as a single dose (macrolide resistance has been reported).
- Penicillin-allergic pregnant women should be considered for penicillin desensitisation. Otherwise they can be treated with erythromycin 500 mg four times a day for 2 weeks. As a result of lower efficacy and poor placental transfer of this drug, it is recommended that babies are examined and retreated at birth with benzylpenicillin and the mother retreated with doxycycline after breastfeeding has ceased.
- Warn patients about the Jarisch–Herxheimer reaction which may need cover with paracetamol and bed rest for 24 hours.
- Partner notification (contact tracing) should be initiated at diagnosis.
- RPR/VDRL serial measurements should be performed at 1, 3, 6 and 12 months post-treatment. A post-treatment fall in the RPR/VDRL of a least 2 titres should be seen by 6 months.

Mycoplasma genitalium

- *Mycoplasma genitalium* is now established as an STI in men and women and can cause a similar spectrum of disease to *C. trachomatis*.
- In women *M. genitalium* is associated with cervicitis and urethritis and can be detected in the endometrium of women with PID. Serological studies suggest a strong association between past infection with *M. genitalium* and tubal factor infertility.
- NAATs for *M. genitalium* are becoming available and should guide clinicians as to the local epidemiology and expand knowledge about its clinical associations.
- The role of screening for infection is currently unknown, but testing and treatment of symptomatic individuals are recommended.
- Current evidence supports the use of azithromycin as first-line therapy for *M. genitalium*, although longer courses seem to be needed to clear infection reliably and some persistent infections have required moxifloxacin therapy to eradicate the organism.

Human immunodeficiency virus infection

HIV (human immunodeficiency virus) is a human retrovirus that causes the acquired immune deficiency syndrome (AIDS). Through the action of reverse transcriptase, the RNA virus is able to make a double-stranded DNA copy of its genetic material that can be inserted into human DNA and establish latent infection. The virus is reproduced whenever the infected cell multiplies. The virus uses the CD4 receptor and a number of co-receptors (CCR5, CXCR4) to enter susceptible cells, which can include lymphocytes, macrophages and microglial cells. A substantial number of HIV-infected individuals will have longstanding asymptomatic infection before progressing to symptomatic HIV infection and AIDS.

The presence of antibodies is used in diagnosis of the disease but they are not protective. Currently, there is no effective vaccine against the virus.

Transmission occurs through infected body fluids being in contact with the body fluids of the recipient in the presence of a break in the integrity of the exposed mucosal surface. Another major route of infection is blood borne, through either sharing needles for intravenous drug use or transfusion of whole blood and concentrated blood products. Blood products are currently tested for HIV antibodies and so new infections rarely occur through this route now. At the start of the HIV epidemic in developed countries, most cases of HIV were detected in men who had sex with men, people with haemophilia and those who injected recreational drugs. Currently in the UK, the greatest increases in newly diagnosed cases are occurring in heterosexual men and women, most of whom are thought to have acquired their infection sexually in high prevalence countries, particularly sub-Saharan Africa (Fig. 6.5).

Symptoms and signs

• Seroconversion illness is often missed in practice but presents with a glandular fever-type illness that may be associated with a rash and orogenital ulceration. Neurological manifestations such as Guillain–Barré syndrome and encephalitis have been described.
• Asymptomatic infections by definition are detected only by screening.
• Symptomatic HIV infection may present with non-specific weight loss, fatigue, lymphadenopathy, diarrhoea and night sweats. Clues may come from recurrent vulvovaginal or oral candidiasis, recurrent and extensive genital warts, shingles, worsening eczema and psoriasis, facial molluscum contagiosum or oral hairy leukoplakia on the tongue.
• AIDS is determined by the onset of certain opportunistic infections or AIDS-related malignancies. Examples include tuberculosis, *Pneumocystis jiroveci* pneumonia (PCP—*P. carinii* pneumonia —former name), cryptococcal infection, cryptosporidiosis, Kaposi's sarcoma and lymphoma.

Investigations

• Diagnosis of HIV infection is established by the detection of anti-HIV antibodies in the serum by ELISA. Newer fourth-generation tests detect HIV antigen as well as anti-HIV antibodies. The window period (the interval between acquisition of the virus and appearance of anti-HIV antibodies detected by the test) is still quoted as 3 months but, in practice, 4–6 weeks appears sufficient to detect new infections with the latest assays due to the presence of HIV antigens.
• Confirmation is obtained using different ELISAs (usually two more).
• Western blots can be performed in reference laboratories to investigate discrepant results in reference centres.
• Plasma HIV viral load gives an estimation of the amount of HIV viral replication.
• The immune status of the patient is estimated by sequential CD4 counts and CD4 percentages.
• It is important to screen for other common STIs.

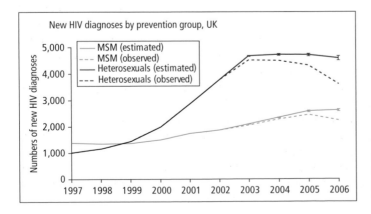

Figure 6.5 New HIV diagnoses in the UK by exposure categories (1997–2006). (Data from the Health Protection Agency.)

When to treat HIV infection?

- In the UK, highly active antiretroviral therapy (HAART) is recommended for all patients with:
  — a CD4 count of $<200 \times 10^6$/l, regardless of the presence or absence of symptoms
  — an AIDS-defining illness regardless of CD4 count. The notable exception to this is pulmonary TB which can occur in patients even with a relatively intact immune system.
- In the UK, treatment should be considered in patients with a CD4 count between 200×10^6/l and 350×10^6/l, but the optimum time to start treatment is still debated. Symptomatic HIV infection, HIV nephropathy, co-infection with hepatitis B or C and a rapidly falling CD4 count are circumstances when HAART would be considered at higher CD4 counts. A recent study has shown that risk of mortality and disease progression is less in those who are on HAART compared with those who start and stop HAART based on CD4 count regardless of the nadir CD4 count, ie even in those whose CD4 count was never $<350 \times 10^6$/l. This suggests that there will be benefit in starting patients at higher CD4 counts, especially as toxicity and tolerability of HAART have improved in recent years. This has to be balanced against the risk of acquiring resistance to HAART, the risk of which increases with the duration of treatment.
- Currently the benefits and optimal duration of HAART for seroconversion illness remain uncertain. Patients undergoing HIV seroconversion are not routinely treated unless serious complications such as meningoencephalitis occur or within the context of clinical trials.

HIV treatment options

- The aim of HIV treatment is to stop viral replication. To achieve this, a combination of three active HIV drugs from at least two different classes is needed to form a HAART regimen. Viral eradication is currently not achievable because the virus is incorporated into the host DNA of some resting cells that are long living. This reservoir of infection is unaffected by treatment as it is not actively replicating, but retains the capacity to do so when drug pressure is removed.

- Monitoring of the efficacy of treatment is done by measuring HIV RNA viral load, which should be undetectable (<40–50 copies/ml depending on the assay) if the patient adheres to the HAART regimen. Once viral replication has been controlled, immune function will be restored, most easily measured by improved CD4 counts and percentage.
- Adherence is crucial to the success of HAART. Adherence levels <95% have been associated with treatment failure. Resistance to antivirals rapidly ensues if patients do not adhere meticulously to their regimens. The virus starts to replicate and mutate in the presence of subtherapeutic drug levels in the blood.
- Antiretroviral resistance can be detected using genotypic assays to look for the mutants that have evolved under drug pressure, but is best done while patients are taking the drugs in question.
- Most patients have wild-type virus archived in sanctuary sites. This virus will replicate and replace resistant virus once drug pressure has been removed as resistant virus strains tend to be less fit.
- The causes of poor adherence should be addressed. Side effects of HAART should be discussed with the patient and minimized. Factors such as pill burden, dosing schedules and dietary restrictions have been shown to affect adherence. Adequate counselling on the importance of adherence and support has to be provided. Issues such as stigma, non-disclosure to partners and psychosocial factors can contribute to adherence problems.
- Current classes of antiretroviral drugs include nucleoside analogues (NRTIs), nucleotide analogues (NtRTIs), non-nucleoside analogues (NNRTIs), protease inhibitors (PIs), integrase inhibitors, and entry inhibitors that include fusion inhibitors targeting HIV gp41 protein on the virus and CCR5 co-receptor blockers:
  — NRTIs include AZT, 3TC, FTC, ddI, d4T, ddC and abacavir
  — NtRTIs include tenofovir
  — NNRTIs include efavirenz, nevirapine and etravirine
  — PIs include nelfinavir, saquinavir, lopinavir, ritonavir, indinavir, fosamprenavir, atazanavir, tipranavir and darunavir

— T20 is the first of a new class of fusion inhibitors that need to be given by subcutaneous injection

— co-receptor CCR5 blocker maraviroc and integrase inhibitor raltegravir have recently been licensed for use in the UK.

• Some HIV drugs are available in combination tablets to help with adherence, eg Combivir (AZT + 3TC), Kivexa (abacavir + 3TC), Truvada (tenofovir + FTC) and Atripla (tenofovir + FTC + efavirenz).

• Most PIs require boosting with low-dose ritonavir (a potent cytochrome p450 inhibitor) to achieve sufficient and sustained drug levels in body fluids.

• It is important to be aware of drug interactions when co-prescribing HIV drugs and other medications to avoid reduced drug exposure and toxicity.

• Prophylaxis against opportunistic infections is necessary until immune recovery occurs on HAART. Co-trimoxazole can be given for PCP and primary toxoplasmosis prophylaxis. Prophylaxis against HSV and *Mycobacterium avium-intracellulare* can be considered in certain circumstances.

• There have been trials assessing the efficacy of interleukin-2 (IL-2) therapy as an immunotherapeutic agent but the clinical benefits remain unclear.

HIV in pregnancy is considered in Chapter 11.

HIV prevention and partner notification

• Partner notification (contact tracing) should be initiated at diagnosis.

• The importance of using condoms for sexual intercourse must be explained to all HIV-positive patients in order to prevent new infections.

• The patient should avoid acquiring drug-resistant HIV from other sexual partners because this may compromise future therapeutic drug interventions.

• Injecting drug users should be provided with sterile needles through needle exchange services and referred to drug treatment programmes.

• Blood and blood products as well as organ donations need to be screened for HIV before use.

• Health-care workers should take precautions to ensure that they do not become infected through sharps injuries or contact with potentially infectious body fluids of patients.

• Surgical instruments should be autoclaved satisfactorily and inspected for possible contamination before use in operating theatres.

• There is no effective HIV vaccine available at the present time, although trials are ongoing.

Sexual problems

Many students do not like considering patients' sexual problems, because they feel that they have hardly sorted out their own sexual lives and are therefore ill equipped to help others. A more open discussion of this subject helps the student to be at ease when discussing sexuality later with patients. It helps the students to become more aware of their attitudes and how these may influence the future doctor–patient relationship.

Patients often consult their doctors about sexual problems and expect them to have the knowledge and skills to help them. It is necessary for a doctor to know the interrelation of sexually related matters and their treatments to general diseases such as heart disease and hypertension.

The facts of human sexuality have not always been known but, by proper analysis, assessment and randomized controlled trials of various therapies, more is becoming comprehensible.

History and examination

As with the rest of medicine, a systematic approach to sexual problems can help make a diagnosis. A full general and gynaecological history should be taken including details of past gynaecological events, the type of contraception used and obstetric history.

The sexual problem should be discussed, allowing the woman or man to use their own phrases, preferably in their own time. If they wander, pointed questions drawn from the following material may be needed to bring them back to the point.

Questions

• Duration and frequency of intercourse
• Factors making the problem better

- Factors making the problem worse
- Problem happens with other partners
- Other associated factors such as alcohol, work or drugs—prescribed or recreational
- Other life events at the time of onset
- The relationship of the partners
- History of previous sex knowledge
- Family background to sex education in childhood
- Past sexual relationships
- Possible child abuse
- Present sexual history
- Details of usual sex activities, eg position and foreplay
- Sexual fantasies.

Examination

This is usually unrewarding:
- In the male, obvious abnormalities of the penis and testes should be excluded.
- In the female, the ease of allowing a pelvic examination may be helpful in assessing the degree of the problem. Any structural abnormalities of the vulva, vagina, cervix or uterus should be excluded. The examination can be used positively as an opportunity to educate about genital anatomy. The use of a mirror to help a woman identify her clitoris can be helpful.

It is important to detect general physical abnormalities that might make intercourse difficult or painful before exploring the possibility of psychosexual problems. The patient's comfort or discomfort with his or her own body and specifically genitalia can give useful information.

The male

Although this is not strictly part of gynaecology, anyone dealing with sexual problems must have a knowledge of the male partner and his problems.

Failure to ejaculate

The inability to produce semen is not always associated with the sex drive itself or the ability to have an erection.

Causes
- Sympathectomy.
- Psychosexual features:
  — anxiety related to sexual performance, often with a new partner
  — past humiliating sexual rejection
  — fear of a pregnancy in partner
  — past maternal domination
  — repressive sexual teaching as a child
  — doubts about sexual orientation

Treatment
Sympathectomy aspects can be treated with drugs:
- Thioridazine
- Indoramin.

The psychological aspects may require long-term psychotherapy, because many cases are a result of the man avoiding depositing semen in his partner's vagina; this produces further anxieties.

Lesser degrees can be dealt with by sympathetic handling by the woman and extravaginal sexual techniques. The encouragement of the use of erotic material can help if there is loss of control at the point of ejaculation.

Premature ejaculation

Ejaculation that occurs with minimal stimulation or before or shortly after penetration and before either party wishes it. Ejaculation is under sympathetic control mediated by adrenoreceptors. It probably means that the mediated system enhances this while the serotonin balance is inhibitory. These equilibria may be over-ridden by behavioural patterns.

Causes
Behavioural patterns are associated with:
- inexperience
- adolescent conditioning to rapid response
- rejection by other partners.

Treatment
Men can be treated individually or with their partners. Sympathetic handling by the partner is important. Male confidence must be generated as he learns to recognize the point of ejaculatory in-

evitability and to control stimulation to delay ejaculation until the time of his choosing. A squeeze technique applied by the partner to the penis at the moment before ejaculatory inevitability can produce a delay in ejaculation.

If a programme is embarked on over a course of weeks or months, this produces good results.

Drugs are occasionally helpful if there is poor response to the psychological approach:

- Clomipramine
- SSRI (selective serotonin reuptake inhibitor) antidepressants may be helpful.

Erectile dysfunction

Erectile dysfunction in men may be primary or secondary. The former is nearly always psychological as a result of problems in the family background/upbringing whereas secondary impotence may be physical or psychological, and is often a combination of the two. A careful history will give clues to the cause, allow discussion of patients' expectations and worries, and assess fitness to resume sexual activity.

Causes
Structural
- After major pelvic operations/trauma/radiotherapy
- Pudendal vein thrombosis
- Hypospadias
- Peyronie's disease (curvature of the penis secondary to fibrotic plaques around the corpora cavernosa).

Endocrine disease
- Diabetes
- Hypogonadism
- Hypothyroidism
- Pituitary tumour
- Cushing's syndrome.

Medical problems
- Peripheral vascular disease
- Hypertension
- Cerebrovascular disease

- Multiple sclerosis
- Spinal cord injury
- Increasing age.

Drugs
- Smoking
- Alcohol
- Antihypertensives
- Antidepressants
- Antipsychotics
- Hormones, eg for body building
- Psychostimulants.

Psychological features
- Stress
- Performance pressure
- Parental influence
- Ignorance of sexual matters
- Poor self-image or body dysmorphic disorder
- Guilt
- Anger
- Relationship problems
- Depression
- Alcoholism
- Gender identity issues.

It is important to differentiate the psychogenic from the organic causes. The former tend to be associated with:
- rapid onset
- a recent depression
- life or family stress
- normal erections:
  — on waking
  — with masturbation
  — in response to erotic material
  — with a different partner.

Investigations
- BP
- Urinalysis to exclude diabetes
- Testosterone to exclude hypogonadism; if testosterone is low, prolactin, LH/FSH (luteinizing hormone/follicle-stimulating hormone)
- PSA (prostate-specific antigen) if over age 50.

Treatment
The patients' expectations and objectives should be discussed. Modifiable lifestyle factors should be

addressed. If psychosexual factors are the predominant cause, referral to a psychosexual therapist is helpful. Use of pharmacological treatments may complement this. Psychological treatment starts with reassurance and education leading on to non-demand, touching exercises based on Masters and Johnson's sensate focus programme.

Erection can be produced by pharmacological means:

- Papaverine injected into the corpus cavernosum works by smooth muscle relaxation.
- Other injectable drugs are phentolamine and prostaglandin E_1, the latter also being available in an intraurethral gel. These work particularly for men with spinal cord injuries or severe erectile dysfunction not responding to oral agents, although priapism can occur.
- Oral phosphodiesterase inhibitors such as sildenafil, vardenafil and tadalafil are effective in most men, although they have a slower onset of action than injectables and need to be taken before the onset of sexual activity. Side effects include flushing and headache. Contraindications include use of nitrates, hypotension, hereditary degenerative retinal disorders and recent stroke or myocardial infarction.
- Problem medications such as antihypertensives or antidepressants may be changed to others with less effect on erectile function.

The female

Superficial dyspareunia

Vulval or vaginal pain during intercourse may be due to a variety of causes. Physical causes of superficial dyspareunia include:

- infection of the vulva or vagina
- dermatological disease of the vulva or vagina
- postmenopausal atrophy
- painful perineal scar from episiotomy
- an undilated hymen —this is very rare and mostly related to women who maintain virginity into their late 30s
- Vulvodynia or vulval pain caused by vestibulitis.

Treatment

Dealt with according to the cause. Surgical reconstruction may be required for a badly healed episiotomy or a rigid undilated hymen.

Deep dyspareunia

This is where discomfort is felt higher up in the vagina and in the pelvis. It often lasts for some hours after intercourse and can be reproduced at vaginal examination by pressing over relevant parts of the female pelvis.

Causes

- Acute or chronic pelvic infection (see Plate 7)
- Endometriosis
- Pelvic tumours
- Fixed uterine retroversion trapping ovaries behind, eg in endometriosis
- Pelvic congestion/pelvic vein varices
- Bladder or bowel pathology
- Failure of arousal response: superficially this results from failure of lubrication and deeply from failure of vaginal ballooning during coitus.

Treatment

Treatment should focus on the basic cause; results depend on the responsiveness to the treatment of physical problems.

Results where no pathology is demonstrated are variable. In these women, dyspareunia may be caused by intra- or interpersonal conflicts. The use of lubricants and delay of penetration until the woman is fully aroused can be helpful.

Vaginismus

Spasm of the superficial and deep pelvic muscles prevents the introduction of the penis and is apparent at a pelvic examination.

Causes

There may be an organic cause but usually it is a psychological result of apprehension and fear. It may be part of a conditioned response to an adverse physical or psychological stimulus. A cycle occurs when subsequent fear and anticipation of pain result in muscle spasm, which results in pain on attempts at penetration. Physical causes include sexual infections (eg genital herpes and recurrent candida infection), trauma, surgery (eg episiotomy), vestibulitis or atrophy of the vagina. Sexual abuse, dysfunctional relationships and poor arousal with poor lubrication can be other causes.

Treatment

A sympathetic approach to examination can help, but no force should be used. Attempts should stop before pain is caused and the woman should feel in control at all times.

Occasionally examination under anaesthesia may be required to exclude structural causes and thus be able to reassure the woman that she is anatomically normal. Usually this is not necessary because she is likely to respond to gradual desensitization techniques. To this end, the use of graduated vaginal trainers is often helpful. Fingers or tampons are sometimes preferred. Referral to a trained sex therapist may be needed. Pelvic floor exercises and relaxation exercises can be used.

Anorgasmia

This is not uncommon in women. It is nearly always psychological, but in a small percentage it is physical.

Causes

A failure to:
- receive stimulation—psychological in origin
- respond to stimulation—often caused by family upbringing/background;
    Other causes:
- Performance pressure from partner or self
- Doubts about sexual orientation
- Fear of pregnancy
- Dyspareunia
- Debilitating disease
- Chronic constipation.

Treatment

Mechanical and organic causes should be treated appropriately. Psychological causes require the attention of a sex therapist, who would discuss the problem fully with the individual or the couple.

A woman can be labelled as frigid all too easily and then accepts this as a part of life. Up to 50% of women are not orgasmic during penetrative sex, but are orgasmic with clitoral stimulation. Understanding this can help remove pressure from both partners to achieve coital orgasm on every occasion.

Treatment usually involves helping the woman to achieve orgasm through masturbation and learning to lose control. The use of erotic material or a vibrator can help. Progress to coital orgasm is then made. Use of vibrators may also help with coital orgasmic problems.

Sexual assault

Sexual assault includes rape, which is now classified as penetration by the penis of somebody's vagina, anus or mouth, without their consent. In the case of vaginal rape only the slightest penetration of the vulva by the penis is required. Issues of whether the hymen is intact or if semen has been deposited in the vagina are irrelevant.

Rape of women is unfortunately all too common and, although the woman may report it to the police, sometimes a day or so later, most cases go unreported. A doctor may be called to examine the victim of alleged rape. The practitioner should ensure that he or she has the authority and consent for the examination and has the equipment for taking the appropriate specimens properly. This would usually best be achieved at a local sexual assault referral centre if available.

A history of what happened is taken and careful notes made. Examination is made of the general demeanour of the woman and of her clothing. Any external bruises or scratches, particularly around the upper arms, lower abdomen, thighs and vulva, should be noted, preferably in a diagrammatic form. The vulva should be examined in detail for bruising or tears. Specimens should be taken from the vulva and vagina for the detection of semen and DNA, placed in appropriate containers and labelled fully in the presence of a woman police constable (WPC) and the complainant. This should then be handed to the WPC for transport to forensic laboratories and a receipt should be received or the chain of evidence may be questioned in any subsequent legal enquiry.

Other swabs and blood may be taken at the time and in follow-up to exclude STIs. Although these often have no legal standing, they may be important in the medical management of the woman's future.

Many police forces have a sexual assault investigation team who are able to satisfy both the law and the psychological needs of the woman who is in this situation. Knowledge of the procedures involved is helpful to all practitioners.

Criminal abortion

One of the outcomes from modern laws about therapeutic termination of pregnancy in England, Wales and Scotland has been the massive reduction in criminal abortions. Not a single death was reported in the 23 years covered by the Confidential Enquiries into Maternal Deaths (1982–2005). This is a very satisfactory situation in the UK but criminal abortion still takes place throughout the world. It is estimated that, of the half a million women who die every year of maternity causes, about a quarter of these do so from incompetently performed illegal abortions.

If a doctor is asked to examine a woman who may have undergone a criminal abortion, he or she must first obtain her consent if she is conscious.

History

This should be taken but may be only partly truthful.

Examination

The woman may be pyrexial with dull pain in the lower abdomen. Pelvic examination may show the cervix to be soft and the os dilated. Blood or pregnancy tissue may be present in the os. There may be signs of the bite of a vulsellum (toothed forceps) on the anterior lip of the cervix and there may be an offensive endocervical discharge. Damage to the genital tract may occur, eg the posterior fornix is commonly perforated by incompetent abortionists who force their instruments into the cul-de-sac of the vagina and penetrate it, breaching the peritoneal cavity.

Treatment

The woman should be admitted to hospital. Broad-spectrum antibiotics should be given urgently, as well as other supportive measures, depending on her clinical status and the severity of sepsis. If the woman is still bleeding from the uterus, curettage may remove septic products from the cavity and hasten healing. If the bleeding still persists or is very heavy, hysterectomy may be required for infection that has entered the substance of the uterus.

Although the confidentiality of the patient is of prime concern to the doctor, if the woman becomes seriously ill or approaches death, legal authorities may be involved. Take advice about this from the legal department of the hospital or relevant medical insurance society. Keep accurate notes and be prepared to take, or act as witness to, a dying declaration.

Part 3

The Reproductive Years

Chapter 7

The mother and fetus in pregnancy

For most women, childbearing is a major event in their lives. The basic changes of pregnancy are covered in this chapter; the rest of pregnancy and childbirth are discussed in Chapters 8–14 and a short chapter, Chapter 15, covers those aspects that the obstetrician should know about the newborn child.

Maternal changes in pregnancy

Pregnancy causes alterations not just in the mother's pelvis and abdomen but in the whole body. Adaptations in the function of various systems occur to minimize the stresses imposed and are interlinked smoothly so that the function of the whole organism does not deteriorate.

Vulva and vagina

During pregnancy, oestrogen increases the vascularity and progesterone permits muscular relaxation and softening of the connective tissue sheath of the vagina by an increase in fluid. Over 38 weeks the tube becomes much more stretchable so that, by full term, the vagina and vulva permit the passage of an infant with a head diameter of approxi-

Lecture Notes: Obstetrics and Gynaecology, 3rd edition. By Diana Hamilton-Fairley. Published 2009 by Blackwell Publishing. ISBN: 978-1-4051-7801-3.

mately 10 cm. The perineum, with the squamous epithelium in the region of the fourchette, does not always stretch so readily and so may tear on occasions.

Uterus

The uterus grows through hypertrophy of the myometrial cells rather than by an increase in myometrial cell numbers. From 28 weeks the lower third of the uterus thins and becomes less vascular, forming the lower segment of the uterus (hence lower segment caesarean section).

The branches of the uterine artery increase in size, number and diameter from each side of the uterus. The placental site gets a preferential blood supply. Penetrating branches pass through the myometrium, under the surface of the decidua. They become spiral arteries and penetrate the decidua. In early pregnancy their exits into the placental bed pool are narrow, but trophoblast invasion normally widens them into deltas so reducing resistance and improving flow by 16 weeks. This allows time for transfer of nutrients and fetal waste products across the placenta. By term, 1 litre of blood can be in the uterine vasculature with 500 ml/min reaching the uterus. If invasion is incomplete, flow is restricted so that, in late pregnancy, the fetus gets fewer nutrients for growth.

The higher pressure in the system may allow clots to form in the maternal placental bed and further reduce flow which causes a build up in pressure which feeds back into the systemic circulation causing pregnancy-induced hypertension and/or pre-eclampsia.

In addition, in labour, the fetus gets less O_2 and so fetal distress follows more readily.

Metabolism

Increased to provide for:

- growth of fetus and placenta
- increased growth of the uterus
- increased growth of support systems
- preparation for lactation.

Weight increase (Table 7.1)

Usually 10–14 kg (22–30 lb) in whole pregnancy. For example:

- 0–14 weeks: 2 kg (4.5 lb)—may be a loss because of vomiting
- 13–28 weeks: 5 kg (11 lb)
- 28–40 weeks: 5 kg (11 lb).

The rest is extracellular fluid, fat and protein storage—6 kg.

A sharp increase in the mother's weight gain in late pregnancy may indicate increased water retention. Maternal weight gain or loss is not a good predictor of fetal outcome and so is not routinely measured.

Protein

The fetus needs little protein in early pregnancy so the woman is in negative balance.

Table 7.1 Breakdown of approximate weight increase during pregnancy

	Weight	
	kg	lb
Fetus	3.5	7
Placenta	0.5	1
Amniotic fluid	1.5	2
Uterus	1.0	2
Blood increase	1.5	3
Breasts	1.0	2
Total	**9.0**	**17**

Two-thirds of the fetal protein is acquired in the last 12 weeks (a half in last 4 weeks). Also the maternal uterus and breasts use much protein in growing tissues and storage occurs for lactation. Approximately 12 g nitrogen/day are needed for the development of these and the fetus.

Carbohydrate

Pregnancy induces insulin resistance and is therefore diabetogenic with a slightly increased calorie need.

Fat

The fetus accumulates fat late, from 2% of the fetal body weight at 32 weeks to 12% at term. Fetal neolipogenesis accounts for most of the baby's fat, with a low transfer rate of precursors across the placenta. Much of the fat is stored as brown fat, particularly around the baby's liver. During the third trimester the liver occupies two-thirds of the baby's abdominal cavity and is the greatest contributor to the abdominal circumference. If the supply of nutrients is reduced for whatever reason, the baby will use the brown fat to sustain itself and so become thinner (see Chapter 9, intrauterine restricted growth). The mother has a higher circulating lipid and lipoprotein level.

Calcium

The fetus utilizes calcium late, taking from the long bones of the mother. If the stores are insufficient the fetus still utilizes calcium, leading to maternal osteopenia. Maternal serum calcium levels stay steady. After pregnancy the mother will regain her bone density if she eats a balanced, healthy diet.

Iron

Iron is mostly passed to the fetus in the last weeks of pregnancy. It is stored in the liver. The mother may have poor iron stores because of:

- too little in diet, so give supplements
- poor absorption.

Cardiovascular system

Load

Pregnancy is an increased load, so more work is required by the heart:
- Growing fetal tissues that have high O_2 consumption rates
- Hypertrophied uterus and breasts require more O_2
- Increased muscular effort by mother to cope with weight gain of 10–14 kg (22–30 lb)
- In the last weeks of pregnancy, the placental bed may act like an arteriovenous fistula. More work is required to overcome this shunt.

Cardiac output

Increased needs are met by increasing cardiac output. In pregnancy, the pulse rate is raised but most increase in output comes from larger stroke volume with enlarged heart chambers and muscle hypertrophy.

The output increases rapidly in the first trimester by up to 40% and steadies for the rest of pregnancy (Fig. 7.1).

During labour, cardiac output can increase by a further 2 l/min in association with uterine contractions.

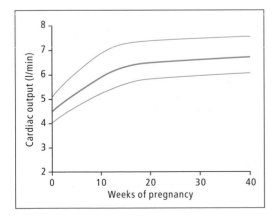

Figure 7.1 Cardiac output in pregnancy in normal women. The lines on the graph represent the mean ± 2 standard deviations.

Systolic and diastolic pressure is much lower in early and mid-pregnancy, rising in the last trimester. Peripheral resistance is decreased and, as cardiac output is raised, pulse pressure is increased.

Blood volume

Return of blood to the heart is maintained by an increased blood volume. Plasma volume increases more than red cells so that relative haemodilution occurs. This used to be called physiological anaemia. As a result all blood values for urea and electrolytes and packed cell volume are reduced. This is normal for pregnancy and it is important to remember this when interpreting results; as a result the normal range for the non-pregnant woman may be abnormal when she is pregnant, eg a creatinine of 120 μmol/l is abnormal in pregnancy but not in the non-pregnant state.

Heart changes

Pregnancy is a hyperkinetic state. The heart is:
- enlarged
- pushed up
- unfolded upon aorta.

These changes produce electrocardiogram (ECG) and radiological changes that are normal for pregnancy, but may appear pathological if interpreted with no knowledge of pregnancy.

There are also sometimes extra murmurs, normal hypervolaemic sounds such as the systolic ejection murmur and the murmur over the internal mammary arteries supplying the breasts.

Respiratory system

Pressure of the growing uterus forces the diaphragm up and lower ribs out, but vital capacity is not reduced in late pregnancy.

Raised progesterone levels increase respiratory rate.

Urinary tract

Renal function

- Renal plasma flow increases by 30–50%
- Glomerular filtration rate increases by 30–50%

- Tubular reabsorption increases by 30–50%
- Patchy glomerular leak happens occasionally (eg glucose).

Lower urinary tract

- Bladder more irritated as growing uterus pushes on it
- Ureters:
  — longer, wider, lower tone because of progesterone effects
  — stasis in ureter and pelvis of kidney may lead to infection.

Alimentary tract

- Teeth more susceptible to spreading caries and gingivitis because of increased cortisone levels
- Nausea and vomiting
- Hypomotility of gut may lead to constipation
- Hypochlorhydria: regurgitation of alkaline chyle (from the duodenum) into stomach
- Slow emptying of gallbladder
- Increased gastro-oesophageal reflux.

Early fetal development

Fetal development is well documented in most mammalian species including the human.

As many women cannot time the precise act of coitus at which fertilization occurred, it is conventional to date pregnancy in weeks from the first day of the last normal menstrual period (LNMP). The difference in the clinical timing of pregnancy and biological age (from conception) is readily understood on realizing that no one becomes pregnant in the first half of a menstrual cycle/before the egg is released. The first 14 days of pregnancy do not relate to the gestation of the fetus using the first day of the LNMP as a method of timing (Fig. 7.2), but as this is the most accurate date that the woman will know, 14 days is added to the true gestation period. If a woman has irregular periods this makes the prediction of the expected date of delivery even more difficult and should be done by measuring the crown–rump length of the baby between 8 and 12 weeks' gestation.

The following milestones are particularly important.

Four weeks (from LNMP) or 14 days biological life

- Sac 2–3 mm
- Ectoderm
- Mesoderm formed
- Endoderm
- Yolk sac formed
- Ultrasound scan—may see sac ± yolk sac.

Six weeks (from LNMP)

- Sac 20–25 mm; embryo 10 mm
- A cylinder with head and tail end formed
- Pulsation of heart tube
- Body stalk (umbilical cord) formed

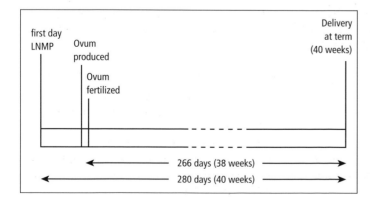

Figure 7.2 The differences between the actual length of gestation and the calculated length of pregnancy from the last normal menstrual period (LNMP).

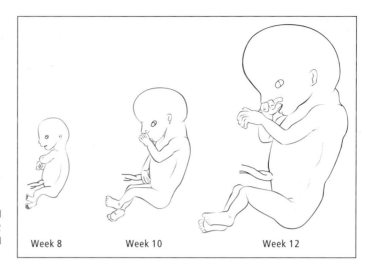

Figure 7.3 Different stages of fetal growth. The fetus at 8, 10 and 12 weeks shown as two-thirds actual size.

Week 8   Week 10   Week 12

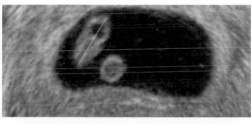

(a)

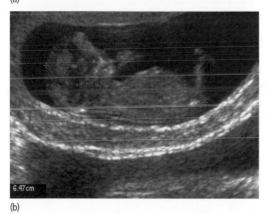

6.47 cm

(b)

Figure 7.4 Different stages of fetal growth: ultrasound scan showing (a) a sac at 6 weeks with yolk sac to the right; (b) a sac and fetus at 12 weeks.

- Villi appear in cytotrophoblast
- Ultrasound scan: embryo visible with yolk sac; able to measure it; usually see pulsating heart. (See ultrasound scan 6 weeks with yolk sac)

Eight weeks (from LNMP)

- Sac 30–50 mm; fetus 20 mm (Figs 7.3 and 7.4)
- Sex glands differentiated
- Limbs well formed, toes and fingers present.
- Centres of ossification present
- Ultrasound scan: embryo clearly visible; able to see limbs and clear head versus rump; may see movement; heart movements clearly visible and demonstrable with Doppler ultrasonography.

Twelve weeks (from LNMP)

- Sac 100 mm; fetus >90 mm
- Primary development of all organ systems
- Nails on fingers and toes
- Ultrasound scan: fetus actively moving; limbs including toes and fingers clearly visible; neural tube defects detectable; nuchal thickness measured as part of antenatal screening (see Chapter 9).

Early placental development

The placenta (Fig. 7.5) is formed from:
- chorion covered by amnion (the membranes)
- decidua basalis.

Villi are buds from the chorionic plate. At first they are made of cytotrophoblast tissue only. Mesoderm appears *in situ* in the centre of the core of each villus (Fig. 7.6).

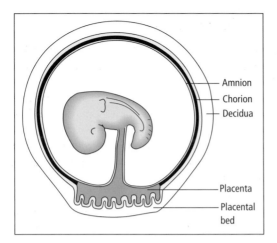

Figure 7.5 Formation of placenta in relation to fetus and fetal membranes.

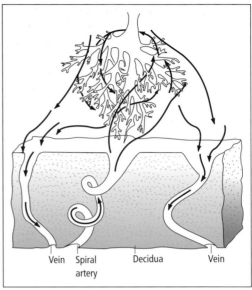

Figure 7.7 Circulation of maternal blood around fine exchange villi.

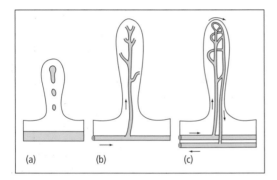

Figure 7.6 Development of blood vessels in the villi: (a) mesoderm appears *in situ* in the core of a villus of proliferating trophoblast cells; (b) blood vessels form and join up with those in the mesoderm layer; (c) capillaries from arterial side circulate blood back to veins.

In this mesodermal core, angioblastic strands are formed. The cells on the edge of these become the endothelium of the blood vessels, and the central cells become the red blood cells. The vessels of the villus join the vessels formed in the mesoderm. By 22 days, the fetal heart pumps blood and a functioning circulation starts.

By 8 weeks, the villi are 200 μm in diameter with a well-organized circulatory system and a double layer of epithelium (cytotrophoblast covered by a cellular syncytiotrophoblast).

Further demands of fetal metabolism require swifter exchanges at the placenta. These come as a result of:
- greater surface area—longer and branching villi
- thinning of epithelium so that syncytiotrophoblast is in direct contact with blood capillary
- nuclei in syncytiotrophoblast that migrate from areas over capillaries where exchange actually occurs
- Localized dome-like swellings occurring on the villi protruding into the intervillous space. These areas are especially thin walled and are probably the site of much of the gas exchange.

Villi are like fronds of seaweed under water as the maternal blood circulates around them (Fig. 7.7). As the placenta grows, fetal size is proportional to the surface area available for exchange. The number of stem villi does not increase after week 12, so the number of lobules is now fixed. The rest of growth is by proliferation and growth of peripheral villi.

At term the placenta is a disc measuring about 25 cm in diameter, with a fetal side where the umbilical cord inserts; the fused amnion and chorion cover the surface. The maternal surface is made up of lobules (each having one stem villus feeding it from the fetus) with the divisions of that stem forming cotyledons. At delivery of the placenta this surface is checked to make sure that all the lobules/cotyledons are present. If one is left behind the woman can bleed immediately after the birth or some days later. It can also be a focus of postpartum infection.

Fetal physiology

The major functions will be reviewed particularly where they differ from adult physiological patterns.

Cardiovascular system

The heart is beating by 22 days from conception and can be detected with vaginal ultrasound at 5 weeks (from LNMP).

There are bypasses in the system as the lungs are not used; <10% of blood goes through them (Fig. 7.8). These bypasses include:
• the foramen ovale between the right and left atria so that most of the oxygenated blood passes straight to the left side of the heart
• the ductus arteriosus from the pulmonary artery to the aorta, so that only a small amount of blood from the right side of the heart goes into the lungs and the rest can use the bypass into the aorta.

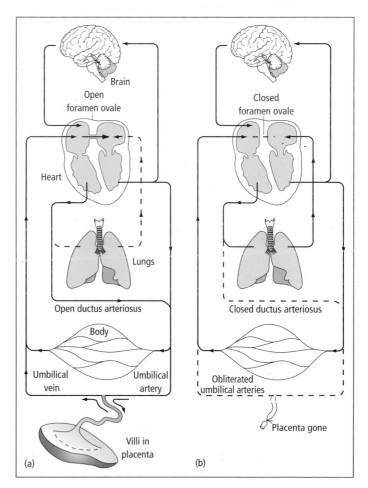

Figure 7.8 (a) The fetal circulation; (b) the neonatal circulation. Note closure of bypasses after birth.

Umbilical blood flow increases with fetal weight. This increase is disproportionate, but, with enhanced O_2-carrying capacity of the fetal blood, the total O_2 transport is increased. Flow is about 100 ml/kg per min, as measured experimentally, but may be greater in vivo.

In the embryonic circulation the umbilical **vein** carries the oxygenated blood from the placenta and the two arteries carry deoxygenated blood, similar to the adult pulmonary vein and artery. (Veins are the way into the heart!)

Fetal haemoglobin

HbA (adult haemoglobin) differs from HbF (fetal haemoglobin) by a 25% alteration of amino acid radicals in the β-haemoglobin chains. At any given PO_2, the O_2 dissociation curve of HbF is to the left of HbA, so it has greater O_2 affinity (Fig. 7.9). The fetus has higher Hb concentration than the adult (18 g/dl in the blood compared with 13 g/dl), allowing further O_2 uptake at the placenta and greater release to tissues. Production of HbF diminishes before birth and has usually ceased by the age of 1 year (Fig. 7.10).

Respiratory system

Within 1–2 minutes this has to adjust from an intrauterine to an independent state. Vascular loops occur in the lungs by 18 weeks and alveoli by 22 weeks.

Surface tension of alveolar epithelium is decreased by surfactant lipoproteins, which are not present in the immature fetus. Hence, if they are born preterm it is difficult for them to open up their lungs and respiratory distress syndrome occurs. Production of surfactant increases after 34 weeks.

Before birth, the alveoli are closed and the trachea is filled with lung fluid. This is different from amniotic fluid and is secreted from glandular cells in the

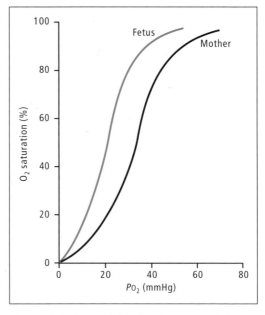

Figure 7.9 Oxyhaemoglobin dissociation curves for human maternal and fetal blood at pH 7.4 and 37°C.

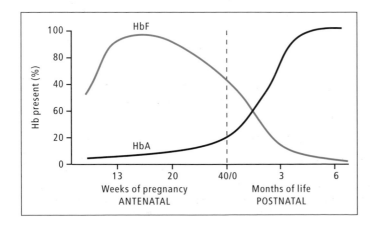

Figure 7.10 Proportion of HbF and HbA present at different stages of fetal and postnatal life.

periphery of the bronchiolar system. Small spontaneous chest movements occur, but, if the fetus is made hypoxic, larger efforts are made; then (and only then) is amniotic fluid drawn into the trachea. Most non-stressed infants are born with a respiratory tract filled with lung fluid, not amniotic fluid.

Fetal growth

Fetal development is mostly by growth (Fig. 7.11); most congenital defects that are going to occur will have been formed by 10 weeks. The critical periods in the development of the human embryo are shown in Fig. 7.12.

Growing from one cell to six billion demands organization of cells into functioning systems so that all can metabolize under optimal conditions. The rate of growth is greatest in the first weeks. Cellular increase is under the control of maternal and fetal hormones; at first, oestrogens are most influential then, later, insulin-like growth factors. In very early pregnancy oestrogens regulate the supply of nutrients in uterine fluid. Later they regulate the course of the blood supply to the placental bed.

After mid-pregnancy, growth is also determined by placental transfer. This could be impaired by the following:

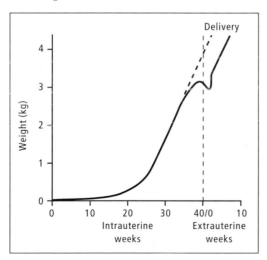

Figure 7.11 The weight gain of the fetus and newborn child. The growth potential falls off in the last few weeks of pregnancy. Note that, after the immediate weight drop, neonatal growth continues at the same incremental rate as it did in the uterus.

• A low environmental supply from the mother of:
— oxygen—only has effect in last weeks, eg living at high altitudes
— nutrients—shows with extremes of specific deprivation or general starvation.
• Reduced blood flow to the placental bed. This follows lack of normal invasion of the arcuate arteries by trophoblasts at 16–18 weeks. This can sometimes be demonstrated by Doppler ultrasonography of the uterine arteries at 20 weeks and later the umbilical artery.
• Poor exchange across the syncytiotrophoblast membrane; if this should be reduced a smaller baby results.

Overall growth is determined by:
• genetic factors inherited from both parents
• placental transfer of nutrients dependent on:
— placental bed flow rates
— placental membrane transfer.

Changes that occur in the fetus at birth

• Closure of the ductus arteriosus: occurs with the first breath so that 100% of deoxygenated blood passes through the lungs
• Closure of the foramen ovale
• Obliteration of the umbilical arteries and veins (see Fig. 7.8b)
• Haemolysis of red blood cells containing HbF and manufacture of red blood cells containing

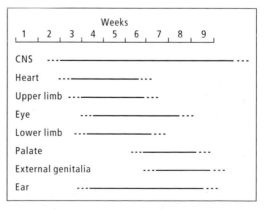

Figure 7.12 Critical periods of various areas of the human embryo. Abnormalities are likely to follow if appropriate teratogens act on tissues at these sensitive times.

HbA. If haemolysis is excessively fast then neonatal jaundice may occur.

Placental physiology

Exchange

The placenta is the fetal exchange station. Compare (a) and (b) of Fig. 7.13: Fig. 7.13a is an adult with organs of homoeostasis (kidney, skin and lung) communicating with the outside environment—the air in the case of humans; Fig. 7.13b shows the fetal situation where these same homoeostatic organs communicate only with the amniotic sac—a closed cavity. All exchange must take place via the placenta to the mother and thence (using her kidneys, skin and lungs) to the outside. The placenta is called the lung of the fetus but is also its liver and kidneys. Transfer of nutrients, waste products, etc occur predominantly by diffusion but active transport mechanisms exist for larger molecules.

Placental hormones

The placenta has a second set of functions—those of an endocrine organ making hormones that regulate the following:
- Rate of growth of fetus.
- Activity of uterus to:
  — prevent premature expulsion of fetus
  — encourage labour contractions at correct time.
- Activity of other organs:
  — breasts
  — ligaments of pelvis in pregnancy.

The hormones made by the placenta are as follows.

Chorionic gonadotrophin
- Made in: cytotrophoblast
- Function: prolongs corpus luteum (early); may control progesterone metabolism (late).

Oestrogens
- Made in: all tissues of placenta
- Function: stimulate uterine growth and development.

Progesterone
- Made in: cytotrophoblast
- Function: damps down intrinsic uterine action in pregnancy.

Human placental lactogen
- Made in: syncytiotrophoblast
- Function: alters glucose and insulin metabolism; may initiate lactation.

Placental tissues age. Maximum efficiency is at 37–38 weeks; many functions deteriorate after this.

Beware extrapolations between transfer and endocrine functions of the placenta. Correlations may not be valid.

The fetus and placenta at term

The fetus

The anatomical features of the fetus that most concern the obstetrician are those found in the mature

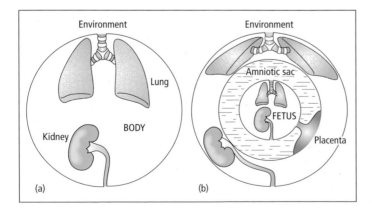

Figure 7.13 (a) Non-pregnant woman; (b) the fetal environment in the pregnant woman.

fetus after 36 weeks' gestation. The most important area is that which is largest, hardest and most difficult to deliver—the head.

The head

Certain measurements should be remembered (Fig. 7.14). These diameters engage in the maternal pelvic brim at different degrees of flexion of the fetal head on the neck.

The intracranial arrangement of the meninges is important (Fig. 7.15) because, under stress, it can be damaged to produce intracranial haemorrhage.

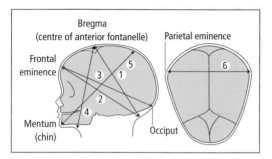

Figure 7.14 The important diameters of the fetal head of a 3-kg baby:
1 Suboccipitobregmatic, 10 cm: vertex presentation
2 Suboccipitofrontal, 11 cm: various flexions of cephalic presentations
3 Occipitofrontal, 12 cm
4 Submentobregmatic, 10 cm: face presentation
5 Mentovertical, 13 cm: brow presentation
6 Biparietal, 10 cm.

The body

The rest of the fetus will usually pass where the head leads. The width of the shoulders is about 10 cm but can be a problem in macrosomic fetuses where the head is normally grown but the abdomen is above the 90th centile causing shoulder dystocia (see Chapter 13).

Placenta

A discoid with 15–20 lobules packed together:
• *Fetal surface*: covered with amnion (not chorion, which fuses with the placental edge). Fetal vessels (arteries paler than veins) course over it, diving into each lobule as an end vessel.
• *Maternal surface*: lobules of compressed villi (like seaweed out of water) separated from each other by sulci.

Maternal side of the placental circulation

Maternal blood is in vessels except in the placental bed where it is in contact with foreign tissues (syncytiotrophoblast of villi). Spiral arteries (about 200) lead blood from the uterine arteries to the placental bed pool. Maternal blood spurts under arterial blood pressure, loses way against a mass of villi and passes laterally, pushed by passive flow to the placental bed veins scattered over the floor of the placental bed.

Measurement of blood flow to the placental bed has been very difficult because it involves direct measurement in animals (unphysiological) or indirect methods with electromagnetic flow meters in

Figure 7.15 Arrangement of the meninges showing how cerebral veins traverse them. If much intracranial movement occurs, the arachnoid moves with the brain but the dura stays with the skull. Hence the vein can be torn at the arrowed sites.

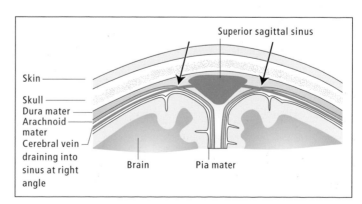

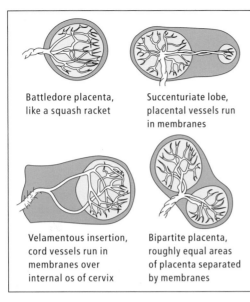

Battledore placenta, like a squash racket

Succenturiate lobe, placental vessels run in membranes

Velamentous insertion, cord vessels run in membranes over internal os of cervix

Bipartite placenta, roughly equal areas of placenta separated by membranes

Figure 7.16 Types of umbilical cord insertion.

humans (imprecise). Now indirect measurements with Doppler ultrasonography allow more precise, non-invasive flow studies in humans.

Maternal blood flow to the uterus is 100–150 ml/kg per min in late pregnancy, of which 80–85% goes to the placenta.

Abnormal implantation

- *Placenta accreta*: villi penetrate decidua just into the myometrial layer; difficulty in separation.
- *Placenta increta*: villi penetrate deeply into myometrium; even more difficult to separate.
- *Placenta percreta*: villi penetrate to subperitoneal myometrium; impossible to separate.

The three diagnoses above cannot usually be differentiated clinically. They are pathological ones made at sectioning a uterus after removal.

- *Placenta praevia*: implantation in the lower segment of the uterus.

Umbilical cord

At term the umbilical cord is about 50 cm long and 2 cm in diameter. It contains two arteries and a

Box 7.1 Diagnostic uses of checking amniotic fluid

- Chromosome content of amniocytes and fetal skin cells in genetic diseases
- Rhesus effect measuring bilirubin breakdown products
- Metabolic upset of the fetus
- Infection of the amniotic cavity in premature rupture of membranes
- Respiratory maturity by measuring the lecithin:sphingomyelin ratio

vein, which is derived from the left umbilical vein of the embryo. (The right one usually disappears.) For types of cord insertion, see Fig. 7.16.

Arteries spiral and give a cord-like appearance. Possibly their pattern wrapped around the vein allows their pulsations to help massage blood back along the umbilical vein. The vessels are packed and protected by a viscous fluid—Wharton's jelly.

There are no nerves in the cord or placenta. Hence ligation and cutting the umbilical cord does not hurt the fetus.

Amniotic fluid

This surrounds the fetus.
- Produced:
  — in early pregnancy: from amnion over placenta and sac
  — in late pregnancy: from fetal urine as well.
- Volume: increase to 38 weeks; 500–1500 ml.
- Osmolality: decreases in late pregnancy.
- Creatinine: increases in late pregnancy.
- Acid–base: normally accumulation of CO_2 and fixed acid causes a slight reduction in pH (about 7.15–7.20).

Amniotic fluid can be removed at amniocentesis and used to diagnose a number of factors (Box 7.1).

Chapter 8

Bleeding in pregnancy

Miscarriage or abortion

A miscarriage is defined as the spontaneous expulsion of the products of conception before week 24 of pregnancy. The word abortion was used for miscarriage but is often considered by women to be a procured termination of pregnancy, legal or criminal. Hence, the softer term 'miscarriage' is better used for the spontaneous event. The nature of miscarriages differs according to the time at which the loss occurs. An early miscarriage is defined as one in the first trimester (before 12 weeks) and a late one between 12 and 24 weeks of gestation. A simple classification is helpful in understanding the various terms used (Fig. 8.1).

In early pregnancy we have become more sophisticated in our ability to monitor and predict the outcome of pregnancy. Ultrasound scans now accurately measure the volume of the gestational sac and the crown–rump length of babies from 6 weeks, and show the fetal heart, allowing us to date the pregnancy accurately and to look for signs of normal progress. In addition serum measurements of human chorionic gonadotrophin (hCG) and progesterone are useful indicators of the progress of the pregnancy. The hCG should rise by more than 60% every 48 hours up to 12 weeks. A rise of less than 60% may indicate a failing pregnancy and it is essential to identify the location of the embryo in order to exclude an ectopic pregnancy that may be life threatening. If a scan therefore shows an empty uterus and the woman is asymptomatic it is reasonable to take a baseline measurement and repeat it after 48 hours. If the level is falling the pregnancy is failing and. even if it is ectopic, the woman is at low risk of experiencing a ruptured tube. If it is rising suboptimally the possibility of an ectopic pregnancy has not been ruled out and she should be managed accordingly.

The progesterone level done at the first visit can be helpful. A level >60 nmol/l usually suggests an ongoing pregnancy, and between 15 and 60 nmol/l the pregnancy may be ongoing, failing or wrongly located. If the level is <7 nmol/l the pregnancy is failing.

Blood levels are therefore useful indicators but not diagnostic, so clinical skill and ultrasound are still key in making the right diagnosis.

Causes of spontaneous miscarriage

These are maternal, fetal and possibly paternal or genetic.

Maternal causes

General
- Age
- Obesity
- Acute febrile illness

Lecture Notes: Obstetrics and Gynaecology, 3rd edition. By Diana Hamilton-Fairley. Published 2009 by Blackwell Publishing. ISBN: 978-1-4051-7801-3.

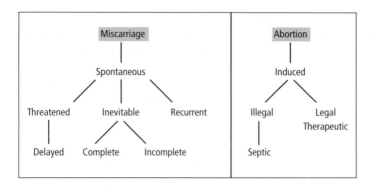

Figure 8.1 A simple classification of the terms used.

- Septicaemia with infection of the fetus
- Severe hypertension or renal disease
- Diabetes
- Hypothyroidism
- Trauma
- A surgical operation

Drugs such as ergot, quinine and lead may be taken to induce abortion. They are not very effective and the risk of poisoning is great.

Local
- Uterine fibroids, particularly submucosal ones
- Congenital uterine malformations
- Adenomyosis
- Incompetence of the internal os:
  — congenital
  — acquired after difficult dilatation of the cervix
- Hormone deficiency:
  — progesterone: the corpus luteum usually produces progesterone, which helps the embedding of the embryo
  — antiphospholipid syndrome (APS)
  — systemic lupus erythematosus (SLE).

Fetal causes

- Genetic abnormalities
- Congenital malformations
- Faulty implantation.

Congenital and genetic malformations

Examination of the chromosomes in material from spontaneous abortion shows gross abnormalities in over half. Most are chromosomal abnormalities such as Turner's syndrome or any of the major trisomies (21, 13, 16, 18). Often the embryo has failed to develop or has been absorbed. In these cases, miscarriage usually takes place between 6 and 8 weeks. Ultrasound shows that the amniotic sac contains no embryo or an embryo that is small for gestation and has no fetal heart movement (delayed miscarriage). In other cases, gross malformation of the fetus is shown.

Faulty implantation

The embryo may become implanted in an unfavourable site in the uterus, eg in the isthmus, cervical canal or the uterine cornu. Most of these cases end in spontaneous miscarriage; rarely the pregnancy continues and may be dangerous.

Incidence of spontaneous miscarriage

The frequency depends on the definition:
- In clinically diagnosed pregnancies 15–20% will miscarry in early pregnancy
- Non-development of the blastocyst within 14 days occurs in up to 50% of conceptions.

Clinical features and management of spontaneous miscarriage

Threatened miscarriage

Symptoms
- Scanty uterine bleeding preceded by symptoms of pregnancy.
- Pain is usually absent; there may be backache or slight uterine contractions.

Examination
- The breasts may be active (enlarged and tender).
- The uterus is enlarged corresponding with dates of amenorrhoea.
- The cervix is closed.
- There is no pelvic tenderness.

Differential diagnosis
- Delayed miscarriage when the uterus is smaller than expected. Check with ultrasound.
- Ectopic pregnancy when pain generally precedes bleeding.
- Dysfunctional uterine bleeding—where no signs of pregnancy.

Ultrasound can show a sac (from 5 weeks), an embryo and the fetal heartbeat (6 weeks). The hCG can be measured in blood or urine.

Treatment
Treatment is usually rest until fresh bleeding has ceased, although there is no evidence that this makes a difference to the outcome.

After bleeding has ceased, the woman should resume her normal life with advice on a balanced diet.

Inevitable miscarriage

Symptoms
Bleeding and pain are characteristic; bleeding is heavier than in threatened miscarriage. There may be crampy, low abdominal pains, and the passage of the sac and placental tissue or an escape of amniotic fluid if beyond 12 weeks.

Examination
- Uterus enlarged.
- The internal os of the cervix is open. Products of conception may be felt in the cervical canal. Once this has occurred, miscarriage is inevitable.
- In second trimester miscarriages the woman can present in significant pain with very heavy bleeding. Commonly this is associated with a low blood pressure and pulse rate (around 50) due to vasovagal shock.

Treatment
Remove any products from the open os to reduce the bleeding and pain/restore a normal blood pressure and pulse.

Before 12 weeks' gestation, evacuate the uterus under general anaesthesia in an operating theatre to stop the bleeding.

After 12 weeks, allow miscarriage to take place spontaneously, but be prepared to evacuate the uterus if it is incomplete. If bleeding is severe, Syntometrine should be given, 5 units/0.5 mg i.m.

Incomplete miscarriage

An incomplete miscarriage occurs when some of the products of conception are retained in the uterus. These are usually parts of the placenta or chorionic tissue attached to the uterine wall.

Symptoms
- Continued bleeding after a period of amenorrhoea
- Previous crampy pains/heavier bleeding commonly with clots.

Differential diagnosis
- Threatened miscarriage
- Ectopic pregnancy
- Dysfunctional uterine bleeding.

Ultrasound may help to clarify the diagnosis.

Treatment
- Conservative management
- Use of prostaglandins to evacuate the products
- Evacuation of the uterus in the operating theatre.

Complete miscarriage

If all the products of conception have been passed and the uterus is empty, the miscarriage is complete. There is little bleeding, and the uterus is small with the cervix closed or merely patulous in a multiparous woman.

No treatment is required provided that the differential diagnosis of ectopic pregnancy has been excluded (see p. 108).

Delayed or missed miscarriage

The embryo dies in early development and is retained there and/or the sac continues to develop. The early embryo is commonly reabsorbed leaving an empty sac—a blighted ovum (a term with unpleasant connotations for the parents and best avoided when talking to the patient and her partner).

Symptoms
• At first those of pregnancy, but these disappear
• The breasts become soft
• Dark-brown vaginal discharge.
The cervix is closed and the uterus smaller than would be expected; hCG levels drop in 7–10 days.

Differential diagnosis
• Hydatidiform mole
• An incomplete miscarriage
• A complete miscarriage.
Ultrasound will confirm the diagnosis.

Treatment
• Surgical evacuation: this should be offered if an embryo with an equivalent size of >8 weeks is present.
• Medical treatment: evacuation of the uterus can be successful in 50% of cases by giving vaginal or oral prostaglandins 600 μg ov 200 μg every 3 hours until miscarriage takes place.
• Expectant management: this is usually safe and effective if the sac is empty or the embryo is <8 weeks in size. The sac usually reabsorbs with minimal bleeding but it may take several weeks and patients should be offered regular follow-up until miscarriage is complete.

Recurrent miscarriage

Three consecutive spontaneous miscarriages constitute recurrent miscarriage. This may be primary, when the woman has borne no viable child, or secondary. The most important associations are:
• Maternal:
— APS (40%)
— polycystic ovaries (see Chapter 3) (50%);

— incompetence of the cervix (5%)
— trauma of the cervix
— previous difficult labour
— repeated dilatation of the cervix
— surgery of the cervix
— congenital malformation of the uterus (1%)
— genetic: most commonly a balanced translocation in one parent (3%).

Management
This depends on the time in pregnancy when it occurs. She is wise to abstain from exertion, intercourse and travelling until after week 14. The pregnancy should be monitored by ultrasound to ensure that the fetus is present and developing normally. Late recurrent miscarriage after week 12 is often a result of incompetence of the cervix which may require prophylactic suturing (Fig. 8.2).

If the woman is found to have APS, treatment with aspirin and heparin during pregnancy up to 36 weeks improves the take-home-baby rate from 10% to 40%. This lower success rate is due to the increased risk that these women have of developing pre-eclampsia which may be early onset (before 37 weeks) and severe, affecting the growth of the baby and/or leading to premature delivery because of fetal, maternal or fetomaternal reasons.

Investigations
1 APS: lupus anticoagulant and anticardiolipin antibodies are measured and repeated after 6 weeks. Two positive results are needed to confirm the diagnosis. For a true positive result both the anticoagulant (prolonged international normalized ratio or INR) and antibodies need to be present. The significance of only having one of these is not fully understood.
2 Polycystic ovarian syndrome (PCOS), luteinizing hormone (LH), follicle-stimulating hormone (FSH), testosterone (days 3–8), ultrasound scan.
3 Cervical incompetence and congenital abnormalities: hysterosalpingography and transvaginal ultrasound scan may show an incompetent cervix or uterine anomaly. In pregnancy, transvaginal ultrasound is usually helpful in showing the same deficiency and/or changes in the cervical length and dilation.

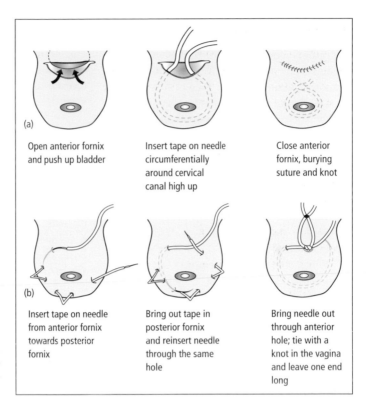

(a)

Open anterior fornix and push up bladder	Insert tape on needle circumferentially around cervical canal high up	Close anterior fornix, burying suture and knot

(b)

Insert tape on needle from anterior fornix towards posterior fornix	Bring out tape in posterior fornix and reinsert needle through the same hole	Bring needle out through anterior hole; tie with a knot in the vagina and leave one end long

Figure 8.2 (a) The Shirodkar and (b) Macdonald sutures, performed under general anaesthetic. If they work, they should be removed at 38 weeks.

4 Karyotype of both parents.

Between pregnancies hysterosalpingography or three-dimensional ultrasound with an echo-poor fluid may show an incompetent internal os. This may also reveal a congenital malformation of the uterus.

Counselling after miscarriage

Counselling is often needed because a spontaneous miscarriage may lead to bereavement even though the event was too early in pregnancy for a viable baby to be born. The woman and her partner should receive an explanation of what happened and of the possible cause of the miscarriage if it is known. If there is a treatable cause, such as uterine fibroids, treatment of this should be discussed even though the operation itself may be best postponed for about 3 months.

The couple are often anxious to have another pregnancy. In most normal cases, where no serious

Table 8.1 Chances of a live birth in a subsequent pregnancy

No. of miscarriages	Percentage
1	85
2	75
≥3	60
Unless APS diagnosed	
No treatment	10
Aspirin and heparin	40

cause is identified, there is no reason why they should not immediately, ie as soon as the woman has had a normal period or two. Commonly given advice to wait 3–6 months has no basis in evidence. A recent study has shown an increased risk of miscarriage if the woman conceives within 6 months of a live birth.

Parents find it helpful to know the chances of a successful pregnancy next time (Table 8.1).

Criminal abortion

Under the Offences Against the Person Act 1861, any attempt to procure abortion by the woman herself or by another person is a felony, irrespective of whether she is in fact pregnant. The position of termination of pregnancy under the Abortion Act is considered in Chapter 5. Abortion may be procured by:
- drugs
- instruments passed into the uterus (knitting needles or other long sharp instruments)
- foreign bodies—slippery elm bark introduced into the cervix
- injections of soap or douching with soap or antiseptic solutions.

Criminal abortion is dangerous:
- Drugs may cause poisoning
- Infection can easily be introduced
- Risk of severe haemorrhage can occur
- Embolism with air or soap solution.

The doctor called to deal with a woman who has had a criminal abortion is bound to respect her confidence. He or she should not inform the police or any other person unless the woman dies or appears likely to do so, when a dying declaration should be obtained. Deaths must be reported to the coroner (see also p. 87).

Septic abortion

Infection of the uterine cavity after an abortion leads to septic abortion. It can occur after spontaneous miscarriage, but most cases result from criminal interference with non-sterile instruments.

Spreading infection leads rapidly to salpingitis, pelvic peritonitis, pelvic cellulitis, septicaemia and pyaemia. Infection with *tetanus* will give the typical features of the disease and can be fatal. Infection with *Clostridium perfringens* is not uncommon in criminal abortions; the picture is that of severe infection with shock and tachycardia. Such cases need prompt and efficient treatment preferably in an intensive care unit.

Symptoms

- A history of abortion, often criminal
- Pelvic infection and septicaemia
- Fever
- Pelvic tenderness with foul discharge from the uterus and bleeding
- Neutrophil leukocytosis found on the blood count
- The haemoglobin level may be reduced.

Treatment

- Admission to hospital.
- Swabs should be taken for cultures from the cervix and blood culture taken in seriously ill patients.
- Adequate doses of antibiotics should start at once; a combination of amoxicillin, clindamycin and metronidazole may be used initially. A change of antibiotic may be needed when the cultures and sensitivities become available.
- Full intravenous supportive measures and steroids may be needed.
- If the products of conception are retained, the uterus should be evacuated. This should be done at once if there is severe bleeding; otherwise it is preferable to wait 24 hours to allow the antibiotics to take effect.

The incidence of septic abortion/miscarriage is now very low in the UK since the introduction of the Abortion Act 1967 and many lives have been saved. Unfortunately in many parts of the world women do not have access to legal and safe abortion and turn to unqualified and ill equipped clinics for help.

Ectopic pregnancy

Ectopic pregnancy is one outside the uterine cavity, the most common site being the fallopian tube. It may also occur, although rarely, in the:
- uterine cornu
- ovary
- cervix
- abdominal cavity
- broad ligament.

For practical purposes, ectopic pregnancy will be considered as a tubal pregnancy.

Incidence

Estimates of the incidence of tubal pregnancy vary. In the UK it is 0.5%. In other countries, especially in Africa, it may be as high as 1% because of the higher prevalence of chronic tubal disease.

Causes

The ovum is fertilized in the fallopian tube and reaches the uterus in about 5 days. Anything that delays the passage of the fertilized ovum to the uterus can result in tubal pregnancy, such as an intrauterine device (IUD) and progesterone-only pill (POP) (Box 8.1).

Salpingitis is the most common predisposing cause. This may not be so severe as to cause complete closing of the tube, but it may destroy tubal cilia, kinking or narrowing the tube. *Chlamydia* sp. is now the most common organism associated with tubal damage. The woman is often unaware that she has had a tubal infection. *Tuberculous salpingitis* is an important but, in the UK, rare cause, because it damages the tube but often leaves it patent.

Congenital malformation of the tube may lead to crypts and diverticula providing sites for ectopic implantation (very rare).

Pathology

The muscular walls of the tube do not allow the embryo to grow beyond a certain size. The trophoblast gradually invades and erodes the tubal wall which, unlike the endometrium, is not prepared for implantation. Blood vessels are damaged and eventually bleeding takes place.

Box 8.1 Risk factors for ectopic pregnancy

Pelvic inflammatory disease
Previous pelvic surgery
Previous ectopic pregnancy
Intrauterine device
Progesterone-only pill
Depo-Provera
Emergency contraception
Sterilization

A tubal pregnancy may terminate in a number of ways:

- *Absorption*: in a few cases it is possible that absorption of a very early tubal pregnancy occurs. The embryo dies in the tube, with a small amount of bleeding, and is partly absorbed.
- *Tubal abortion*: part or all of the products of conception are expelled from the tube into the peritoneal cavity.
- *Tubal rupture*: this is the most dramatic and best known outcome of a tubal pregnancy, though in fact it is less common than absorption or tubal abortion. There is acute intraperitoneal haemorrhage from erosion of an artery. The pregnancy is often implanted in the narrower isthmus of the tube.
- *Secondary abdominal pregnancy*: this is the rarest outcome of all. The embryo is expelled complete from the tube and acquires a secondary attachment in the peritoneal cavity. It can occasionally go on to a full-term abdominal pregnancy. Many cases of children delivered from the peritoneal cavity by laparotomy have been reported, particularly in the West Indies.

Clinical features

The following is the picture of ectopic pregnancy:

- *Amenorrhoea*: this can be 4–8 weeks' duration, but may present before amenorrhoea is noticed.
- *Pain*: typically constant and often unilateral due to spasm of the tubal muscle. There may be referred shoulder pain via the phrenic nerve from blood in the abdominal cavity.
- *Vaginal bleeding*: when a pregnancy implants in the tube, the uterine endometrium is still converted into decidua. When the embryo dies, the decidua in the uterus separates. The bleeding is usually scanty, less than a normal period and dark brown in colour.
- *Faintness* or even *shock* with an acute rupture.

Unruptured ectopic pregnancy

This may present with:

- lower abdominal pain, often unilateral
- slight tenderness over one side of the uterus.

On bimanual examination, the uterus is slightly enlarged and the cervix is soft. There may be dark blood oozing from the external os. The pregnant tube is usually not palpable. There will be cervical excitation (see p. 23) with tenderness on the side of the ectopic.

On bimanual examination, the tubal mass is rarely felt as a diffuse boggy swelling. If it is of any size, it displaces the uterus to the opposite side of the pelvis.

Acute rupture of a tubal ectopic

This presents as an acute abdominal emergency with:
- collapse
- severe abdominal pain
- pallor, rapid pulse and hypotension
- blood that may track up under the diaphragm giving shoulder pain
- an abdomen that is slightly distended, tender and rigid
- on vaginal examination, uterus that is soft and may be enlarged but very tender
- a tender tubal mass that may not be palpated because of extreme tenderness and guarding
- the patient should be taken straight to the theatre for a laparotomy.

Investigations

- *Ultrasound* is helpful. Although it may not always show the embryo or its sac in the tube, findings may include:
  — an empty uterus with thickened decidua
  — fluid (blood) in the pouch of Douglas
  a multi-echo mass in the region of the tube.
- *Progesterone levels* are commonly low because the pregnancy is failing.
- *Serum β-hCG* is usually lower than expected for gestation and on serial measurements increases by <60% over 48 hours.
- *Laparoscopy* is the ultimate investigation to make the diagnosis with direct vision.

Differential diagnosis

The diagnosis is from any other acute abdominal event such as rupture of a viscus or acute peritoni-tis. The clinical picture is so typical that in most cases diagnosis presents no difficulty. Other diagnoses that may confuse are:
- inevitable miscarriage
- bleeding with an ovarian cyst
- pelvic appendicitis
- acute salpingitis.

Treatment

The treatment of tubal pregnancy is normally removal of the pregnancy and sometimes the affected tube by laparoscopy or laparotomy. If the tube is patent and not seriously damaged, it may be possible to conserve it and thus leave the woman with a chance of conception later in life. Increasingly medical treatment is being offered and accepted by women.

Laparoscopy techniques exist to:
- kill the embryo with a direct injection of methotrexate or mifepristone allowing absorption, so requiring no surgery on the tube (rarely done and can be done ultrasonically)
- incise the swollen tube over the ectopic pregnancy, aspirate the embryo and achieve haemostasis (salpingostomy).The woman should be followed up with serial hCG levels to ensure that all the pregnancy tissue has been removed.

In a case of severe haemorrhage, the patient must be taken immediately to the operating theatre. Little time should be wasted in attempting resuscitation, which can prove useless and may only increase bleeding. An intravenous drip should be set up and a blood transfusion given as soon as possible. It is sometimes possible at operation to collect the extravasated blood from the peritoneal cavity with a Cellsaver and return it to the circulation.

In most cases the affected tube should be removed; an exception may be made if the woman desires children and the other tube is already missing or seriously diseased. The disadvantage of conservation is the increased risk of recurrence of ectopic pregnancy.

Tubal pregnancy and normal intrauterine pregnancy may occur simultaneously in rare circumstances, most commonly after assisted conception.

Medical treatment with methotrexate can be used if the hCG level is <5000 IU/l and the ectopic mass is <4 cm in diameter on ultrasound scan. There should be no symptoms or signs of rupture.

Counselling after an ectopic pregnancy

The woman should allow herself time to recover from her operation or treatment. If she has received methotrexate she should be put on contraception for at least 3 months. The oral contraceptive pill is ideal. As her tubes are damaged the IUD and POP or depo preparations should be avoided.

Her chances of a successful intrauterine pregnancy depend to some extent on the findings at operation. If the contralateral tube looked normal and there were no pelvic adhesions/signs of chlamydia infection (Fitz-Hugh–Curtis syndrome), she has a 70% chance of a successful pregnancy if the affected tube was removed. If she has a positive history of PID, an abnormal tube at laparoscopy, a previous ectopic or had a salpingostomy, her chances are significantly lower than this.

All the women should be told to attend an early pregnancy clinic or have an ultrasound scan at 6 weeks in a subsequent pregnancy to check the location of the pregnancy as early as possible, to minimize the risk of her presenting with a ruptured tubal ectopic pregnancy in the future.

Hydatidiform mole

Hydatidiform mole is a benign tumour of both parts of the chorion; the cytotrophoblast and the syncytiotrophoblast may be found in varying proportions. The villi undergo cystic or hydropic degeneration and a certain amount of bleeding almost always occurs.

Hydatidiform moles vary greatly in their rate of growth, the amount of chorionic gonadotrophin produced and the level of invasion of the uterine wall.

Only rarely can a fetus be found, but hydatidiform degeneration may occur in the placenta. The birth of a living fetus with a hydatidiform mole has been described.

Incidence

In the UK one in 2500 pregnancies, but much more common in the Far East.

Clinical features

The typical clinical features are amenorrhoea followed by continuous or intermittent vaginal bleeding. The other symptoms of pregnancy occur, often exaggerated; vomiting may be severe and early pre-eclampsia can develop. The uterus is often larger than the dates would suggest and feels very soft and boggy. Theca lutein cysts may develop in the ovaries.

Vesicles of the mole may be passed spontaneously and this is diagnostic of the condition.

Investigations

Chorionic gonadotrophin excretion in urine is often greater than other pregnancies; while levels of 40000–60000 IU/l are common, concentrations of over 100000 IU/l are generally diagnostic of a mole. Ultrasonic examination is reliable in showing the absence of a fetus with the characteristic picture of snowflakes or soap bubbles (bright sunlight shining through washing-up water).

Treatment

The uterus must be emptied completely in all cases. If there seems to be spontaneous evacuation, the uterus must still be carefully aspirated and curetted, the specimen being sent for histology examination.

A complate mole may be dealt with by suction evacuation under cover of continuous oxytocin intravenous drip, curetting gently to remove the entire mole. Intravenous Syntocinon must be given to minimize bleeding. Suction evacuation is safest and carries less risk of perforation than curettage.

Dangers include:
* haemorrhage which can be profuse
* sepsis
* perforation of the uterus

- air embolism
- incomplete evacuation of the uterus.

A second aspiration or curettage may be needed 2 weeks later to be sure that the mole has been completely removed.

Follow-up

The woman should be followed up by regular estimations of urinary hCG for at least a year and avoid pregnancy for 6 months after hCG levels have returned to normal. Tests should be carried out monthly for the first 6 months and after that every 2 months. Persistence of hCG after 1 month may suggest incomplete evacuation of the uterus or malignant change. Persistence is an indicator for chemotherapeutic treatment with actinomycin D or methotrexate to prevent choriocarcinoma.

During the period of follow-up, the woman should not take the contraceptive pill but use barrier methods of contraception.

In the UK, follow-up is undertaken in specialist centres.

Invasive mole

In some cases of hydatidiform mole, there may be great trophoblastic activity with penetration of the uterine wall. This can still be a simple invasive mole causing uterine enlargement and bleeding with a positive pregnancy test; this may require hysterectomy.

In more severe cases trophoblast penetrates into the parametrium and leads to internal haemorrhage. The level of hCG is very high. These cases require urgent hysterectomy.

Choriocarcinoma

This malignant tumour invades the uterine wall and metastasizes widely through the bloodstream. Rarely primary tumours are found in the ovary or testis as a form of teratoma.

It is fortunately an unusual tumour; about 40% follow hydatidiform mole, 40% follow abortion and 20% follow pregnancy at term. Conversely, a hydatidiform mole may go on to choriocarcinoma in 4–5% of women with a mole, compared with 0.0002% after normal pregnancy.

Clinical features

Uterine bleeding is the most common symptom. Secondaries may appear rapidly and are most often found in the lungs, uterus and vagina, but they can involve the liver and the central nervous system. The levels of hCG are very high, often >100 000 IU/l.

Choriocarcinoma is sensitive to cytotoxic drugs and is now curable in most patients. Those with low-grade disease treated with methotrexate can retain their fertility and have further successful pregnancies. Assay of hCG in serum or urine is used as a tumour marker and reduction in its levels is a test of cure.

Chemotherapy is best given in units that specialize in its use and various combinations of drugs are given; cisplatin is the first line of attack and may be combined with methotrexate, vincristine, cyclophosphamide and actinomycin D.

With modern treatment, hysterectomy is now rarely indicated except with massive tumours causing severe bleeding or when the response to chemotherapy is poor.

Chapter 9

The antenatal period

It must be remembered that pregnancy is a physiological process, which for most women will progress normally and end with a live healthy baby being born to a healthy mother.

The aims of antenatal care are to bring the mother and child to labour in the best possible condition. They are:

1 A screening process applied to the entire pregnant population to detect subgroups at higher risk for complications of pregnancy.

2 Suitable diagnostic procedures to determine those who are really at risk.

3 The provision of appropriate management for high-risk pregnancies.

4 The educational preparation of the couple for childbirth and the rearing of the infant.

Diagnosis of pregnancy

Symptoms

Amenorrhoea

The monthly shedding of the endometrium is prevented by higher progesterone levels from the persistence of the corpus luteum. Pregnancy is dated from the first day of the last normal menstrual period (LNMP) even though conception does not occur until about 14 days later. Any bleeding after the LNMP should be considered as abnormal.

Nausea and vomiting

Nausea occurs in 80% of nulliparous and 60% of multiparous women. For many pregnant women this is the first sign of pregnancy with the symptoms occurring even before the first period is missed.

The nausea and vomiting usually disappear by 16 weeks' gestation and lessen in severity after about 12 weeks. Although some women are sick first thing in the morning, it is not unusual to find that vomiting may occur at any time of the day. Commonly some biscuits or sweets help prevent nausea.

There is usually no accompanying metabolic upset, women do not feel ill all the time and it does not affect their daily activities. They do not usually require hospitalization. Specific causes may include urinary tract infection or ingestion of iron tablets.

Breast symptoms

Breast enlargement accompanied by tingling of the skin and nipples. Montgomery's tubercles develop from between 6 and 8 weeks' gestation

Lecture Notes: Obstetrics and Gynaecology, 3rd edition. By Diana Hamilton-Fairley. Published 2009 by Blackwell Publishing. ISBN: 978-1-4051-7801-3.

and colostrum may be secreted from the nipples after about 12 weeks' gestation.

Urinary symptoms

From 6 weeks' gestation onwards, many women experience increased frequency of micturition, as a result of:
• increased renal blood flow in the early stages
• pressure on the bladder from the growing uterus in later pregnancy.

Signs

Uterus

• An increased softness and enlargement of the uterus can be felt on bimanual vaginal examination from 6 weeks to 8 weeks' gestation.

Breasts

• Increased in size and feel warm
• The areolae darken
• Montgomery's tubercles develop
• Tortuous skin veins dilate.

Investigations

Pregnancy test

Animal pregnancy tests and early crude immunological tests have now been replaced by accurate, sensitive tests involving monoclonal antibodies. Human chorionic gonadotrophin (hCG) is a glycoprotein hormone that contains two carbohydrate side chains: alpha (α) and beta (β). The α subunit is identical to that of follicle-stimulating hormone (FSH), luteinizing hormone (LH) and thyroid-stimulating hormone (TSH). The β subunit is immunologically specific. The hCG is secreted by the trophoblast cells of the fertilized ovum and later by the definitive placenta.

Modern tests can detect hCG levels as low as 25 IU/l, before the time of the missed menses. Such tests can be performed in 2 minutes and are unaffected by urine contaminated by proteinuria or bacteria. Only a few drops of urine are required. The tests come in a variety of kits that can be bought in any chemist and are based on a colour change occurring if hCG binds to the monoclonal antibody embedded in the absorbent paper. Two main sorts are available: a double band of blue or a central spot of pink indicates a positive test whereas a single band of blue or absence of a pink spot indicates a negative pregnancy test.

Ultrasound

Real-time ultrasound machines will detect an intrauterine gestation sac from 5 weeks of amenorrhoea, with fetal heart activity becoming visible at 6 weeks and a fetal pole at 7 weeks.

Transvaginal probes enable a better resolution image than transabdominal ultrasound, allowing the diagnosis of an intrauterine pregnancy to be made 1 week earlier (5–6 weeks).

Antenatal visits

The current method of antenatal care was established 80 years ago but is now subject to change. In particular, the visits in mid-pregnancy (12–34 weeks) may be reduced.

Traditionally, the woman is seen monthly from the booking visit until 28 weeks, fortnightly until 36 weeks and then weekly until delivery. A reduction in the number of visits does not affect the outcome of pregnancy (Table 9.1) and is very popular with women. The expectation is that women will receive their first appointment before week 12 of pregnancy and be seen on a minimum of eight further occasions provided that no complications arise.

The aim of the visits is to screen the low-risk population by means of history, examination and investigation; then antenatal care for high-risk women may be carried out on a more frequent basis.

The following scheme applies to all women and is an attempt to identify risk factors.

Table 9.1 The spacing of antenatal visits by traditional and by modern care

Traditional (gestation in weeks)	Modern
6–12	8–12
16	
20	20
24	
	26
28	
30	
32	32
34	
36	36
37	
38	38
39	
40	40
41	41

Box 9.1 Establishing the expected date of delivery (EDD) from the LNMP (last normal menstrual period)

		Example
1	Take date of first day of LNMP	21 September 2008
2	Take away 3 months and add a year	21 June 2009
3	Add 7 days	28 June 2009
4	This is the EDD	

Do not use if
- Dates uncertain
- Cycle not regular (ie outside range of 24–35 days)
- Been on oral contraception within 2 months

The first visit

Ideally the booking visit should be at 8–12 weeks' gestation. More frequently now the woman's history is being taken in her own home by a community midwife. Increasingly women are being cared for by a named midwife or case-load midwife who will look after the woman during the pregnancy and labour, and postnatally. This has been shown to increase the normal delivery rate, reduce the rate of postnatal depression and increase breastfeeding rates. Satisfaction surveys have shown that this is a very popular model of care among women and their midwives. The women also report feeling more confident about themselves during the pregnancy and labour, as well as being better able to look after the baby in the first few weeks.

History

The woman carries her own maternity notes in the UK so that all aspects of her care can be communicated in one place regardless of where she is seen—hospital clinic, community clinic, GP surgery, ultrasound or other maternity units when on holiday. Some aspects of the history may have to be recorded separately if the father of the baby or the woman's family are unaware of previous opera-

tions or that she is HIV positive. These are usually recorded using an agreed code that makes sense to the health professionals but is obscure to a layperson.
- Establish the reliability of the LNMP (Box 9.1):
  — Was the woman sure of the dates?
  — Was the cycle regular?
  — Was the woman on oral contraceptives within 2 months?
  — Was there bleeding in early pregnancy?
  Any of the above circumstances render prediction of expected date of delivery (EDD) from LNMP unreliable and later ultrasound examination is needed to determine dates.
- History of maternal disease, eg hypertension, diabetes mellitus, previous thromboses, epilepsy, thyroid disease, anaemia, congenital heart disease.
- Family history, eg diabetes mellitus, tuberculosis, hypertension, multiple pregnancy or the birth of a congenitally abnormal baby, inherited disorders.
- Past obstetric history: this involves listing all the pregnancies in chronological order together with the following details (Box 9.2):
  — deliveries after 24 weeks regardless of outcome
  — miscarriages and ectopic pregnancies:
  — first trimester (<12 weeks) or second trimester
  — if second trimester, were they:

115

— relatively painless, associated with early rupture of the membranes suggesting cervical incompetence?

— associated with pain and bleeding suggestive of premature placental separation?

— associated with the delivery of a dead, macerated baby—an intrauterine death?

— list all therapeutic abortions, their reason, gestation and method by which they were performed.

- Drug history: note all drugs taken in the pregnancy so far.
- Allergies: note allergies to medication, food or Elastoplast.
- Social history: detail:

— the woman's alcohol, tobacco and illicit drug intake giving appropriate advice

— the woman's marital status, her occupation and that of her partner

— the living conditions

— social support: family, friends.

Routine questioning about domestic violence is now recommended using open questions such as 'Do you feel safe at home?'. The incidence of domestic violence increases in pregnancy and up to 10% of women disclose at this time. It is essential that the midwives have training in handling a positive response and that there is access to suitable agencies to provide help and support to women. Ideally this questioning should be repeated during the second trimester because it is common for women to deny on first questioning and then reveal when asked again.

Examination

In the absence of a relevant history and with the routine use of ultrasound, there is little need to examine the pregnant woman's pelvis. Most doctors and midwives, however, would still perform the following examinations:

- Maternal blood pressure (essential).
- Maternal height and weight as a body mass index (BMI) > 30 kg/m^2 places a woman at increased risk of developing gestational diabetes and she should be referred for a glucose tolerance test at 28 weeks. She should be advised to reduce her carbohydrate intake and try to maintain a constant weight through pregnancy because all other pregnancy-related risks are increased (hypertension, caesarean section, intrauterine death).
- The breasts to check for:

— lumps

— inverted nipples, which may require advice for breastfeeding.

- The spine for kyphosis or scoliosis.
- The abdomen looking for scars, masses and, if the pregnancy is sufficiently advanced, the size of the uterus.
- The legs looking for varicose veins.
- Vaginal examination is not recommended at antenatal visits unless clinically indicated. If a cervical smear is due then this should be performed 6 weeks postnatally.

Investigations

Urine

- Proteinuria: infection or renal disease
- Glucose: diabetes
- White blood cells: response to infection
- Nitrite: bacteria.

Blood

- Haemoglobin
- Red cell indices, particularly for the mean corpuscular volume (MCV) } Anaemia

- ABO and rhesus (Rh) group (if negative, need for anti-D)
- The presence of atypical antibodies
- Haemoglobin electrophoresis for sickle cell disease or thalassaemia
- Test for hepatitis antigens and antibodies
- Test for rubella antibodies
- Human immunodeficiency virus (HIV) test; all women after appropriate counselling should be offered an HIV antibody test but the following patients are at high risk:
  — women from or with partners from sub-Saharan Africa
  — drug abusers or partners of drug abusers
  — women who have bisexual partners
  — women with haemophiliac partners
  — women who have had a blood transfusion overseas.
  With the increasing prevalence of HIV among women universal testing is performed with an opt-out policy
- Screening tests for syphilis (usually Venereal Disease Reference Laboratory [VDRL] test); if positive, more specific tests are required (see Chapter 6).

General advice for healthy pregnancy

- Establish a rapport between the woman and the antenatal clinic staff.
- Show the woman where she can discover more about her pregnancy and delivery from:
  — books available
  — parentcraft classes
  — relaxation classes
  — video and TV programmes.
- Discuss the social welfare benefits available.
- Make arrangements for the medical social worker to see the woman if there are any difficulties, such as care of the other children or housing.
- Advise a visit to the dentist reasonably soon, as dental care in pregnancy is free, and there is an increased prevalence of tooth decay and gingivitis in pregnancy.
- Give dietary advice: this should be simple advice as most people in the UK have a more than adequate diet. The idea of eating for two should be discouraged and, in general, pregnant women need

only an additional 500 kcal (2100 J) a day to ensure normal fetal growth.

Vegans may require specialized advice from the dietitian in order to ensure adequate nutrition throughout the pregnancy, especially for certain amino acids. Similarly, some Asian women may need dietary advice or supplements of vitamin D as a consequence of living in the cloudy northern hemisphere.

- Advise the woman to stop smoking because it increases the risk of intrauterine growth retardation (IUGR) and delayed fetal maturation.
- Advise the woman to stop drinking alcohol or cut down on her intake.
- Advise the woman to avoid unpasteurized products, soft cheese and paté because these have been associated with intrauterine death secondary to listeriosis.
- Advise the woman to be careful when dealing with cats' litter by avoiding emptying the tray and using rubber gloves because of the risk of acquiring toxoplasmosis, which may lead to learning difficulties in the fetus.
- Consider providing iron supplementation. The routine of prophylactic iron supplements in pregnancy is controversial. Many obstetricians provide iron only if the woman has a haemoglobin <10.5 g/dl or a MCV <84 fl at the booking visit. Additional indications may be for multiple pregnancies or the previous pregnancy within 2 years. Most women's haemoglobin level will fall by about 1 g/dl due to haemodilution which occurs in pregnancy.

If iron is given, it should be taken with meals because it is absorbed only in the ferrous state and this is best achieved in the presence of vitamin C. In the non-pregnant state, about 10% of iron is absorbed and this is thought to double in pregnancy. When supplementation is given, you should aim to give at least 100 mg elemental iron a day.

- Vitamin supplements: these are not usually required by women receiving an adequate diet. An exception is folic acid because it is often only barely sufficient in many diets. The requirements in pregnancy rise from 50 µg/day to 300 µg/day. Many women are therefore given prophylactic iron tablets that also contain folic acid (500 µg/day.)

Folic acid supplements have been shown to reduce the incidence of neural tube defects (NTDs) when taken preconceptually and up to 14 weeks' gestation.

Subsequent visits

To be performed at all visits

• Check the history of recent events including pain, bleeding, loss of fluid, and pain in legs or chest, and ensure that the baby is moving.
• Examine the following:
— Blood pressure.
— The growth of the uterus and its contents can be assessed by measuring the symphysiofundal height (SFH; Fig. 9.1)—the fundus of the uterus is palpated by placing the right hand flat on the abdomen below the xiphisternum and moving it stepwise down the abdomen until the uterus is first felt in the midline; one end of a tape measure is placed and held there while the tape is extended over the fullness of the uterus to the top of the symphysis pubis in the midline. The distance is then read in centimetres. Normal growth is 1 cm/week ± 2 cm, eg at 32 weeks the SFH should be 30–34 cm. Less than 30 cm may indicate growth retardation or oligohydramnios; >34 cm may indicate a multiple pregnancy, polyhydramnios or macrosomia. Clinical assessment by palpation is rather a crude method with only 40% of small babies accurately detected and of these only 60% will still be small for dates at birth (Fig. 9.10).

Beyond 26 weeks the following should be noted in the notes:
— lie (longitudinal, oblique, transverse) (Fig. 9.2)
— presentation (cephalic, breech, none) (Fig. 9.3)
— engagement (fifth's palpable, see p. 172)
— liquor volume (normal, polyhydramnios, oligohydramnios)
— fetal heart auscultation with hand-held Doppler ultrasonography (from 14 weeks) or pinard stethoscope (beyond 30 weeks). The rate should be between 110 and 160 beats/min.
— Test the urine with a dipstick for protein, glucose, leukocytes and nitrites.
— Check all results from previous visits.

Additionally at 26–28 weeks

• Check the haemoglobin.
• If the woman is rhesus negative also check for the presence of Rh antibodies. Give prophylactic anti-D.
• Ensure that high-risk women (obese, family history of late-onset diabetes) are referred for a glucose tolerance test. Some now screen for gestational diabetes by doing random blood sugar at 28 weeks' gestation.
• Check the lie and presentation of the fetus.

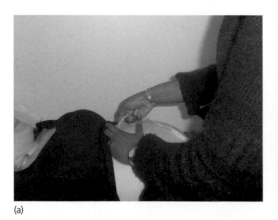
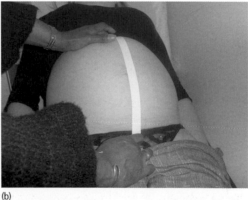

(a) (b)

Figure 9.1 Measuring the symphysiofundal height (SFH). (a) Palpate the fundus and place start of tape (b) Take tape (face down) to symphysis.

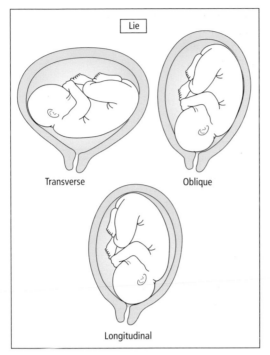

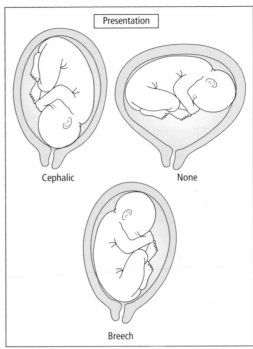

Figure 9.2 Diagrammatic representation of the possible lies of a baby.

Figure 9.3 Diagram of the possible presentations of a baby.

Additionally at 34 weeks

- Check haemoglobin level.
- If the patient is Rh negative, check for the presence of antibodies. Give prophylactic anti-D.
- If the presentation is cephalic, is the head engaged?

Between 41 and 42 weeks

Examine the cervix to assess the chances of success of induction if this is needed and do a membrane sweep if the cervical os is open; 70% of women will go into spontaneous labour within 48 hours. Arrange induction of labour for 41 weeks +5 days to 42 weeks, because there is a small increased risk of intrauterine death beyond 42 weeks. It is important to be sure of the woman's dates before doing this because inducing before this time increases the risk of an operative delivery for failed induction.

Advice to mothers

Apart from the dietary and social welfare information that should be available to the woman when she books, the following should be enquired about specifically.

Intercourse

There is no restriction to intercourse during pregnancy unless the woman bleeds from the vagina or has placenta praevia. Mechanical problems may occur in late pregnancy so that alterations in the position of intercourse may become necessary, eg the woman may be more comfortable on top.

Alcohol

Alcohol crosses the placenta readily and so can affect a fetus as much as an adult. Excessive drinking in pregnancy is associated with the fetal alcohol syndrome, characterized by a short nose with a low bridge, small eyes with a narrow palpebral fissure and learning difficulties.

No ill-effects have been described with an alcohol intake below 4 units a week.

Rest and exercise

Even in normal pregnancy, the extra weight carried by the woman may increase her sense of tiredness and lethargy. Sensible exercise such as walking and swimming or organized exercise to which the woman is accustomed (eg aerobics) should be allowed in pregnancy.

Travel

The woman should travel only over distances that are comfortable to her.

Air travel is probably better than train for long distances, but airlines can refuse to carry women over 34 weeks' gestation for international flights and over 36 weeks' gestation for domestic travel. They are the final arbiters, not the travel agents.

Clothes

Women should be advised to wear what looks good and feels comfortable.

Maternity brassières are often not required until late pregnancy, but women should be advised to move into them as soon as they feel that their present brassière is inadequate for support.

Bathing

The woman should bathe as she wishes. Avoid vaginal douching in pregnancy.

Bowels

Pregnancy tends to make women constipated because of the progestogenic effect of relaxing smooth muscles. This is best overcome by increasing fluid intake, fresh fruit and the use of foods rich in fibre. Laxatives should not be used unless the constipation becomes symptomatic.

Onset of labour

Many nulliparous women have no idea what to expect; up to 10% of women who present with pains are subsequently proved not to be in labour.

Advise that the onset of labour is usually accompanied by one of the following:
• Regular painful contractions coming from the small of the back and radiating to the lower abdomen. Nulliparous women are usually advised to come into hospital when such contractions are occurring once in every 5–10 min.
• A bloody or mucous show. This is not necessarily a sign of labour. If accompanied by uterine contractions women should be advised to contact their midwife or delivery unit.
• Rupture of the membranes recognized by a gush of amniotic fluid. In this case, women should be advised to come into hospital because of the risk of cord prolapse.

Increasingly the woman is visited in her home by the midwife and advised what she should do. This avoids unnecessary journeys to the hospital. It should be emphasized that it is much better for a woman to come into hospital if she thinks that she is in labour or is worried. Even if she is not, many of the causes of uterine pain may be serious and should be evaluated in the maternity unit.

Psychological preparation

Pregnancy and delivery are a worry to most women. Commonly there is a fear of:
• the unknown
• the pain that accompanies labour
• something going wrong during labour and ending up with a child with learning difficulties
• losing control because of the pain or the health professionals 'taking over' unnecessarily

• loss of dignity, particularly being naked and vulnerable in front of strangers, and for some cultures the presence of unknown men (doctors, midwives and other staff such as cleaners and caterers).

Many women's fears can be alleviated by proper antenatal preparation and by encouraging them to ask questions at the antenatal clinic. Women and their partners should be encouraged to attend talks about childbirth and subsequent rearing of their children. The antenatal clinic is a busy place, but doctors and midwives should never appear to be rushed and should encourage women to express their fears or anxieties and to ask questions.

Parentcraft classes

The aim of these classes is to help women and their partners to prepare for labour, delivery and the care of their newborn baby. Couples should be encouraged to attend together.

The following areas are covered:
• Stages of labour
• Possible abnormalities of labour
• Methods of delivery
• Pain relief:
  — natural methods: teaching the woman relaxation exercises:
    — in the first stage, slow breathing between contractions and quick shallow breathing during contractions
  In the second stage, women are taught expulsive breathing that involves fixing the diaphragm and the upper abdomen
  — inhalational gases (N$_2$O)
  — transcutaneous electrical nerve stimulation (TENS)
  — regional local anaesthesia: epidural
  — acupuncture/hypnotherapy
  opiates: these are no longer recommended
• Place of birth:
  — hospital 90%
  — GP/midwifery unit 5%
  — home 5%.

Five per cent choose in early pregnancy to deliver at home but only 2% actually deliver there in the UK, although this varies across the country from less than 1% to 17%. Forty per cent of primigravidae will be transferred in labour because of failure to progress in the first or second stage. This can be very distressing for all concerned. They must be counselled that regional anaesthesia will not be available, and that resuscitation of the newborn and treatment of a postpartum haemorrhage will be more difficult compared with delivery in hospital.

Women in their first pregnancy often have very high expectations of having a normal labour and delivery, which can be unrealistic. They may write detailed birth plans (virtually never written by women in their second or third pregnancy) outlining their desired management of labour. It is important to try to make their expectations realistic, otherwise the mother (and her partner) may experience profound disappointment, anger and a sense of failure if things do not go as planned, which may both affect her ability to care for her newborn baby and increase her risk of postnatal depression.

Assessment of fetal well-being

The obstetrician is responsible for the care of two patients in pregnancy, one of them being the fetus. The hidden patient is guarded by the following barriers:
• *Anatomical*: these can be overcome to some extent by ultrasonography.
• *Physiological*: these need an understanding of the interaction between fetal and maternal physiology.
• *Psychological*: these need an explanation to the mother, her relatives, and often medical and midwifery staff to overcome the in-built resistance to investigating the unborn.

Screening for NTDs and Down syndrome

Neural tube defects (NTDs) account for 50% of congenital abnormalities. The incidence of NTDs varies across the country, with the highest rates traditionally in Norfolk and Glasgow. The discovery that folic acid supplements in early pregnancy significantly reduce the risk has led to a reduction in the incidence of these abnormalities within the western world. Some hospitals offer a blood test at 15–17 weeks to measure maternal serum α-fetoprotein, although most of these defects are now detected by high-resolution real-time ultrasound routinely performed at 18–20 weeks' gestation. Serious NTDs such as anencephaly, cystic hygromas or melingomyelocoele should be detected at the 12-week scan which is now recommended.

The rate of Down syndrome is most heavily influenced by maternal age. The risk at 20 is 1:1500, at 30 1:800, at 35 1:270, at 40 1:100 and at >45 1:50. The serum and ultrasound tests described below use a computer-generated algorithm to try to give a more specific risk for each pregnancy. It is very important to recognize that these tests are only an indicator of the relative risk of having a baby affected by Down syndrome and not a diagnosis of Down syndrome. In the UK a risk of >1:250 is used as the cut-off for offering an invasive diagnostic test because the risk of miscarriage for these tests is between 1 and 3%, depending on which one is performed. The algorithm used is heavily weighted by age because of the rapid increase in risk with age; this makes it difficult for a woman over 40 to reduce her risk enough to be advised not to have an invasive test and, vice versa, makes it very hard for a woman of 25 to increase her risk to a level that allows her to undergo invasive testing. The introduction of these tests has led to an increase in the number of terminations being performed for Down syndrome with no overall decrease in the number being born, most to women under the age of 35 and usually undiagnosed antenatally.

The couple therefore needs to be carefully counselled before undergoing these tests as the results can lead to unnecessary anxiety, unnecessary invasive testing and the potential loss of a normal baby after invasive testing. Early diagnosis on ultrasound of very abnormal babies can lead to early termination when spontaneous miscarriage over the next few weeks is the most likely outcome and may have been easier for the couple to accept. Offering such tests makes assumptions about the nature of the condition that tend to be negative, leading professionals to almost expect couples to wish to terminate babies with Down syndrome when the diagnosis is made. Occasionally professionals may refuse to do an amniocentesis for a couple who would not have a termination if the baby was abnormal, even though it is perfectly legitimate for couples to want to prepare themselves for a less than perfect outcome in advance. Society can also drift into expecting all babies to be perfect and become intolerant of even minor, correctable abnormalities such as a cleft lip, and request termination. This is an ethical and moral minefield that requires very careful and skilful communication in order to ensure that couples fully understand all the possible consequences of the decisions that they are taking.

Screening tests for Down syndrome

The tests for Down syndrome include two modalities, a blood test which measures two, three or four of the following agents:
- α-fetoprotein (AFP)—low in Down syndrome, high in NTD
- hCG—raised in Down syndrome
- unconjugated estriol—lowered in Down syndrome
- inhibin-A—high levels in Down syndrome
- pregnancy-associated plasma protein A (PAPP-A)—raised in Down syndrome.

Ultrasonography is performed at 11–14 weeks to measure the skin thickness behind the baby's neck (Fig. 9.4) and again at 20–22 weeks to detect heart and other structural abnormalities. This scan has the added advantage of providing a more accurate estimated date of delivery than the later anomaly scan.

The tests can be divided into those for the first trimester and those for the second trimester.

First trimester screening
Fetal nuchal translucency (FNT) measures the nuchal pad at the nape of the fetal neck. Ultrasonographers have to be specially trained to do this test and it is dependent on the baby being in the right position. It has a 20% false-positive rate (FPR)

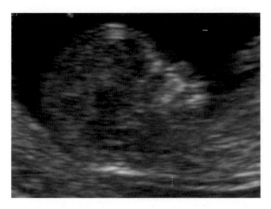

Figure 9.4 Ultrasound scan at 11–14 weeks to measure skin thickness at back of neck (nuchal translucency).

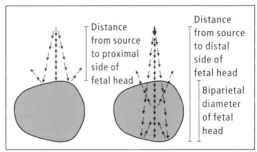

Figure 9.5 From the combined source and receiver, the transducer, the ultrasound impulses go out in straight lines. Only those that strike reflective surfaces at right angles will return along the same path. Hence the highest and lowest points of the fetal skull may be determined. The distance between them can be measured to a sensitivity of 1 mm.

for an expected 85% detection of Down syndrome, but also detects major cardiac anomalies and other trisomies. At 10–14 weeks a depth of >3 mm is associated with an increased risk of abnormality and a chorionic villous sampling or amniocentesis can be offered. The larger the measurement, the greater the risk of abnormality. If the karyotype is normal the woman should be offered a specialist fetal cardiac scan between 22 and 24 weeks (Fig. 9.4).

Serum tests alone: measurement of hCG and PAPP-A (double test) at 10 weeks has a false-positive rate of 12% or the serum integrated test done with PAPP-A at 10–13 weeks and the quadruple test (see below) at 15–16 weeks

Combined test: FTN with hCG and PAPP-A has a FPR of 6% for a detection of 85%. If the second trimester quadruple test is added the FPR reduces further to 1.2%.

Second trimester screening

Serum screening:
- The triple test: AFP, unconjugated estriol, hCG. FPR 9.3% for an 85% diagnostic rate.
- The quadruple test, AFP, unconjugated estriol, HCG and inhibin-A. The FPR is 5% for an 83% diagnostic rate and is replacing the double and triple tests.

The integrated test may be the most cost-effective because the more expensive investigations are offset by the lower FPR, so reducing the number of invasive tests.

Routine anomaly ultrasound scanning (18–20 weeks)

Most hospitals in the UK now offer a routine ultrasound examination at 18–20 weeks' gestation. The aim of this ultrasound examination is to:
- establish gestational age
- exclude major structural abnormalities of the fetus
- diagnose multiple pregnancy.

A small pulse of ultrasound is sent into the tissues and a recorder in the same transducer then detects the echoes. The distance between tissue boundaries can be assessed by determining the differences in time taken for the echoes to return from each boundary (Fig. 9.5).

At the 18- to 20-week routine ultrasound visit, the following are assessed:
- The biparietal diameter (BPD; Fig. 9.6)
- The head circumference (HC)
- The abdominal circumference (AC)
- Femur length (FL).

These measurements are used to confirm the gestational age of the fetus. The EDD may be changed if the measurements are more than ten days greater

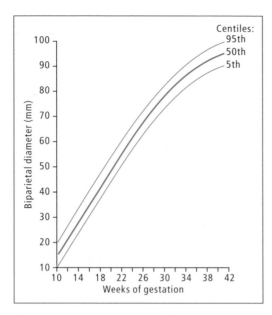

Figure 9.6 Growth measurement of the biparietal diameter to determine the gestational age.

or smaller than the 50th centile at 18–20 weeks. The later the scan is done the less accurate dating by ultrasound becomes, and caution should be exercised before changing the EDD if the first scan is done after 22 weeks.

The ultrasound scan will detect the following if not already detected at 12 weeks:

- Multiple pregnancy
- Placental site: particularly low-lying placenta (5% at 20 weeks but 0.5% at 34 weeks when the scan should be repeated)
- Fetal congenital abnormalities:
  — anencephaly (absent top of the head and brain)
  — spina bifida
  — double bubble of dilated stomach and duodenum in duodenal atresia (common in Down syndrome)
  — some cardiac abnormalities (Fallot's tetralogy, ventricular septal defect [VSD], atrial septal defect [ASD])
  — hydrocephaly
  — renal pelvic dilatation (outflow obstruction—urethral valves in boys)

— sacral agenesis (in type 1 diabetes)
— major limb defects (dwarfism)

The ultrasound scan is the first time that parents see their baby and it is known to increase the bonding that they feel towards it.

The ultrasound scan is also an opportune time to look at the blood flow to the uterus because a notch in the down side of the wave helps to identify a group of women more likely to develop hypertension in pregnancy. It may affect one or both of the uterine arteries and the significance of this is not fully understood.

Third trimester assessment

Maternal assessment of fetal movement

The mother counts 10 fetal movements entering them on a chart. She is asked to start counting fetal movements from 9.00am and then to record the time by which she has felt 10 movements. If this is later than 9.00pm she is asked to report for further examination with a cardiotocograph (CTG).

Current evidence suggests that maternal appreciation of fetal movements is of value in high-risk pregnancies but does not seem to prevent unexplained stillbirths in pregnancies thought to be at low risk. The use of the Cardiff kick chart has reduced over recent years because the subjective reporting of reduced fetal movements by mothers is just as accurate.

Biochemical tests

These tests have been replaced by biophysical methods of monitoring fetal health because of:

- a wide range of normal values obtained in pregnancy
- the errors in laboratory measurement
- the need, in most cases, for serial testing.

These tests used to include measurement of estriol and human placental lactogen (hPL) but are never used in modern obstetric units.

Biophysical methods

These may be considered as:

- Short-term methods:
  — the biophysical profile

— the CTG

— Doppler studies of the fetal circulation

• Medium-term methods:

— measurements of fetal growth

— Doppler measurements of the uteroplacental circulation.

Short-term methods

The biophysical profile

Ultrasound examination of the following features composes the biophysical profile:

• Fetal movements

• Fetal breathing movements

• Fetal tone

• The amniotic fluid volume

• The CTG.

Each element is scored 0, 1 or 2 over 40 minutes, giving a maximum possible score of 10. A score of <6 is evidence of fetal compromise and delivery should be considered.

The biophysical profile is not used routinely in the UK, but is useful in high-risk pregnancies, particularly after intrauterine growth retardation has been detected. Measurement of the amniotic fluid volume is one of the most sensitive measures of fetal well-being and a significant reduction is associated with a poor outcome for the baby.

The Cardiotocograph (CTG)

An antenatal record of the fetal heart rate is recorded with Doppler ultrasound. In addition, fetal movements and uterine activity are measured by an external pressure transducer. A mnemonic, DR C BRAVADO, has been developed to ensure a more standard evaluation of the CTG by doctors and midwives. The date (D) and reason/risk (R) for doing the CTG should be recorded on the CTG printout as well as the name, date of birth (DOB) and hospital number of the patient. In antenatal assessment of fetal well-being a 20-minute trace is performed.

The following are the essential features of the CTG:

• *The baseline rate* (BR): between 110 and 160 beats/min, with a variability of 5–15 beats/min; rates outside these limits are extremely rare antenatally:

— baseline bradycardia usually suggests congenital heart disease

— fetal tachycardias are seen in the presence of anything that causes a rise in the maternal pulse rate such as a maternal pyrexia. In the absence of a maternal cause, the fetal tachycardia should be taken as a sign of fetal distress.

• *Acceleration* (A): in a 20-minute recording, the fetus normally produces an acceleration (Fig. 9.7). An acceleration is a rise in fetal heart

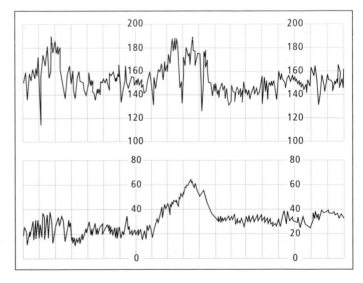

Figure 9.7 Acceleration of fetal heart rate (above) with uterine contraction (below).

rate of 15 beats/min above the baseline that is sustained for more than 15 seconds.

A CTG that shows two or more accelerations in a 20-minute period is considered normal. If there are no accelerations within the 20 minutes and the woman is not in labour a biophysical profile or amniotic fluid index and Doppler ultrasound should be performed.

• *Variability* (VA) (Fig. 9.8): the fetal heart rate from 26 weeks is controlled by a balance between the sympathetic and parasympathetic nervous system resulting in a natural variability of 5–15 beats/min.

Baseline heart rate variation of <5 beats/min is rarely seen antenatally, although it may follow drugs such as diazepam or night sedation. In the absence of drugs it may indicate fetal distress.

• *Decelerations* (D): antenatal decelerations in the fetal heart rate that are not associated with contractions are of serious significance and should indicate delivery taken in association with other factors.

• *Overall impression* (O): reassuring, suspicious or pathological. This final conclusion leads the doctor or midwife to make decisions about the management of the pregnancy. Senior medical staff must be involved in the decision-making if the CTG is suspicious or pathological because it may reflect fetal distress. It should be remembered that the CTG is only one of many parameters for assessing fetal well-being and even pathological CTGs are sometimes associated with a perfectly healthy, well-oxygenated, baby. Examples of pathological CTG traces are shown in Chapter 13.

There is no universal agreement as to how frequently the CTG should be performed. As with many other things in obstetrics, it should be planned and interpreted in the light of the woman's circumstances, eg if there has been a small unexplained antepartum haemorrhage (APH) only a daily CTG is required, but a growth-retarded baby in a woman with severe hypertension may warrant two or even three CTGs per day.

At present, the predictive value of a normal CTG is in doubt.

Doppler waveforms from the fetal circulation

If sound is aimed at a moving target, the echoes that return from the target will have shifted in frequency—the Doppler shift. The blood cells moving in the umbilical artery can be readily detected by Doppler ultrasound and in normal pregnancies produce the waveform shown in Fig. 9.9a.

If resistance increases in the placenta, eg in pre-eclampsia, Doppler ultrasound-shifted frequencies are not recordable in the last part of diastole (absence of end-diastolic frequencies). Figure 9.9b demonstrates this phenomenon.

In a few babies, there may be a reversal of frequencies in end-diastole (Fig. 9.9c), indicating that blood, which should be flowing towards the placenta for exchange of O_2 and nutrients, is flowing backwards towards the baby. This means that the baby may die soon and delivery should be expedited.

Doppler ultrasound examination of the wave from the umbilical artery (coming back from the baby) can be performed weekly in high-risk pregnancies. Other arteries within the baby can also be looked at—the middle cerebral and hepatic vein—which demonstrate shifts in flow that the

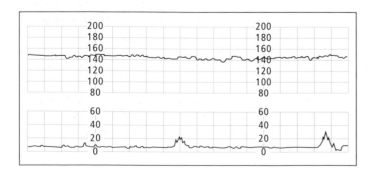

Figure 9.8 Antenatal CTG showing loss of baseline variability.

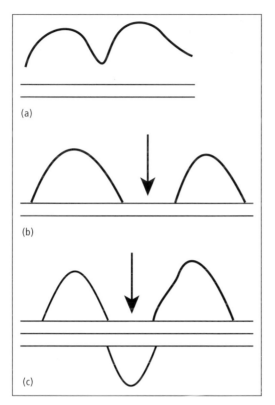

Figure 9.9 Doppler waveforms from the umbilical artery reflecting resistance to flow (impedance) in the fetal vessels of the placenta: (a) normal; (b) loss of end-diastolic frequencies (arrowed)—increased resistance; (c) reversed frequencies (arrowed)—much increased resistance.

baby may be making in order to maximize the oxygenation of the brain and heart.

Medium-term methods

Measurements of fetal growth

Measurements of fetal growth are best achieved by measurements of the head circumference and the abdominal circumference every fortnight from 26 weeks in high-risk babies or from the detection of a reduced symphysiofundal height or 4-weekly in multiple pregnancies, because growth of each individual cannot be measured clinically. Real-time ultrasound can be used to determine fetal growth in one of three ways:

1 To determine size when the fetus is thought clinically to be small.

2 As a screening test for small babies: some hospitals now offer a second ultrasound examination at 30–34 weeks' gestation to measure the fetal abdominal circumference. If this is not low, the baby only has a small chance (approximately 10%) of being small for gestational age (SGA) at birth.

3 Serial measurements of fetal growth: women at risk of having a SGA fetus should have serial ultrasound (fortnightly) to document the growth velocity of their babies.

Doppler waveforms from the uteroplacental circulation

Waveforms may be recorded from the maternal arcuate arteries, the first branches of the uterine arteries.

Failure of invasion results in a persistence of a high-resistance waveform (a notch) rather than the development of the usual low-resistance waveforms. Women with persistently high-resistance waveforms have a high probability of developing pre-eclampsia and an asymmetrical SGA fetus.

Definition of terms

There is much confusion in the obstetric literature over the terms used to signify that the baby is small:

• *Low birth weight (LBW)*: this term is used for a baby with a birth weight <2500 g. It is most useful on a worldwide basis where gestational age at delivery is often unknown. It is obvious that a baby who is <2500 g at birth may be preterm, small or both. Neonatal paediatricians have extended this classification to very-low-birth-weight (VLBW) babies which indicates a birth weight <1500 g and extremely low-birth-weight (ELBW) babies with a birth weight of under 1000 g.

• *Intrauterine growth restriction (IUGR)*: IUGR is the presence of a pathology that is slowing fetal growth, which if it could be removed would allow the resumption of normal fetal growth. There are no tests available antenatally or postnatally to determine whether a baby has truly suffered from IUGR although the HC:AC ratio on ultrasound scan may help.

- *SGA*: this is a statistical definition used if the infant's birth weight is below a certain standard for the gestational age. There is no universally agreed standard and such lower limits as the 10th, 5th and 3rd centile, or two standard deviations from the mean, have all been used. As the definition is statistical, one should expect, for example, that 10% of the normal population of babies have birth weights <10th centile. To interpret the birth weight, it is necessary to have charts derived from the local population being measured.

The term SGA is also applied antenatally when the growth or size of the fetus falls below statistically determined limits on population-derived charts.

The IUGR fetus

In broad terms, impairment of fetal growth can be the following:
- Symmetrical IUGR (Fig. 9.10): in this case the measurements of the fetal head and abdominal circumference are equally small. The baby is a miniature baby. The majority of these babies represent the biological lower limits of normal. Causes of symmetrical SGA are shown in Table 9.2.
- Asymmetrical IUGR (Fig. 9.11): this is a rarer form of impaired fetal growth, the causes of which are also shown in Table 9.2. The abdominal circumference slows its growth relative to the increase in head circumference. This is secondary to the fetus using the stores of brown fat normally laid down around the liver for nutrition of the baby in the first few days of life. In many cases, abnormal growth is associated with absence of end-diastolic flow in the umbilical circulation. Such babies are at risk of antenatal hypoxia, which may result in stillbirth, neonatal death or major learning difficulties.

The differential growth patterns in these fetuses result from a redistribution of fetal blood flow. In response to underperfusion in the intervillous space, there is an increase in resistance to blood flow within the fetal circulation. This means that blood returning from the placenta to the fetus takes the path of least resistance and is diverted to the fetal brain, coronary arteries and adrenals. Initially, this is to the benefit of the fetus but, if it continues for too long, the fetal bowel, kidneys and liver become ischaemic, resulting in the complications of asymmetrical IUGR babies: necrotizing enterocolitis, renal failure and failure of coagulation caused by insufficient production of coagulation factors by the liver.

Management of IUGR

Symmetrical IUGR

Most IUGR fetuses represent the biological lower limits of the normal range and require only serial

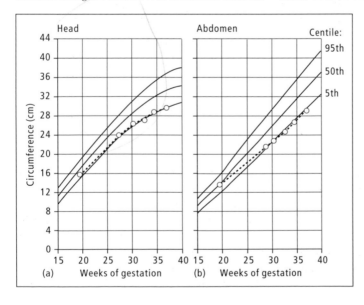

Figure 9.10 Symmetrical small for gestational age SGA measurements of (a) fetal head circumference (HC) and (b) fetal abdominal circumference (AC). HC:AC ratio = 1.0.

Table 9.2 Causes of babies who are small for gestational age (SGA)

Symmetrical IUGR (60%)	Asymmetrical IUGR (40%)
Race (white > black > Asian)	Poor maternal response to:
Sex (boy > girl)	pregnancy
Maternal size	pre-eclampsia
Toxins:	poor trophoblast invasion
alcohol	Essential hypertension
cigarettes	Cigarettes
heroin	Drug abuse
methadone	Chromosomal and
	congenital abnormalities
Congenital infections:	
cytomegalovirus	
parvovirus	
rubella	
syphilis	
toxoplasmosis	
Malnutrition	

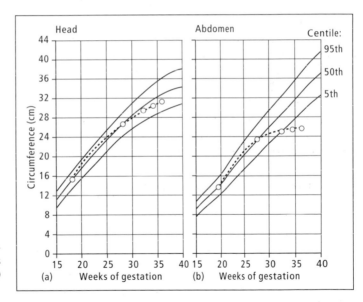

Figure 9.11 Asymmetrical small-for-gestational-age (SGA) measurements of (a) fetal head circumference and (b) fetal abdominal circumference.

measurements of ultrasound growth performed on a fortnightly basis. If the baby demonstrates normal growth (see Fig. 9.10), no further action is necessary.

The only problem posed for the obstetrician is to recognize those few babies who are congenitally abnormal or infected. The following actions are recommended:

• Check maternal blood for infections that are known to cross the placenta (syphilis, toxoplasmosis, rubella, parvovirus and cytomegalovirus).

• Search the fetus carefully with ultrasound looking for structural markers that may suggest a chromosome abnormality. If these are present the baby should be karyotyped, usually by means of a fetal blood sample obtained from the umbilical cord (cordocentesis). This is of value even in the third trimester because it is well known that fetuses with trisomies are prone to fetal distress in labour or intrauterine death before term. If the trisomy is lethal then, after discussion with the parents, a caesarean section may not be advised should such distress develop.

Asymmetrical IUGR

Management should be as follows:

• Fortnightly ultrasound measurements of head circumference and abdominal circumference to determine growth rate. The amniotic fluid volume should be measured by determining the height of the largest column of fluid or the addition of a column from the four quadrants of the uterus giving an amniotic fluid index. The former is normally between 2 and 8 cm; <2 cm suggests increasing fetal compromise.

• Doppler waveforms from the umbilical circulation. If these are normal they should be repeated on a weekly basis. Delivery is not indicated in the presence of normal umbilical artery waveforms. Absent end-diastolic flow should indicate delivery in a fetus that is considered to be viable, >24 weeks, >500 g.

• In the absence of Doppler waveforms, immediate fetal well-being should be monitored by daily CTGs and maternal counting of fetal movement. Delivery is indicated for cessation of fetal growth over a 4-week period, for abnormalities of the CTG and significant reduction in fetal movements.

Chapter 10

Diseases of pregnancy

Hyperemesis gravidarum

Incidence

Less than 1 : 1000 pregnancies in UK; a rare condition in the endogenous population.

Aetiology

- Hormonal: rapid increase in human chorionic gonadotrophin (hCG) and progesterone; hypothyroidism.
- Reflex: a chemosensitive trigger zone that stimulates the vomiting centre.
- Ketosis: after excess vomiting, build-up of ketones exacerbates the vomiting and a vicious circle develops.
- Hydatidiform mole: very high hCG levels.
- Multiple pregnancy: higher hCG and progesterone levels.

Progress

Can lead to:
- dehydration
- hypovolaemia
- electrolyte depletion

- vitamin deficiency, particularly thiamine
- haematemesis due to tears in the oesophagus from excessive vomiting
- death from liver failure or the end processes of the above.

Presentation

- Cannot retain food or fluid
- Weight loss because of loss of body fluid and burning up of fat
- Haemoconcentration and unstable acid–base balance
- Ketosis.

Management

- Exclude other diseases:
  — thyroid disease
  — urinary infection
  — hiatus hernia and gallbladder disease
  — obstructive gut lesions
  — central nervous system (CNS)-expanding lesions.
- Exclude obstetric cause:
  — multiple pregnancy.
  — hydatidiform mole.
  — acute yellow atrophy of the liver (very rare).
- Restore fluid and electrolyte balance intravenously
- Specific anti-vomiting drugs, eg cyclizine, prochlorperazine or metoclopramide

Lecture Notes: Obstetrics and Gynaecology, 3rd edition. By Diana Hamilton-Fairley. Published 2009 by Blackwell Publishing. ISBN: 978-1-4051-7801-3.

- Thiamine to prevent Wernicke's encephalopathy
- Steroid therapy: being assessed
- Psychological treatment: most respond to suggestion; if not, formal psychotherapy is needed
- Therapeutic abortion: very rarely required.

Hypertensive disorders of pregnancy

Hypertension has these risks:
- In the mother:
  — cerebrovascular accident
  — renal failure
  — heart failure
  — coagulation failure
  — liver failure
  — adrenal failure
  — eclampsia: a generalized convulsive disorder similar to epilepsy but which occurs only in pregnancy associated with hypertension and proteinuria
- In the fetus:
  — asymmetrical intrauterine growth restriction (IUGR)
  — placental abruption
  — iatrogenic preterm delivery.

Definitions

The currently internationally agreed definition of hypertensive disease in pregnancy is: pregnancy-induced hypertension (PIH) is hypertension occurring for the first time after 20 weeks' gestation.

Hypertension in pregnancy is defined as one of the following:
- Blood pressure of 140/90 mmHg on two occasions more than 4 hours apart.
- A rise of more than 30 mmHg in systolic blood pressure over the booking blood pressure.
- A rise of more than 15 mmHg in diastolic blood pressure over the booking figure.

If it is associated with new proteinuria of >300 mg/24 hours it is classified as pre-eclampsia. Women who develop PIH are more likely to go on to develop pre-eclampsia. PIH may be classified as:

- *Mild*: a blood pressure up to 140/100 mmHg without proteinuria.
- *Moderate*: a blood pressure up to 160/110 mmHg without proteinuria. In the absence of proteinuria PIH is rarely dangerous to mother or fetus but requires antihypertensive medication. In the presence of proteinuria it is called pre-eclampsia and carries significant risks to the mother and baby.
- *Severe*: a blood pressure of more than 160/110 mmHg; and the presence of proteinuria (pre-eclampsia/pre-eclamptic toxaemia [PET]).

Prevalence

This varies with the population, but in the UK 10–15% of primigravid women will develop some form of hypertension. Of these, about 6% may be considered as suffering from PIH and 2% will develop pre-eclampsia.

PIH is almost entirely a disease of primigravidae. Pre-eclampsia occurs only in multigravid women under the following conditions:
- Those who have had it severely in the first pregnancy.
- Those who have changed their partner between pregnancies.
- Pregnancies complicated by hydatidiform mole.
- Multiple pregnancies.
- Gestational diabetes.
- Those with antiphospholipid syndrome.

There are no good predictive tests for which women may develop pre-eclampsia in their first pregnancy; those at increased risk include women with:
- pre-existing hypertension
- body mass index (BMI) >30 kg/m^2
- multiple pregnancies
- pre-existing renal disease
- antiphospholipid syndrome
- microvascular disease secondary to type 1 diabetes.

Aetiology

The precise mechanism is unknown; the following are recognized:

- Women who develop pre-eclampsia have a failure of the second wave of trophoblastic invasion.
- This failure probably leads to a local alteration of the prostacyclin : thromboxane ratio. Both these prostaglandins are produced by trophoblasts and exert opposite effects. In PIH, the balance of the ratio appears to favour thromboxane. This leads to local vasoconstriction and platelet agglutination on already undilated vessels.
- The combination of the above two factors is associated with failure of the initial fall in peripheral resistance, so blood pressure in mid-pregnancy is maintained—it normally shows a marked fall during the second trimester. Subsequent narrowing or clotting of the abnormal blood vessels leads to a further increase in peripheral resistance and hence hypertension.
- The narrowing of the blood vessels also leads to decreased perfusion of the intervillous space and hence the development of a fetus with asymmetrical IUGR.

Clinical course

PIH usually presents in primigravidae in the late third trimester. It usually requires either no treatment or antihypertensive therapy alone while awaiting the onset of labour. Occasionally this progresses to the development of pre-eclampsia.

A few women present with the symptoms and signs of pre-eclampsia and occasionally this can occur in the late second or early third trimester. The presence of symptoms—headache, blurred or altered vision with a rising blood pressure or increasing proteinuria—heralds the onset of fulminating pre-eclampsia and requires prompt treatment and delivery to prevent the development of eclampsia and renal/cerebral damage (Table 10.1).

Oedema associated with hypertension and proteinuria is a sign of worsening pre-eclampsia. Oedema alone is of little significance.

Table 10.1 Pregnancy-induced hypertension

	Mild	Moderate	Severe (pre-eclampsia)
Symptoms	None	Mild headache	Frontal headache
		Oedema	Oedema
			Visual disturbance
Signs			
BP	<140/100	<160/110	>160/110
Proteinuria	None	None	++ or +++
Reflexes	Normal	Normal	Hyperreflexia/clonus
Fundi	Normal	Normal	Occasional papilloedema
Renal	Normal	Normal	Decreasing urinary output
Bloods			
FBC	Normal	Normal	Rising or falling Hb
			Decreasing platelets
Urate	Normal	Slightly raised	Increasing
LFTs	Normal	Normal	Increasing
Clotting	Normal	Normal	Prolonged
Fetus	Normal	Normal/SGA	Asymmetrical SGA
Treatment	None	Antihypertensives	Antihypertensives
			Anti-epileptics/MgSO$_4$
		? Delivery	Delivery

FBC, full blood count; LFTs, liver function tests; SGA, small for gestational age.

Mild disease

Women with mild PIH may be discharged from hospital and assessed as outpatients if:
- the blood pressure remains below 140/100 mmHg
- they do not develop proteinuria
- the fetus does not demonstrate asymmetrical IUGR.

The woman's blood pressure should be monitored at least twice a week and fetal growth should be monitored fortnightly by ultrasound with or without other tests of fetal well-being such as regular Doppler ultrasonography of the umbilical artery, cardiotocograph (CTG) monitoring and a biophysical profile. If the condition does not deteriorate, it is difficult to justify induction of labour, although few obstetricians would be prepared to let these women go past 40 weeks' gestation.

Moderate disease

All primigravidae who have a sustained blood pressure of 140/90 mmHg or more should be monitored regularly in a day assessment unit or in hospital because the subsequent course of their disease cannot be predicted. In the absence of rapidly progressive disease, the following management features are relevant.

Maternal

The women should be asked about any symptoms regularly to watch for signs of worsening pre-eclampsia.
- *Measurement of blood pressure*: there is no evidence that treating maternal blood pressure with antihypertensive drugs alters the course of the pre-eclamptic disease process or improves the prognosis of the fetus, but treatment is indicated to protect the maternal circulation. Sustained blood pressures of more than 160/100 mmHg would therefore indicate treatment, unless delivery was imminent. The current choice of therapy is oral methyldopa, nifedipine or labetalol.
- *Assessment of maternal renal function*: all patients should have assessment of:

— urinary protein (daily)
— plasma urea and electrolyte estimation (weekly)
— plasma urate levels (weekly)
— total urinary protein excretion (once)
— liver function tests (twice weekly)
— full blood count and clotting screen.

Once the urinary protein exceeds 300 mg/24 hours the woman has pre-eclampsia. Most units would admit her at this point but increasingly units are waiting until the protein levels reach 500 mg.

The following changes in blood results indicate worsening disease and consideration should be given to delivery. This is always a balancing act of the risks of prematurity for the baby and the risks of pre-eclampsia to the mother:
- A rising urate (>0.35)
- A falling platelet count
- A rising haemoglobin level that indicates haemoconcentration
- A rising creatinine and/or urea is a sign of worsening renal function.

These are signs of fulminating pre-eclampsia and delivery should be considered. Rising liver enzymes (aspartate transaminase [AST], alanine transaminase [ALT]) and a falling haemoglobin (Hb) and/or platelets are signs of the development of HELLP syndrome (**h**aemolysis, **e**levated **l**iver enzymes, **l**ow **p**latelets) and are an indication for immediate delivery because these women are at high risk of developing eclampsia and liver failure.

Fetal well-being
- Real-time ultrasound assessment of fetal size. If this indicates asymmetrical IUGR then carry out:
— daily or twice daily CTGs (minimum 1 hour each time)
— a weekly examination of the umbilical circulation by Doppler ultrasound
— Doppler waveforms from uteroplacental circulation.
- In moderate disease, delivery is indicated for:
— progression to pre-eclampsia
— declining maternal renal function
— fetal distress, which usually means an abnormal CTG or absence of end-diastolic flow in

the Doppler measurement of the umbilical circulation

— placental abruption.

In the absence of the above features, most obstetricians would consider inducing the pregnancy after 38 weeks' gestation, if the cervix is favourable and neonatal facilities are adequate.

Severe or fulminating pre-eclampsia

Symptoms

● *Frontal and often occipital headache* caused by cerebral oedema. The headache is dragging or throbbing in nature and is worse when the woman is supine. It occurs classically first thing in the morning and resolves to some extent during the day if the patient is mobile.
● *Visual disturbances* due to oedema of the optic nerve or the retina, consisting of black holes in the visual field or double vision.
● *Epigastric pain* caused by stretching of the liver capsule.

Signs

● *Hyperreflexia and clonus*: caused by the cerebral oedema; gives the clinical picture of an upper motor neuron lesion.
Hyperreflexia, in obstetric terms, is defined as the ability to obtain the reflex away from the tendon that usually causes it, eg the knee jerk reflex occurs by tapping the anterior surface of the tibia rather than the infrapatellar tendon.
Clonus in obstetric terms is considered serious only if it is sustained for more than four beats.
● *Papilloedema*: checking the fundi is important because papilloedema is a sign of imminent eclampsia or cerebrovascular haemorrhage.
● *A rapid rise in blood pressure.*
● *Rapid increase in proteinuria.*
● *Decreasing urine output.*

Treatment

This disease process starts to reverse as soon as the placenta is delivered and hence the solution to ful-minating pre-eclampsia is to end the pregnancy. Before this happens, the maternal condition must be prevented from worsening:
● Control the maternal blood pressure with intravenous magnesium with additional nifed-ipine orally or hydralazine or labetalol i.v. as required.
● Prevent maternal fits with magnesium sulphate.

Having controlled the blood pressure and reduced the risk of fitting, the baby should be delivered, preferably vaginally, but indications for caesarean section are:
● An unfavourable cervix
● An abnormal fetal position such as a breech presentation
● Fetal distress
● Abruption of the placenta
● A failed induction
● Difficulty in controlling the maternal blood pressure.

Prognosis

Maternal

In the absence of eclampsia, maternal mortality should be low, but it must be remembered that pre-eclampsia is one of the leading factors of maternal death, even in developed countries ($7.5/10^6$ UK maternities, 2003–05). The woman should continue the magnesium sulphate for up to 24 hours after delivery. The urine output should be monitored closely because these women commonly become severely oliguric or even anuric. Despite this they should be fluid restricted because they have a lot of fluid in their extravascular space, which will return to the circulation over the first 48 hours. Giving fluid challenges to improve the urine output can precipitate pulmonary oedema. Recovery is often indicated by a diuresis. Their blood profile should be repeated regularly because they can develop HELLP syndrome and acute fatty liver within the first 24–48 hours after delivery, which may necessitate support in a high dependency unit. If the woman is properly cared for over the first 48 hours after delivery, the disease rapidly gets better. Usually no permanent long-term renal or vascular damage follows pre-eclampsia.

Many women require antihypertensive therapy for the first days and sometimes weeks after delivery. Eclamptic fits can occur in the hours and up to 1 week after the birth, not solely antenatally.

Fetal

The perinatal mortality rate (PNMR) increases with the severity of the disease, but may be summarized as follows:
- Mild: no change in PNMR
- Moderate: slightly increased depending upon gestation at birth
- Severe: double PNMR
- Severe pre-eclampsia superimposed on PIH: treble PNMR.

The morbidity to the baby is difficult to quantify because it depends upon the gestation at delivery and the fetal size (see Chapter 23).

Eclampsia

Eclampsia is characterized by epileptiform fits associated with hypertension of a moderate-to-severe degree. In the UK it is rare with a prevalence of about 1:3000 deliveries. Worldwide it is usually preceded by pre-eclampsia, but the quality of antenatal care in the UK now is such that three-quarters of cases of eclampsia occur without pre-existing recorded evidence of hypertension.

Prevalence

In the UK the disease is rare for the following reasons:
- Better antenatal care which has led to earlier recognition of pre-eclampsia.
- More aggressive treatment of pre-eclampsia which has lessened the incidence of subsequent eclampsia:
  — the rate of eclampsia may be taken as a guide to antenatal care—to its availability, usage and quality
  — less than 1% of women in the UK with moderate or severe PIH will go on to develop eclampsia.

Aetiology

- Cerebral oedema
- Cerebral vasoconstriction
- Cerebral hypoxia.

These lead to cerebral ischaemia and thence to fits.

Clinical course

At present in the UK about 25% of women with eclampsia will have a fit before labour; most of the rest are likely to have a fit in the postpartum period. The character of the fit is very similar to an epileptic fit with a typical fit consisting of the following:
- Twitching: 30 seconds
- Tonic phase: 30 seconds
- Clonic phase: 2 minutes
- Coma: 10–30 minutes.
  Such fits may repeat frequently.

Treatment

Aims
- Keep the woman alive during the fit.
- Prevent more fits.
- Deliver the baby.

Prevention
Magnesium sulphate reduces the incidence and severity of fits.

During the fit
- Turn the woman on her side.
- Maintain the airway.
- Stop the fit by giving intravenous magnesium sulphate and diazepam.

After the fit
- Prevent further fits; this is usually done by giving a continuous infusion of magnesium sulphate.
- If the woman is not in hospital, arrange an emergency transfer, giving adequate anticonvulsants to cover the journey.
- Lower the blood pressure by use of intravenous hydralazine, labetalol or magnesium sulphate.

• Deliver the baby. As with fulminating PIH, such women are best if the baby is delivered vaginally, because this speeds the recovery process. The indications for caesarean section are those listed in the section on pre-eclampsia.

Prognosis

Maternal mortality

In the UK death from eclampsia is rare with the woman more likely to die from the hypertensive effects on the cerebral circulation from a cerebrovascular accident.

Fetal mortality

During an eclamptic fit: 300/1000. Overall: 150/1000 intrauterine deaths from hypoxia or neonatal death from prematurity.

Rhesus (Rh) incompatibility (Box 10.1)

Rh genes

The Rh genes are carried on a pair of chromosomes. There are six Rh antigens (C, D, E, c, d, e) of which D and d are the most important, because upon these depend whether a person is designated Rh positive or Rh negative.

The individual making these gametes may be heterozygous if some of the gametes contain c, d, e and others C, D, E, or the person may be homozygous if all gametes carry c, d, e.

There is no problem if the woman is Rh positive, even if her partner is a Rh-negative man; if homozygous, all her children will be Rh positive; if heterozygous, she may have a Rh-negative child but that is no problem.

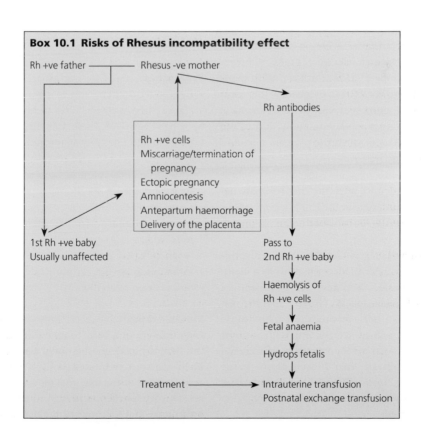

Box 10.1 Risks of Rhesus incompatibility effect

Should she be Rh negative and her partner homozygous Rh positive (35% of the male population), she will always have a Rh-positive child and there may be problems.

The partner may be heterozygous Rh positive (65% of the male population) producing equal numbers of Rh-positive and Rh-negative gametes, with equal chances of giving his Rh-negative partner a Rh-positive or Rh-negative child.

Immunization

A Rh-positive mother cannot be immunized against the Rh factor and so there are no problems for her and her baby.

The Rh-negative woman can be affected if she is inoculated with Rh-positive blood. The Rh gp antigens evoke an antibody response against the Rh gp (most marked against the *D* antigen—anti-D).

In Rh-negative women the inoculation of Rh-positive cells can occur from:
- the passage of red cells from a Rh-positive baby
- an incomplete cross-matched transfusion.

The former is more likely in a major feto-maternal bleed which may occur in the following situations—antepartum haemorrhage (APH), spontaneous miscarriage, ectopic pregnancy, therapeutic abortion, amniocentesis, external cephalic version (ECV)—but most commonly during the third stage of labour when the placenta separates from the uterine wall.

In most Rh-incompatible pregnancies no antibody is formed until after the first fetomaternal bleed, most commonly in the third stage of labour and, consequently, the baby of the first pregnancy is unaffected.

In subsequent pregnancies, if the fetus is Rh positive, small fetomaternal bleeds may evoke a major secondary antibody response. Large amounts of antibody (immunoglobulin G, IgG) cross the placenta and can cause increasingly severe Rh disease in successive pregnancies if the fetus is Rh positive. The antibody weakens the envelopes of the fetal red cells, which are then broken down in the spleen. Depending on the speed and degree of cell breakdown, this can produce the following:
- Fetal anaemia.

- Hyperbilirubinaemia: *in utero* the excess bilirubin is removed across the placenta to the maternal circulation but after delivery the bilirubin accumulates and so the infant becomes jaundiced.
- Oedema.

Clinical picture

This can vary:
- The fetus may die *in utero* if the anaemia is severe enough.
- The infant may be born grossly anaemic and oedematous with hepatosplenomegaly—*hydrops fetalis*. There is a rapid rise in bilirubin after birth. Jaundice develops rapidly within the first 24 hours of life.
- The infant can be anaemic and continues to break down red blood cells after delivery because the maternal Rh antibodies are still circulating in his blood, and so can become more anaemic and jaundiced during the postnatal period.

Management

Prevention
- Either give 1500 IU anti-D immunoglobulin to all Rh-negative women at 26 and 34 weeks
- Or be selective and give 1500 IU anti-D immunoglobulin after delivery at any gestation, or if she has:
  — a therapeutic abortion
  — a spontaneous abortion/ectopic pregnancy
  — an amniocentesis
  — any bleeding in pregnancy/threatened miscarriage
  — an ECV.

The first is now the recommended programme for prevention of Rh disease.

Variable doses

After delivery of a baby to a Rh-negative mother, the baby's blood group should be checked and Kleihauer's test performed on the maternal blood. Acid is added to the maternal blood; fetal cells are resistant to destruction in acid so the amount of fetal blood that has entered the maternal circulation can be calculated. If the baby's blood group is positive the dose of anti-D is adjusted to ensure that all the Rh-positive fetal cells are destroyed without sensitizing the mother. This prevents the development of Rh disease in the next baby.

Detect at-risk fetus

• Maternal Rh screening, anti-D antibody titres.

• Ultrasound scan to detect hydrops fetalis: oedema of the skin, pleural effusion, ascites, hepatosplenomegaly, cardiac enlargement.

• Amniocentesis or cordocentesis is performed under ultrasound guidance; 10 ml amniotic fluid (AF) or 5 ml fetal blood is removed. The content of bilirubin is measured by spectrometry or directly in the serum and the haemoglobin can be measured in the blood. If the bilirubin is raised in the amniotic fluid the need for a transfusion is calculated from Lilley's at-risk graph.

History

• Check history of:
— previous transfusion
— jaundiced babies
— exchange transfusions
— hydrops fetalis
— stillbirth or neonatal death.

• Check all Rh-negative pregnant women for anti-D and, if above 20 IU/l, perform an indirect Coombs' test. Check:
— on booking
— if negative at booking, at 26 and 34 weeks
— if positive at booking, at 20, 24, 28, 32 and 36 weeks or more frequently if rapidly rising.
— If antibody titre rises above 1 : 8 by 20 weeks, do an amniocentesis.
To reduce risks carry out amnio-/cordocentesis under ultrasound guidance. Remove 10 ml AF or 5 ml fetal blood. Check for haemoglobin and bilirubin.

• Check cord blood immediately after birth for:
— ABO group and Rh group
— haemoglobin
— direct Coombs' test
— bilirubin.

Treatment

• Intrauterine transfusion
• Elect time of delivery
• Exchange transfusion after delivery
• Phototherapy after delivery
• Top-up transfusion.

Intrauterine transfusion

In very severe Rh disease the fetus can die *in utero* from anaemia and hydrops before it can be delivered. An intrauterine transfusion can prolong the life *in utero* of an infant to a gestation where the risks of prematurity are estimated as being less than those of the Rh disease. This can be done by the following:

• An intraperitoneal transfusion guided by ultrasound

• An umbilical vein transfusion guided by ultrasound.

Rh-negative blood is transfused into either the fetal peritoneal cavity under ultrasound control, or an umbilical vein. Repeat as necessary, according to amniotic optical density or fetal haematocrit. The intravenous route is increasingly becoming the preferred method.

Choose time of induction and best method of delivery

Balance the risks of prematurity (too soon) with that of worsening Rh disease (too late). Consider the risks of vaginal delivery and be prepared for a lower segment caesarean section (LSCS). The paediatric team should be in close liaison and a senior paediatrician present at the delivery with fresh Rh-negative blood available.

Resuscitation and exchange transfusion

Good resuscitation is essential. In an anaemic and preterm infant, lung disease is common, caused by:

• Surfactant deficiency at very early delivery
• Pulmonary oedema from anaemia and hypoproteinaemia
• Hypoplastic lungs secondary to pleural effusions.

In severe Rh haemolytic disease of the newborn, an umbilical artery catheter should be inserted as soon as possible to assess and control Pa_{O_2} and pH. Central venous pressure should be measured and pleural effusions and ascites drained at resuscitation.

Indications for exchange transfusion
- *Early:* decision mainly based on cord haemoglobin (in addition consider history of previously affected babies):
  — cord haemoglobin <12 g/dl
  — strongly positive Coombs' test
  — cord bilirubin >85 μmol/l.
- *Late:* usually done for hyperbilirubinaemia. The aims of exchange transfusion are to:
  — treat anaemia
  — wash out IgG antibodies
  — decrease degree of haemolysis
  — remove bilirubin
  — prevent kernicterus.

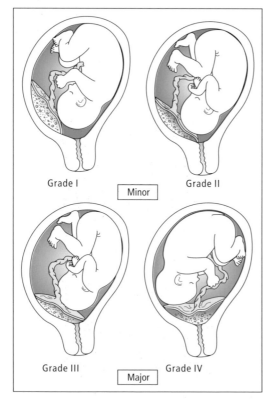

Figure 10.1 Grades of severity of a placenta praevia (see Box 10.2).

Continuous phototherapy
For jaundice from birth, until bilirubin falling.

Top-up transfusion
A late anaemia can develop. If haemoglobin falls <7 g/dl, give top-up transfusion. Prophylactic oral folate will be required.

Genital tract bleeding in late pregnancy

Antepartum haemorrhage is defined as bleeding from the genital tract after week 24 of pregnancy and before the onset of labour. (Before 24 weeks it is defined as a threatened miscarriage.)

Incidence

Five per cent of all pregnancies.

Causes

Maternal
- Placenta praevia: 30%
- Abruptio placentae: 35%
- Local cause in the vagina and cervix: 5%
- Blood dyscrasias: <1%
- Cause never found: 30%.

Fetal
Vasa praevia: <1%.

Placenta praevia

A placenta that encroaches on the lower segment of the uterus. The lower segment can be defined as that part of the uterine wall that:
- does not contract in labour but is stretched in response to contractions
- used to be the isthmus before pregnancy
- underlies the loose fold of peritoneum reflecting from the bladder
- is covered by a full bladder anteriorly
- is within 8 cm of the internal cervical os at term.

Classification

Box 10.2 shows the classic, contemporary and ultrasound classifications. Figure 10.1 shows the grades of severity of a placenta praevia.

Aetiology

Placenta praevia follows the low implantation of the embryo. The following are associated factors:
- Multiparity
- Multiple pregnancy
- Embryos are more likely to implant on a lower segment scar from previous caesarean section. This increases the risk of placenta accreta/increta/percreta (see p. 102).

Presentation

- Nowadays most cases of low-lying placentas or placenta praevia are diagnosed by ultrasound.
- Recurrent, painless, bright-red vaginal bleeding.
- A persistent malpresentation or high head in late pregnancy.

An ultrasound scan will show the position of the placenta clearly within the uterus (Fig. 10.2). If the placenta lies in the anterior part of the uterus and reaches into the area covered by the bladder, it is known as a low-lying placenta (before 24 weeks) and placenta praevia after 24 weeks.

Management

Asymptomatic low-lying placenta

- About 5% of pregnant women will have a low-lying placenta when scanned at 16–20 weeks' gestation.
- The incidence of placenta praevia at delivery is about 0.5%, so in 9 of 10 women the placenta will rise away from the cervix as the uterus grows.
- All women with a low-lying placenta diagnosed in early pregnancy should be rescanned at 34 weeks' gestation.
- There is no need to restrict work activities or sexual intercourse in women with a low-lying placenta on ultrasound unless they bleed.
- If the placenta praevia is still present at 34 weeks' gestation and is grade I or II, the woman should be rescanned on a fortnightly basis but need not be admitted to hospital unless bleeding occurs. If the placenta is covering the os, many clinicians will admit asymptomatic women from 37 weeks to minimize the risk of a major bleed at home, which is most likely to occur when the woman goes into labour.
- Clinically, a high presenting part or abnormal lie at 37 weeks implies that the placenta is covering

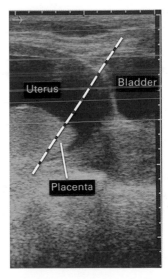

Figure 10.2 Ultrasound scan showing posterior placenta praevia (grade I) at 32 weeks' gestation. Dotted line is the junction of the upper and lower segments of the uterus.

Box 10.2 The classification grades of placenta praevia

I The placenta reaches the lower segment but not the internal os
II The placenta reaches the internal os but does not cover it
III The placenta covers the internal os before dilatation but not when dilated
IV The placenta completely covers the internal os of the cervix even when dilated

Classic	*Ultrasound*
Grade I	} Minor
Grade II	}
Grade III	} Major
Grade IV	}

the cervix and a caesarean section should be performed electively.

Placenta praevia with bleeding

- Admit to hospital.
- Insert a broad-bore intravenous cannula and start an infusion of 0.9% or physiological saline; if the woman is shocked start with a colloid infusion, eg Gelofusin.
- Take blood for cross-matching and haemoglobin estimation. Cross-match at least 2 units depending on how much she has bled/continues to bleed.
- If the woman is anaemic, she is no longer bleeding and the baby is <37 weeks she should be transfused, aiming for a haemoglobin >10.5 g/dl. This can be repeated as necessary until the baby reaches maturity when delivery should be by caesarean section.
- *Avoid all digital vaginal examinations.* A gentle bivalve speculum examination should be performed to determine if blood is coming through the cervical os, especially if a placenta praevia has been suspected but not diagnosed definitely.
- Perform ultrasound as soon as possible because this is more precise.
- Two units of cross-matched blood should be kept permanently available. The transfusion laboratory should be aware that more blood may be needed at short notice if the woman starts to bleed.
- Placental position and fetal growth should be monitored by fortnightly ultrasound scans.
- At 36–37 weeks' presentation, a final ultrasound should be performed and acted upon:
    — grades III and IV placenta praevia (major) should have a caesarean section between 37 and 38 weeks' gestation by an experienced obstetrician particularly if the placenta is on the anterior wall of the uterus
    — if the presenting part is below the lower edge of the placenta in grade I, it is safe to wait until labour and these women can be expected to deliver vaginally.

Prognosis

Maternal

Death from placenta praevia is now extremely rare in developed countries. If women are in hospital caesarean section should be undertaken to prevent death from excessive bleeding. The major cause of death in women with placenta praevia now is postpartum haemorrhage (PPH). PPH is common because the lower segment does not contract and retract as in the upper segment, so maternal vessels of the placental bed may continue to bleed after delivery. This may lead to an emergency hysterectomy if the bleeding cannot be stopped. In women who have previously had a caesarean section the placenta is more likely to be low. If this is anterior, it may implant incorrectly and erode through the scar to varying degrees (placenta accrete/percreta).

Fetal

Bleeding from placenta praevia is maternal in origin. The risk to the fetus therefore mostly depends on the gestation at which it becomes necessary to deliver the baby.

Placental abruption

This is antenatal bleeding from the placental bed of a normally sited placenta. It may occur as an antepartum or intrapartum event.

Classification

Major

This is clinically obvious and may result in the death of the fetus. It is also life threatening to the mother and usually involves separation of more than a third of the placenta.

Minor

Premature separation of small areas of the placenta may result in placental infarcts. Several small abruptions may precede a large abruption. Much of the bleeding that occurs from an abruption is not discharged through the vagina and is known as a concealed haemorrhage. Bleeding that is clinically obvious is revealed haemorrhage. Most times it is obviously mixed.

Aetiology

The causes of abruption are not known but the following factors are associated:

- Proteinuric hypertension
- Multiparity: fourth pregnancies carry a four times risk over first pregnancies
- Trauma: ECV and seat belt injuries (rarely)
- Overstretched uterus (polyhydramnios, multiple pregnancy) at the time that the membranes rupture
- Previous placental abruption: this increases the risk by two to three times
- Raised maternal serum α-fetoprotein in the absence of fetal malformation (6% risk).

Presentation

Major

Women present with abdominal pain and varying degrees of shock. The blood loss that is visible (revealed haemorrhage) is often less than the degree of shock. On examination:

- The uterus is woody hard, due to a tonic contraction.
- The fetal parts cannot be felt.
- The fetus may be dead.

Minor

Minor abruptions are often not diagnosed until after delivery. They may present with:

- mild abdominal pain associated with threatened preterm labour
- unexplained APH
- Tenderness over one area of the uterus only.

Complications

Severe abruption may result in:

- shock from blood loss due to a large retroplacental clot, often concealed
- a disseminated intravascular coagulopathy (DIC)
- oliguria or anuria due to hypovolaemia.

Minor degrees of placental abruption may result in impaired fetal growth and/or hypoxic ischaemic encephalopathy (HIE)—cerebral palsy.

Management

Major placental abruption is a life-threatening condition for both the mother and the baby. If the fetus is still alive the following should be carried out:

- Insert two large-bore intravenous cannulas and infusion of 0.9% saline/colloid.
- Send 20 ml blood for cross-match of 4 units, haemoglobin and coagulation studies. These women are at high risk of developing a DIC.
- Perform an immediate caesarean section if necessary to save the baby's life (high risk of PPH).
- Ensure adequate fluid replacement after the caesarean section.
- Leave an indwelling urinary catheter in to monitor urinary output.
- Consider insertion of a central line to monitor maternal intravascular volume more closely.

If the fetus is dead, the woman should be allowed to deliver vaginally. This usually happens rapidly (within 4–6 hours) as the abruption stimulates labour. If not in labour, rupture of membranes usually leads to a swift delivery. The following are the relevant points of the management of labour:

- Epidural analgesia is contraindicated because of the risk of coagulopathy, but a patient-controlled opiate infusion can be used.
- If a coagulopathy has developed (prolonged APTT [activated partial thromboplastin time], PTT [partial thromboplastin time], increased fibrin degradation products, low platelets) or the woman starts to bleed, she should be managed in the following manner together with a consultant haematologist:

  — Give 4 units of fresh frozen plasma. The haematologist will advise on other clotting factors such as cryoprecipitate, platelets or fibrinogen.

  — Cross-match further whole blood because she is likely to continue bleeding until enough clotting factors have been replaced.

The consumptive coagulopathy begins to improve immediately after the uterus has been evacuated of its contents. Marked abnormalities of the coagulation tests usually resolve within 4–6 hours of delivery of the placenta.

Local causes of bleeding in late pregnancy

Urinary or anal bleeding may be reported as vaginal bleeding in error. They need exclusion and their own treatments.

Cervicitis and vaginitis

- Occasional excessive infection (especially with *Candida*)
- Treat cause.

Cervical polyp

- Scanty bleeding; can be seen with speculum.
- Leave alone in pregnancy and treat later if necessary (often disappears/is delivered with the baby unnoticed.

Cervical ectropion

- Spotting of blood only; can be seen with speculum.
- Leave alone in pregnancy and treat later if necessary.

Varicosities of vagina

- Moderate bleeding in mid-trimester.
- Treat with pressure if close to vulva.
- Only ligate surgically in pregnancy if absolutely necessary; it is difficult.

Cancer of cervix

- Rare but important.
- Irregular bleeding and discharge; confirm diagnosis by biopsy.
- If before 24 weeks, hysterotomy and immediate Wertheim's hysterectomy followed by radiation.
- If after 24 weeks, may await 32 weeks then caesarean section and Wertheim's hysterectomy followed by radiation.

Blood dyscrasias

These are extremely rare. Bleeding may be seen in the following conditions:
- Idiopathic thrombocytopenia
- Von Willebrand's disease
- Leukaemia
- Hodgkin's disease
- Antiphospholipid syndrome.

Management

These conditions are usually known about before pregnancy and are best managed together with a relevant specialist.

Fetal bleeding

This occurs from rupture of vasa praevia when there is a velamentous insertion of cord vessels, which cross the cervical os.

Diagnosis

This condition usually presents with scanty bleeding at the time of membrane rupture. It may be associated with alterations in the fetal heart rate, producing a sinusoidal pattern (see p. 191, Figure 13.8).

Confirmation

If there is time, the blood lost can be checked for fetal haem by its resistance to alkalinization (Kleihauer's test). Alternatively the condition may be suspected when an ultrasound examination reveals the presence of a succenturate lobe on the opposite side of the internal os to the placenta.

Treatment

Deliver the fetus as soon as possible and prepare to transfuse.

Polyhydramnios

Definition: an excess of amniotic fluid detected clinically. The range of normal volumes of fluid present is wide and varies with the duration of pregnancy. *Average* values for amniotic fluid are:

12 weeks: 50 ml
24 weeks: 500 ml
36 weeks: 1000 ml

The normal range at term in a singleton pregnancy is large—500–1500 ml.

Diagnosis

This is either clinical or by simple ultrasound. Other methods of measuring amniotic fluid *in situ* are too complex for routine use and often unreliable.

History

- Tenseness of abdomen
- Unable to lie comfortably in any position
- Dyspnoea, indigestion, piles and varicose veins
- Decreased sensation of fetal movements.

Examination

- Increased symphysiofundal height
- Very tense, cystic uterus bigger than maturity (like a balloon filled with water)
- Difficult to feel any fetal parts.

Investigations

Ultrasound: the deepest column >8 cm or amniotic fluid index greater than the 95th centile.

Differential diagnosis

- Twins: laxer feel to uterus and too many fetal parts felt
- Ovarian cyst: uterus displaced to one side in later pregnancy
- Full bladder.

All are resolved by ultrasound examination.

Associations

Maternal
- Diabetes.

Fetal
- Congenital abnormality; anencephaly; meningomyelocoele; upper alimentary atresia, eg tracheo-oesophageal fistula
- Twins (particularly monozygotic).

Clinical course

Acute
- Painful with tense uterus and oedematous abdominal wall

- Primiparous
- Pre-eclampsia
- Often early (22–32 weeks' gestation).

Chronic
- Slower onset
- Uncomfortable rather than painful
- Last weeks of pregnancy.

Management

Acute
- Bed rest
- Ultrasound to rule out twins or abnormality
- Release fluid from uterus:
  — If *fetus normal*: through abdominal wall with narrow-bore needle. Drain fluid off slowly until the woman is comfortable (500–1000 ml over 4–8 hours)
  — If *fetus abnormal* and viable, consider induction. If not viable, paracentesis.

Chronic
- Bed rest
- Ultrasound to rule out twins and fetal abnormality
- Glucose tolerance test
- Sedation if very painful
- Treat underlying maternal condition
- If fetus normal, induce labour when indicated by fetal state *not* because of the polyhydramnios
- Watch for uterine dysfunction and PPH after labour.

Oligohydramnios

A lack of amniotic fluid; a much rarer condition.

Diagnosis

- Uterus is small for dates (early)
- Uterus feels full of fetus (later)
- Ultrasound shows reduced amniotic fluid index (<2 cm columns).

Fetal associations

- Adhesions from fetal skin to amnion
- Renal agenesis

- Asymmetrical small for gestational age (IUGR).

Clinical course

- Labour often preterm
- High fetal death rate
- High rate of fetal abnormalities (eg dislocated hips and talipes).

Obstetric cholestasis

Obstetric cholestasis occurs only in pregnancy and usually presents in the third trimester. It is more common in multiple pregnancies.

Presentation

- Itching, often generalized but commonly worst on palms and soles of feet
- Absence of rash
- Insomnia
- Right upper quadrant pain
- Malaise
- Intolerance of fatty foods.

Investigation

Liver function tests (LFTs):
- Raised transaminase concentrations (ALT and AST)
- Raised bile salts.

Risks

Maternal
- Increased risk of PPH.

Fetal
- Increased risk of fetal distress
- Increased risk of stillbirth over 38 weeks (18/1000 births)
- Double the incidence of premature labour
- Increased risk of intracerebral haemorrhage.

Treatment

- Prophylactic vitamin K until delivery because of reduced absorption leading to increased risk of PPH
- Antihistamines, calamine, aqueous cream (for itching)
- Ursodeoxycholic acid: effective in reducing itching and usually returns LFTs to normal or near normal. However, it does not alter the outcome of pregnancy, although the symptoms become tolerable allowing the baby to mature to term in most cases (37 weeks).

Monitoring

Maternal
- Weekly LFTs and clotting screen.

Fetal
- Alternate-day CTG
- Weekly liquor volume and umbilical artery Doppler ultrasonography
- Fortnightly growth ultrasound scan.

Delivery

All women should be delivered at 37–38 weeks to try to prevent intrauterine death. Vaginal delivery is indicated in most cases and it is rare for induction to fail even in primigravidae. As there is a theoretical increased risk of fetal distress the fetal heart rate should be monitored continuously electronically (CTG). Syntometrine/Syntocinon must be given with the birth of the anterior shoulder to reduce the risk of PPH.

Recurrence

There is a high likelihood (>60%) of recurrence in subsequent pregnancies.

Chapter 11

Diseases in pregnancy

Most women who become pregnant are healthy and remain so throughout their pregnancy. A few present with pre-existing medical disorders that may affect the pregnancy. Some disorders may arise during the pregnancy. Doctors should be aware of the effect that pregnancy may have on these disorders and their treatment.

Urinary tract infection in pregnancy

During pregnancy the ureters are dilated and kinked because of:
• increased progesterone levels which relax the smooth muscle
• mild obstruction of the lower ureters in late pregnancy.
  This encourages:
• stasis of urine
• reflux of infected urine to the kidney, evoking pyelonephritis.

Asymptomatic bacteriuria

The presence of more than 10^5 bacteria/ml of urine in the absence of symptoms.

Incidence

About 3% of pregnant women—increases with parity and age.

Significance

Asymptomatic bacteriuria is associated with a risk of:
• acute pyelonephritis in pregnancy (30%)
• structural abnormalities in the urinary tract (3–5%).

Screening

In early pregnancy, all women should have urine tested for the presence of:
• either leukocytes and nitrites on a dipstick test in clinic
• or >200 white cells per field and >200 bacteria per field on microscopy.
Then this should be cultured for bacteria.

Treatment

The most common organisms grown are:
• *Escherichia coli*
• *Proteus mirabilis*.
  These are usually sensitive to amoxicillin, cephalosporins, trimethoprim or nitrofurantoin. A 5-day course of an antibiotic to which the organism is

Lecture Notes: Obstetrics and Gynaecology, 3rd edition. By Diana Hamilton-Fairley. Published 2009 by Blackwell Publishing. ISBN: 978-1-4051-7801-3.

sensitive should be prescribed. This will result in a cure in more than 85% of women, but the urine should be recultured a week after treatment.

A renal ultrasound should be performed if this occurs on two or more occasions in pregnancy. An intravenous urogram (IVU) should be performed in pregnancy if a urinary/renal calculus is suspected or 3 months after delivery to exclude a structural urinary tract abnormality.

Symptomatic infections

Incidence

- 1–2%; more common in primigravidae.

Symptoms

- Dysuria (caused by urethritis)
- Increased frequency (caused by trigonitis)
- Backache, loin pains, night sweats and rigors (caused by pyelonephritis)
- Headache, vomiting and muscle aches (caused by pyrexia).

Examination

- The woman is usually pyrexial if the infection has involved the kidneys. In many cases this may be at levels of up to 40.5°C.
- If the woman has pyelonephritis she will be tender in the renal angles.

Investigation

A midstream specimen of urine (MSU) should be sent for:
- dipstick for nitrites and leukocytes
- microscopy for white cells
- culture to determine the organism responsible
- sensitivity of organisms to antibiotics.

Management

All women who have renal angle tenderness or a pyrexia must be admitted to hospital because of the threat of preterm labour. Management consists of the following:

- Ample fluid intake, at least 3 litres a day; if nauseated, give intravenously.
- Start a broad-spectrum intravenous antibiotic such as amoxicillin or, in areas where penicillin resistance is common, a cephalosporin at double the normal dose; this may need to be changed when an organism's antibiotic sensitivities are known.
- If the woman has pyelonephritis, do a renal ultrasound when she has recovered from the infection.
- Keep her in hospital until the renal angle tenderness has disappeared.
- The antibiotics can be given orally once her temperature is normal. At least a complete 5-day course should be given. In cases of pyelonephritis antibiotics should be continued for 2 weeks. The urine should be recultured 5 days after the last dose of antibiotic has been given.

Chronic renal disease

Renal changes in normal pregnancy

- Renal blood flow increases.
- Glomerular filtration rate (GFR) increases.
- Plasma concentrations of urea and creatinine fall in normal pregnancy secondary to the increased GFR and the relative haemodilution in the expanded plasma volume.
- There is an increase in total body water that exceeds the increase in total body sodium, resulting in a decrease in plasma osmolality.
- There is a 25% fall in serum uric acid concentrations during the first two trimesters but this returns to pre-pregnant levels by the third trimester. Watch if using urate to monitor pre-eclampsia.

Prognosis

The outcome of the pregnancy is worse if:
- the woman was hypertensive before pregnancy
- the woman had proteinuria before pregnancy started
- the woman had a creatinine of >120 µmol/l before pregnancy

- there is active progression of renal disease or it is associated with other medical conditions.

Pregnancy probably has no long-term adverse effects on renal disease.

Fetal prognosis

- Normotensive women with chronic renal disease have two to three times greater risk of developing pre-eclampsia. In the absence of pre-eclamptic toxaemia (PET) perinatal mortality is not increased. If PET develops, the risk of fetal death is directly related to the gestation at delivery.
- Women with more severe renal disease have a high incidence of both PET and impaired fetal growth. Among women with pre-existing hypertension and proteinuria, the perinatal mortality rates approach 30%. Cause of death is from preterm delivery and complications associated with small for gestational age (SGA).

Acute renal failure in pregnancy

This may be:
- tubular necrosis: largely recoverable
- cortical necrosis: usually irrecoverable and these patients go on to need long-term dialysis or transplantation.

Presentation

- Oliguria: <500 ml/day (20 ml/h), the minimum volume to remove catabolites
- Anuria: the absence of urine.

Aetiology in obstetrics

- Hypovolaemia:
  — severe pre-eclampsia
  — placental abruption
  — postpartum haemorrhage (PPH)
  — hyperemesis gravidarum
  — miscarriage.
- Gram-negative shock. This may result from:
  — pyelonephritis
  — chorioamnionitis

  — puerperal infections
  — septic miscarriage.
  The usual organism is *E. coli*, but it may be *Clostridium* spp.
- Nephrotoxins: in modern obstetric practice these are rare. Illegal abortions may result in infection followed by haemolysis and renal failure.
- Acute renal failure associated with acute fatty liver of pregnancy. Rare, usually fatal.
- Vomiting in late pregnancy associated with jaundice. The disease occurs in many systems and renal failure, pancreatitis and colitis may occur.

Management

This consists of three consecutive phases:
1 *Oliguria*: lasts from a few days to a few weeks. Complete anuria is rare in acute tubular necrosis and usually suggests acute cortical necrosis or obstruction.
2 *Polyuria*: markedly increased urine production that may last up to 2 weeks. The urine is dilute and metabolic waste products are poorly eliminated. Plasma urea and creatinine may continue to rise for several days after the increase in urinary output. Profound fluid and electrolyte losses can occur in this phase.
3 *Recovery*: urinary volumes decrease towards normal and renal function improves.

General management
- Determine the cause.
- Insert a urinary catheter and maintain accurate fluid balance charts.
- Insert a central venous pressure line and measure the pressure.
In pregnancy, central venous pressure should range from +4 cmH$_2$O to +10 cmH$_2$O. If this is low it suggests that the cause of the renal failure is hypovolaemia, so the volume should be restored with up to 2 litres 0.9% saline followed by a plasma expander. Response of >30 ml of urine in 1 hour should be seen within 1 hour of the fluid load.
- Send baseline investigations, including urea and electrolytes, liver function tests, serum amylase, plasma proteins and coagulation studies and, if required, perform an arterial blood sample for acid–base balance.

- If the patient is not hypovolaemic or does not respond to the fluid load, then the alternatives are as follows:

  — Conservative management: give intravenously the volume of patient fluid output plus 500 ml/day. Monitor electrolytes and start dialysis if or when the patient is uraemic or hypercatabolic.

  — Intensive management using vasodilators and inotropes (renal dose dopamine). This requires the insertion of a pulmonary artery catheter and the monitoring of cardiac output. Vasodilators and inotropes are given and the patient is fluid loaded.

- Involve intensive care physicians and the renal physician at an early stage.

Anaemia

Anaemia can follow:

- Lack of production of blood: haematopoietic
- Increased breakdown of blood: haemolytic
- Blood loss: haemorrhagic.

In pregnancy, most anaemia is haematopoietic when it may result from lack of one of the following:

- Iron: iron deficiency anaemia
- Folic acid: megaloblastic anaemia
- Protein: iron deficiency anaemia.

Normal levels of haematological indices are shown in Table 11.1.

Iron deficiency anaemia (Table 11.2)

Aetiology

Poor intake

- Diet deficient in iron-containing foods.

Table 11.1 Normal haematological values in pregnancy

Blood	Range
Total blood volume (ml)	4000–6000
Red cell volume (ml)	1500–1800
Red cell count (10^{12}/l)	4–5
White cell count (10^9/l)	8–18
Haemoglobin (g/dl)	10.5–13.5
Mean corpuscular volume (fl)	80–95
Mean corpuscular haemoglobin (mg)	32–36
Serum iron (mmol/l)	11–25
Serum ferritin (mg/l)	10–200
Serum folate (mg/l)	6–9
Total iron-binding capacity (mmol/l)	40–70
Platelets (10^9/l)	150–300

Table 11.2 Indices of iron deficiency and megaloblastic anaemia

	Iron deficiency	Megaloblastic
Blood film		
Red cells		
Size	N or ↓	↑
Hypochromia	↓	N
Anisocytosis	+	+
Poikilocytosis	+	+
White cells	N	Leukopenia Hypersegmented
Haematological values		
Hb	↓	↓
MCV	↓	N or ↑
MCHb	↓	N
MCHbC	↓	↑
Serum iron	↓	N
Serum ferritin	↓	N
Serum folate	N	↓
Marrow	↓ Iron stores	↑ Megaloblasts

MCHb, mean cell haemoglobin; MCV, mean corpuscular volume; MCHbC, mean cell haemoglobin C.

Poor absorption

- Vomiting in pregnancy affecting absorption
- Increased pH of gastric juice
- Ferric ions in gut instead of ferrous
- Lack of vitamin C.

Increased utilization

Demands of pregnancy. Total body iron measures about 3500 mg, and includes:

- fetus and uterus: 500 mg
- increased maternal blood volume: 500 mg.

More if:

- multiple pregnancies
- grand multiparity
- pregnancies close together
- mother is vegetarian (particularly if vegan)
- previous heavy periods.

Diagnosis

- Rarely made clinically unless woman is severely affected with shortness of breath/palpitations.
- May show pallor of conjunctivas.
- May have tiredness and oedema.
- Hb estimates must be done on all pregnant women at booking, and twice later in pregnancy, ideally at 26 and 34 weeks.
- If level <10 g/dl, diagnose anaemia, measure ferritin/vitamin B_{12} and folate particularly in areas where α-thalassaemia trait is prevalent; look for other causes and treat.

Treatment

Preventive

Regular iron-bearing foods in diet (Box 11.1). If needed, iron tablet supplements. Daily requirements are 100 mg elemental iron with 300 μg folic acid.

- See that she gets them—give them to her at the clinics.
- See that she takes them—ask at each visit.
- See that they are effective—check Hb levels.

Curative

Depends on the following:

- Degree of anaemia
- Duration of pregnancy

Box 11.1 The iron-rich foods

Animal
Red meat—iron in haemoglobin and myoglobin
White meat }
Fish } iron in the myoglobin

Plant
Lentils
Dark-green leaf
vegetables } moderate amount of iron only
Beans of all sorts } (rich in folates)

- Cause of iron deficiency:
  — mild anaemia: Hb < 10 g/dl
  — severe anaemia: Hb < 8 g/dl.

Mild

1 Check that the woman is being given, and is taking, oral iron.

2 If so, increase oral iron; add vitamin C to aid absorption or try another preparation.

3 If she cannot swallow tablets, use liquid preparation.

4 If change of oral therapy does not improve, use intramuscular or intravenous preparation. Preferred method is to give total dose intravenously as a transfusion on alternate days after a test dose for anaphylaxis (hydrocortisone and adrenaline [epinephrine] should be immediately available). Alternatively, iron dextran 250 mg is associated with a rise in Hb of about 1 g/dl. Give on alternate days, intramuscularly, for six doses, with small test dose first to check anaphylaxis.

Severe and early

1 Admit to hospital and check that anaemia is solely iron deficient:
  — blood film
  — serum ferritin
  — serum folate
  — sickle/thalassaemia status.

2 Treat with oral, intravenous or intramuscular therapy as required.

3 Check that protein and vitamin intake adequate.

4 Check that improvement is maintained for the rest of pregnancy.

Severe and late
1 If after 36 weeks, too late to rely on haematopoiesis: give alternate-day intravenous muscular transfusion for six doses and oral iron or provide red cells in time to cover labour if woman is a poor attender or does not comply with therapy. Transfuse slowly with packed red cell blood.
2 If Hb < 4 g/dl consider exchange transfusion.
3 Build up iron stores for puerperium with intravenous therapy.

Folic acid deficiency anaemia

Aetiology

Folic acid required for building DNA in all tissues. Hence demands are maximal when fetal tissue being made.
1 Poor intake:
- diet deficient in folates
- vomiting in pregnancy.
2 Increased utilization:
- demands of pregnancy
- rapid growth of fetal, placental and uterine tissues
- worse if:
  — multiple pregnancy
  — grand multiparity
  — fetal haemolysis (in Rh effect)
  — infection.

More common in less developed countries and combined with other forms of malnutrition.

Diagnosis

Sometimes made clinically:
- May be tired, breathless, oedematous.
- May have other signs of malnutrition.

Haematology

See Megaloblastic column, Table 11.2.

Treatment

Preventive
Folic acid supplements in last 20 weeks of pregnancy (300 µg/day).

Theoretical risk of masking pernicious anaemia (PA) and its uncommon accompanying subacute combined degeneration (SCD) of the spinal cord. In practice, PA is very rare in those aged under 35 years and SCD almost unknown in the pregnancy age group.

Curative
- Mild or moderate anaemia: folic acid 5–10 mg/day orally only.
- Severe anaemia: folic acid 5–10 mg/day i.m.:
  — with oral iron as Hb will rise faster
  — blood transfusion given with care.

Haemolytic anaemias

These can all be diagnosed before pregnancy at pre-pregnancy consultation.

Haemoglobinopathies

Sickle cell disease
Aetiology
Abnormal Hb: typical original geography.
- HbS (most common): Middle East, Africa, USA, Caribbean and southern Europe
- HbC: Ghana
- HbE: south-east Asia
- HbD: Punjab.

Diagnosis
- Crises or infarcts:
  — chest pain
  — sudden head or abdominal pain
  — joint pains.
- Bone marrow exhaustion.
A crisis could be triggered by:
- infection
- hypoxia
- dehydration
- trauma
- cold.

Haematology
- Low Hb
- Sickling and target cells on blood film
- Electrophoresis shows abnormal Hb patterns.

Treatment
- Detect early
- Hydrate with intravenous fluids
- Oxygen
- Folic acid prophylactically 5 mg/day in pregnancy
- Transfusion of red blood cells
- Diuretic with slow transfusion
- Antibiotics.

If crisis:
- Hydrate
- Check Hb every 4 hours
- Prophylaxis with low-molecular-weight heparin and thromboembolic stockings
- Antibiotics
- Consider exchange transfusion
- If blood pressure rises rapidly, deliver
- Splenectomy for some.

Thalassaemia

Aetiology

Defective genes alter Hb side chains. May be α or β which can be either:
- Homozygous: thalassaemia major—usually fatal before pregnancy age group.
- Heterozygous: thalassaemia minor—most common thalassaemia. α-Thalassaemia minor is the more serious, especially if combined with any other abnormal Hb such as HbS or HbC.

Diagnosis
- Classically women from the Mediterranean countries but now widespread in the Middle and Far East; the woman usually knows about this and will mention it in the history
- Globin chain synthesis studies
- Occasionally a mild anaemia (MCV↓ MCH↓ MCHC=)
- Splenomegaly
- Jaundice

- Pain from bone infarcts (later in life—ulcers of legs).

Haematology
- Increased red blood cell fragility
- Hb level low
- Serum iron raised.

Treatment

1 No use giving iron alone as risk of overload (iron stores often high—check ferritin) but folate helpful.

2 Cover haemolytic crisis with transfusions carefully.

3 Prevent stress if possible (eg hypoxia).

4 Treat infections early.

5 Beware coexistent:
  - malaria
  - glucose-6-phosphate dehydrogenase deficiency
  - other abnormal Hb.

6 Deliver between crises.

Haemorrhagic anaemia

- Rare in temperate climates: recurrent chronic gastrointestinal bleeding (peptic ulcer, piles).
- Commoner in tropics: recurrent chronic bleeding (eg tapeworms, hookworms).

Treatment

- Treat cause.
- Correct anaemia—as above.

Heart disease

Frequency and severity of acquired heart disease in pregnancy are diminishing in women born in this country because:
- most heart disease in this age group is rheumatic in origin
- rheumatic fever is much rarer in childhood with better housing and nutrition
- rheumatic fever is more effectively treated in childhood by chemotherapy.

Rheumatic heart disease should still be asked for in women living in or migrating from endemic areas. However, women with congenital heart disease are increasingly surviving to adulthood and becoming pregnant.

Aetiology

- Rheumatic 20%: mitral valve affected 85%, aortic valve 10%, both 5%.
- Congenital 75%: septal defects and reversed shunts.
- All the rest 5%: ischaemic, thyrotoxic.

Pathophysiology

Pregnancy is a hyperkinetic state and is an extra load on the heart. If the heart is damaged, the following may be associated with a worsening of the underlying condition:

- Anaemia: blood is inefficient at oxygen transport.
- Pre-eclampsia: harder work if hypertension or oedema present.
- Arrhythmia: fibrillation is inefficient at delivering blood.
- Flare-up of rheumatic fever: not common but watch for and treat.
- Acute bacterial endocarditis risk increased because of irregular endothelium over heart valves; hence cover labour, surgery and dentistry with antibiotics.

Cardiac complications in pregnancy

1 With mitral stenosis:
  - Pulmonary oedema
  - Right-sided congestive failure.

2 With aortic stenosis: left-sided congestive failure—associated with syncope and reducing exercise tolerance.

3 Eisenmenger's syndrome: if right-to-left shunt—pulmonary hypertension and high risk of maternal death.

4 Fallot's tetralogy: if right-to-left shunt, risk of cardiac failure.

5 Coarctation of aorta: risk of rupture in late pregnancy or labour. Often repaired before; if well healed, no increased dangers.

6 Artificial valves: thrombosis.

7 Aortic dissection: Marfan's syndrome and other collagen disorders. Rare but may be acute and fatal.

8 Myocardial infarction: rare in pregnancy. Increased risk in sickle cell disease.

Management

In pregnancy

1 Diagnose early:
  - history
  - examination: particularly in women who have recently arrived in the UK because they may never have been diagnosed.

2 Assess severity early: ideally cardiologist and obstetrician to see woman together at same antenatal clinic. Investigations:
  - electrocardiogram (ECG)
  - chest X-ray
  - echocardiography
  - maybe:
    — catheter studies (pressure and blood gases)
    — 24-hour ECG
    Factors:
    — age
    — severity of lesion
    — functional decompensation.

3 Book for hospital delivery and be prepared for admission to hospital.

4 Extra rest at home.

5 Continue anticoagulation if patient already on it. Consider subcutaneous heparin rather than oral anticoagulants unless mechanical valve prosthesis. For these continue on warfarin.

6 Senior cardiologist, anaesthetist and obstetrician make labour plan and write it on hospital records. See that senior staff of each discipline are available to cover labour.

In labour

1 Reduce extra work—good analgesia; probably epidural unless anticoagulated.

2 Nurse head-up: tilt bed or extra pillows.

3 Antibiotics especially if a congenital heart lesion.

4 Short second stage; maybe forceps or vacuum extraction.

5 Give Syntometrine only if high risk of PPH; otherwise give Syntocinon.

6 Manage pulmonary oedema if it occurs:
- tilt head-up 35°
- O_2
- morphine 15 mg
- digoxin if arrhythmia or tachycardia
- diuretics—furosemide.

In puerperium

1 Rest:
- keep in hospital longer
- check home conditions adequate—few stairs if possible.

2 Physiotherapy to legs and gentle exercises.

3 Breastfeeding allowed unless cardiac condition deteriorated in pregnancy. It can be hard work, because only one person can do it and it means getting up at night.

Prognosis

Maternal

Mortality: increased risk of death—cardiac disease is the most frequent cause of maternal death as a result of a medical condition in the UK (9% of all maternal deaths in UK). There is a 50% risk of death in the presence of pulmonary hypertension.

Morbidity: increased risk of deterioration of heart condition. Used to be inevitable. This is not so if proper care is taken.

Fetal

There is a small increased risk of congenital heart disease (CHD) in babies of mothers who were born with it. They should be offered a specialist fetal cardiology scan. Otherwise there is surprisingly little increased risk to the fetus if the mother is kept healthy. Watch for fetal risks from anticoagulation if relevant.

Respiratory diseases

Asthma

In pregnancy

Often emotional factors are involved so asthma may worsen if pregnancy is resented. Thirty per cent of

people with asthma get worse (highest risk among those with brittle asthma); most stay the same and some improve. Continue all treatments started before pregnancy. With the exception of leukotriene antagonists, all drugs used in the treatment of asthma are safe for the fetus and the risks of an asthma attack to the mother and fetus far outweigh the risks of treatment with the use of well-established drugs:
- Bronchodilators
- Antibiotics
- Steroids—inhaled or systemic.

Women with asthma who smoke should be sent to smoking cessation clinics because smoking in pregnancy can increase the likelihood of asthma becoming worse. It is well established that smoking is harmful to babies, causing growth restriction and premature delivery.

Most women with asthma do not deteriorate in pregnancy but may in the puerperium. No obvious correlation with hormone changes.

In labour

Severe asthma attacks are very rare in labour and so they should be treated as normal and given their usual therapy:
- Treat as normal.
- If on regular systemic steroids (>7.5 mg daily), intravenous hydrocortisone is required to cover labour.
- Baby may be small for dates if asthma control was poor.

Pulmonary tuberculosis (TB)

Incidence

Less than 1 : 1000 in UK; rare in endogenous population, higher in immigrants.

Presentation

- History of disease:
  — persistent cough, weight loss, pyrexia of unknown origin
  — recent known contact.
- Pick up on routine chest X-ray.

Management

1 Notify any new cases to public health physician.
2 Continue any antituberculous drugs already started in combination:
- INAH (isonicotinic hydrazide).
- ethambutol
- rifampicin*
- streptomycin.*
3 Bed rest.
4 Surgery if needed in mid-pregnancy, avoiding first 14 and last 10 weeks.
5 Follow up the family.

Labour

Women with TB should be allowed a normal delivery.

Mother

- Allow breastfeeding if no positive sputum bacteriology within 1 year and no signs of recent activity on chest X-ray.
- Continue all drug treatments.
- Suppress lactation if baby has to be separated.
- Rest in hospital longer.
- Check community back-up services to give least effort to mother and ensure compliance with therapy.
- Arrange for follow-up at chest clinic in case of TB flare-up.

Baby

- If mother has had bacteria in sputum within 1 year, separate baby from mother at birth. The mother must be warned during pregnancy that this will happen. If properly explained, she will realize that it is a wise move.
- Give baby isoniazid-resistant BCG 0.05 mg at 7 days (unless preterm). Await positive Mantoux test before allowing baby back to mother (about 6 weeks).
- All babies living in endemic TB areas should be immunized at birth.

* Usually avoided in pregnancy

Endocrine diseases

Thyroid disease

Pregnancy is a hyperdynamic state. Increased oestrogen levels cause enlargement of thyroid gland and an increased output of thyroid hormone. Since this is mostly in the form of protein-bound thyroxine, such patients are not hyperthyroid, for the active fraction is not increased.

Hyperthyroidism

- Difficult to diagnose for the first time in pregnancy so need a measure of free thyroxine (fT_4) level as well as thyroid-stimulating hormone (TSH) to assist in diagnosis.
- If established beforehand, continue treatment, usually carbimazole, but keep dose as low as possible. Treatment in pregnancy includes anti-thyroid medication such as carbimazole and propylthiouracil with β blockers if the patient has palpitations.
- Consider thyroidectomy if disease is increasingly difficult to control.

Surgery is safe if mother is properly prepared. Avoid radioactive iodine testing because of fetal thyroid pick-up and retention. Maternal thyroid-stimulating IgG passes across placenta and may stimulate fetal thyroid, sometimes enough to cause neonatal thyrotoxicosis. This is unusual but can be predicted by testing maternal blood levels of IgG (thyroid-stimulating immunoglobulin, TSI). Women who are clinically euthyroid after Graves' disease can still have affected infants due to thyroid-stimulating antibodies (TSIs).

Pre-eclampsia and intrauterine growth restriction are associated with poorly controlled hyperthyroidism.

Hypothyroidism

- Rarely get pregnant if not on therapy.
- If treated, continue treatment, and be prepared to increase dosage.
- Check thyroid function using TSH and fT_4 at least once in each trimester.

Pituitary disease

Prolactinoma

- Women on long-term dopamine agonists, eg cabergoline/bromocriptine, become pregnant.
- Oestrogen stimulation of pregnancy may cause enlargement of the tumour.
- Prolactin levels are not a reliable means of monitoring the risk of adenoma enlargement.
- If the tumour enlarges it may put pressure on the optic chiasma and threaten vision, so visual fields should be checked during pregnancy.
- Check adenoma with magnetic resonance imaging (MRI) or computed tomography (CT) of the pituitary.
- A few tumours need treatment if they enlarge:
  — first a dopamine agonist
  — then surgery.
- Breastfeeding is safe for women with a prolactinoma unless treatment is urgent because of the size of the tumour.

Hypopituitarism

- Mostly starts in puerperium after pituitary vein thrombosis following PPH.
- Study each pituitary-controlled function separately and treat those who are deficient.
- If mother treated, baby does well.

Diabetes

Diabetes is a metabolic disease that results from an underproduction of insulin by the pancreas. This results in disturbances of carbohydrate, fat and protein metabolism, and leads to a sustained rise in blood glucose.

During pregnancy, diabetes may be one of the following types:

1 Pre-existing diabetes that is usually insulin dependent (type 1) although pre-existing type 2 diabetes is becoming more prevalent as the population becomes more obese.

2 Gestational diabetes or an impaired glucose tolerance discovered for the first time in pregnancy.

Glucose homoeostasis in pregnancy

- In normal pregnancy, fasting glucose blood levels are maintained at 4–5 mmol/l.
- To maintain the glucose level, however, there is a doubling in the secretion of insulin in the second and third trimesters of pregnancy. Pregnancy represents a relatively insulin-resistant state.
- The insulin resistance results from the placental secretion of oestrogen, progestogen and human placental lactogen (hPL), together with a change in peripheral insulin receptors.
- Glucose crosses the placenta by facilitated diffusion, resulting in a fetal glucose level of approximately 1 mmol/l less than its mother.
- The facilitated diffusion system is saturated at maternal levels of 11–12 mmol/l. Therefore the fetus is probably never subject to levels >11 mmol/l.

Established diabetes mellitus

Occurs in 1–2% of pregnant women.

Effects of pregnancy on diabetes

- Insulin requirements increase during pregnancy and rapidly fall to pre-pregnancy levels after delivery.
- Pregnancy aggravates proliferative diabetic retinopathy. Ideally any retinopathy should be treated before pregnancy.
- Women with diabetic nephropathy are more likely to develop pre-eclampsia and to have poorer renal function during pregnancy, but there are few adverse long-term effects on renal function.
- There is a high incidence of asymmetrical SGA and preterm delivery.
- Diabetic neuropathy and vascular disease are rare in pregnancy.

Effects of poorly controlled diabetes on the pregnancy

- Diabetes is associated with an increased risk of first trimester miscarriages.

• Second trimester miscarriages, as a result of fetal death.

• Congenital abnormalities: threefold increase, 50% neural tube defects, 30% cardiac abnormalities. Women with diabetes tend to have babies with multiple malformations of which caudal regression occurs only in babies of women with diabetes.

• Pregnancy-induced hypertension.

• Preterm delivery.

• Polyhydramnios.

• Macrosomic infants, which may result in difficulties at delivery particularly shoulder dystocia.

• Sudden intrauterine death in the last 4 weeks of pregnancy. This appears to be confined to babies who are macrosomic.

• Perinatal mortality increased two to three times. This can be reduced to background levels with good diabetic control.

• Intrauterine growth restriction can occur in women with longstanding diabetes who have microvascular disease (retinopathy, nephropathy).

Effects of diabetes on the infant

• Macrosomia: birth weight for gestational age exceeds the 90th centile.

• An increased risk of birth trauma, because of shoulder dystocia.

• An increased risk of asphyxia during delivery.

• An increased risk of respiratory distress syndrome (RDS) compared with babies of similar gestation.

• Hypoglycaemia: the fetal pancreas secretes high levels of insulin during pregnancy to cope with the passage of glucose from the mother. After delivery, the glucose source is removed, but the pancreas continues to secrete extra insulin, resulting in hypoglycaemia.

• Hypercalcaemia.

• Hypothermia: infants of mothers with diabetes have large surface areas and so lose heat rapidly. Although they have more fat than the normal baby, this is yellow fat and not the thermogenic brown fat.

• Hyperbilirubinaemia: infants of mothers with diabetes are plethoric due to polycythaemia and

the excess red blood cells break down after delivery, causing jaundice.

Management

There is increasing evidence that good control of diabetes around the time of conception, and the first weeks after, reduces the incidence of congenital abnormalities and of miscarriage. Good control throughout pregnancy reduces many of the complications but has little effect on macrosomia (approximately 30%).

Pre-pregnancy care

• All women with type 1 diabetes of reproductive age should take adequate contraceptive precautions until ready for pregnancy.

• Stress the need for pre-pregnancy counselling and planning:

— If they are on oral hypoglycaemic agent they should be changed to insulin.

— Twice-daily insulin regimens are the minimum acceptable for pregnancy. The best control of diabetes is achieved by giving a long-acting insulin at night and then using a short-acting insulin to cover each meal throughout the day.

• Women should be taught to monitor their own blood sugar by BMStix or Dextrostix. The monitoring should preferably be done using an electronic glucose meter.

• Blood sugar should be monitored first thing in the morning, 1 hour before each meal and 1 hour after the biggest meal of the day.

• The aim is to maintain the blood sugar between 4 and 7.5 mmol/l.

• Glycated Hb (HbA1c) level or fructosamine levels should be checked after 6 weeks on the above regimen and should be <8%.

• High-dose folic acid should be taken while trying to conceive and during the first trimester.

Pregnancy management

This should ideally be in a joint clinic in which women are seen by a doctor specializing in diabetes with an interest in obstetrics and an obstetrician with an interest in diabetes:

- The aim is to maintain normoglycaemia as described above, throughout the pregnancy. This may lead to an increase in the number of hypoglycaemic attacks but these are not harmful to the fetus.
- The fetal death rate with hyperglycaemic coma is as high as 25%.
- The woman should be seen 2-weekly throughout her pregnancy.
- Retinal scans should be performed in each trimester in women with type 1 diabetes.
- Management of pregnant women with diabetes can normally be achieved at home, especially if a specialist diabetic nurse is available to give advice over the telephone or to visit the woman's home.
- At each antenatal visit the following should be checked:
  — the woman's diabetic record of home monitoring should be reviewed
  — the blood pressure
  — symptoms suggestive of infection, particularly in the urinary tract
  — fetal growth by clinical means and by reviewing the ultrasound results.
- The insulin requirements will increase markedly during pregnancy. In the first trimester they are usually static but then increase rapidly until 34 weeks, when they may stabilize. Women should be taught to change their own insulin dosage.

Ultrasound investigations

1 At 12 weeks' gestation to confirm the presence of a fetal heartbeat and the number of fetuses. A nuchal translucency screening for neural tube defects/trisomies should be performed because women with diabetes are not suitable for serum screening.
2 At 16–20 weeks' gestation a detailed scan for structural abnormalities.
3 At 22–24 weeks' gestation to look specifically for cardiac abnormalities.
4 Type 1 diabetes alone is not an indication to perform karyotyping.
5 Monthly fetal growth and amniotic fluid volume should be monitored every 4 weeks from 28 weeks. Figure 11.1 demonstrates the pattern of growth that is observed in babies who are destined to be macrosomic.

Delivery

- Women who have type 1 diabetes or poorly controlled type 2/gestational diabetes mellitus (GDM), and those with well-controlled GDM on insulin

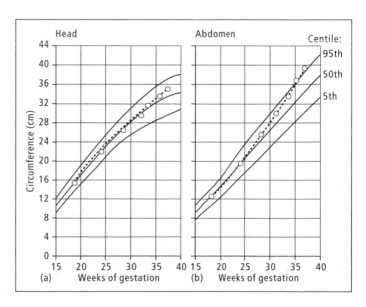

Figure 11.1 Ultrasound growth charts showing a case of fetal macrosomia: (a) head circumference; (b) abdominal circumference.

should be induced at 38 weeks to try to prevent a term stillbirth.

• In women with well-controlled type 2/gestational diabetes aim to allow spontaneous labour but induce within a few days of the expected delivery date (EDD).

• Caesarean section should be carried out only on obstetric grounds.

• Control of diabetes during labour is achieved by intravenous insulin infusion together with intravenous glucose (a sliding scale that alters the insulin dose according to the blood glucose level). The woman's blood glucose is checked every hour by means of BMStix, and should be 4–10 mmol/l.

• The woman should be encouraged to have an epidural because pain and fear release catecholamines, which are gluconeogenic.

• Labour should be accelerated with Syntocinon if readings are more than 2 hours to the right of the partogram (see Chapter 13).

• A senior obstetrician should be present at the delivery because of the risk of shoulder dystocia.

• The incidence of caesarean section in pregnant women with diabetes is 50% (more than double the normal population) regardless of whether the onset of labour is spontaneous or induced but may be due to:

— failed induction
— fetal distress in early labour
— disproportion (macrosomia)
— an abnormal lie.

Immediate care of the baby

A paediatrician should be present at the delivery of all babies of mothers with type 1 diabetes. The following features are important:

• Resuscitate the baby if required.

• Dry the baby and keep it warm.

• Perform a BMStix estimation of glucose from a heelprick at: 30 min, 1 h, 4 h, 8 h, 12 h and 24 h.

• To prevent hypoglycaemia feed the baby early and frequently.

• Treat low values of blood glucose (<1 mmol/l) with an intravenous infusion of glucose. Some babies are resistant and may need to be given intramuscular glucagon.

• Carefully examine the baby for congenital abnormalities.

• Measure the serum bilirubin on the second day because this is when the hyperbilirubinaemia usually starts.

Gestational diabetes

This is defined as the onset of diabetes or the appearance of abnormal glucose tolerance for the first time during pregnancy. A small proportion of these women will remain diabetic after delivery.

Gestational diabetes is not associated with congenital abnormalities. The main effects are:

• development of polyhydramnios
• increase in the incidence of preterm labour
• development of macrosomia.

It can be screened for in the following ways:

1 Oral glucose tolerance test (OGTT) on women at high risk (Box 11.2)

2 Oral glucose load and a single blood sugar estimation 2 hours later

3 Random blood sugar at 28 weeks' gestation 2 hours after the last meal. Women who have high blood sugars are then given an OGTT.

The OGTT

This is a 50-g oral load of glucose in a flavoured drink. Fasting values of >5.8 mmol/l or 2-hour values of >7.8 mmol/l require further testing.

Treatment

There is no consensus view on treatment except that oral hypoglycaemics are currently not used. The following outline is suggested:

> **Box 11.2 High-risk features for abnormal glucose tolerance in pregnancy**
>
> Maternal weight >90th centile (BMI > 30 kg/m^2)
> Previous big baby (>4.5 kg)
> A first-degree relative with diabetes
> Glycosuria:
> • Once at <20 weeks
> • Twice at >20 weeks
> Previous unexplained stillbirth or neonatal death
> Polyhydramnios
> Fetal macrosomia on ultrasound

- Home monitoring by means of an electronic glucose monitor.
- Fasting and 1-hour blood sugar after each meal on at least 2 days a week.
- No treatment required if the fasting blood sugar level is <5.5 mmol/l and the postprandial figures are <9 mmol/l.
- If higher levels are involved, the woman should start a simple carbohydrate-restricted diet. In addition to checking her blood sugars twice a week, also test her urine for ketones.
- If the simple diet does not achieve the required blood sugar levels, start a twice-daily regimen of medium- and short-acting insulin.
- If ketosis occurs the diet should be relaxed and insulin started.
- Ultrasound scan for fetal growth and amniotic fluid volume at least monthly.
- If no evidence of excessive fetal growth and none of the conditions mentioned above exist, spontaneous labour can be awaited up to 42 weeks' gestation. Women with ultrasound signs of macrosomia should be induced at term, although some obstetricians do this earlier at 38–39 weeks' gestation. The outcomes for the baby are the same but the caesarean section rate is higher in the earlier inductions, particularly in primigravid women.
- Control of blood sugar in labour is important. Those on insulin antenatally should have the same intravenous glucose and insulin regimen as people with type 1 diabetes.
- With the delivery of the placenta, the insulin requirements soon disappear.
- There is evidence that women who have gestational diabetes have about a 40% chance of developing diabetes in the next 10–20 years, the risk doubling if the woman is obese. In the latter case, once breastfeeding has ceased, the woman is given strict dietary advice and advised to lose weight.
- Gestational diabetes usually recurs in future pregnancies but this is not inevitable.

Epilepsy

All anticonvulsant medications carry a small risk of teratogenicity. However, the risk of epileptic seizures to the pregnancy outweighs the risk of teratogenicity, although some women may need to change their medication in the first trimester from sodium valproate to carbamazepine in the first instance. A single antiepileptic drug (AED) should be used where possible and the newer drugs, eg gabapentin, lamotrigine and levetiracetam, used with caution because little is known of their teratogenicity/effects in pregnancy.

Management

- To reduce the teratogenic risk, women should be advised to take the higher dose of folic acid (5 mg) preconceptually and throughout pregnancy.
- All women should be offered a fetal cardiology scan to detect congenital heart disease which, together with neural tube defects, is the most common congenital abnormality associated with antiepileptic drugs.
- Vitamin K from 36 weeks to reduce the risk of PPH and haemorrhagic disease of the newborn in women who are taking enzyme inducing drugs (phenytoin, carbamazepine and phenobarbital).
- Consider measuring AED in each trimester to determine whether drug doses need increasing. The physiological increase in plasma volume commonly reduces the circulating drug concentration to below the therapeutic range. This increases the risk of epileptic fits, which can be harmful to the mother and fatal to the fetus. If the level is below the therapeutic concentration the dose is increased and the levels re-checked 2 weeks later.

Abdominal pain in pregnancy

Diagnosis depends mostly on history and examination with very few investigations helping.

Early pregnancy

Pelvic causes

- Miscarriage:
  — spontaneous: crampy pain with contractions and bleeding
  — induced: pain with sepsis.

- Ectopic pregnancy: pain from: stretch, leak of blood from ostium of tube, or rupture.
- Fibroids: pain from red degeneration—most common in mid-trimester.
- Ovarian cysts: pain from: rupture, twisting or bleeding into cyst.
- Ligament stretch: pain from tension or haematoma.
- Impaction of the uterus.

Extrapelvic causes

- Vomiting in pregnancy: pain from abdominal wall muscle overstretch.
- Urinary infection: pain from bladder irritation and back pressure on kidney.
- Constipation: commonly occurs in pregnancy as a result of progestogenic reduction in smooth muscle motility in the large bowel
- Appendicitis (Box 11.3): pain from: peritoneal irritation, peritonitis or rupture.

Late pregnancy

Pelvic causes

- Labour (intermittent): pain from myometrial contractions.
- Hydramnios (constant): pain from stretch.
- Abruptio placentae (constant): pain from myometrial damage and stretch.
- Ruptured uterus (constant): pain from haemorrhage into peritoneal cavity (more common after previous uterine surgery).

Box 11.3 Reasons why appendicitis is a serious concern in pregnancy

1 Underdiagnosed for it is not considered
2 Undertreated due to fear of abdominal surgery in pregnancy
3 Appendix pushed out of right iliac fossa and becomes a general abdominal organ
4 Omentum does not wall off inflamed organ
5 Cortisol levels high, therefore poor inflammatory response.

- Ovarian cyst accident: rupture, haemorrhage, torsion.

Extrapelvic causes

- Rectus haematoma: pain from tissue stretch and irritation of tissues by blood.
- Fulminating pre-eclampsia (epigastric pain): pain from stretch of peritoneum over swollen liver.
- Cholecystitis: pain from gallbladder distension and inflammation.
- Peptic ulcer: pain from associated gastritis and acid irritation of submucosal tissues.
- Appendicitis: see p. 259.
- Pyelonephritis: pain from inflammation of pelvis or kidney.
- Ureteric stone: pain from renal colic caused by obstruction.
- Pancreatitis.

Management of abdominal pain
- Make diagnosis accurately from history and examination and act quickly.
- Use ultrasound with vaginal probe if considered helpful.
- Be prepared to use a laparoscope in early pregnancy.
- Do not consider laparotomy to be dangerous in pregnancy.
- A pregnancy in a woman with an intra-abdominal inflammatory disease will not be harmed by proper surgical treatment. The fetus is more likely to be damaged if the proper operation is delayed.

Infections in pregnancy

Any infection producing pyrexia may cause miscarriage or preterm labour. Three groups of infections are particularly important in pregnancy:
1 Genital tract infections
2 Infections that cross the placenta
3 Urinary tract infections.

Genital tract infections

Syphilis in pregnancy

Syphilis (see also Chapter 6)

All pregnant women are still screened for syphilis because, although the disease is rare, the incidence is increasing. Appropriate treatment can prevent congenital syphilis.

Congenital syphilis may occur in infants born to those women who are infected and book late for their antenatal care, or in whom infection is acquired after their initial booking blood tests have been performed. In pregnant women with untreated early syphilis, 70–100% of infants will be infected. Vertical transmission has been reported in women with untreated syphilis of many years' duration. All pregnant women with positive treponemal serology should be evaluated for clinical evidence of syphilis and treated as for syphilis, even when non-venereal treponematoses are suspected to be the cause of their underlying seroreactivity. Ideally treatment should be initiated before a confirmatory second serology is available, to prevent neonatal complications if the patient defaults follow-up.

Women who had documented treatment for syphilis in the past do not need re-treatment during current or subsequent pregnancies if there is no clinical evidence of syphilis and the non-specific serology (VDRL [Venereal Diseases Reference Laboratory] or RPR [rapid plasma reagin] titre) is negative or serofast in low titre compared with the patient's previous results. Re-infection still needs to be excluded by checking recent sexual partners, and babies should also be followed up by a paediatrician to exclude congenital syphilis.

Serological tests

These fall into two groups:
1 Non-specific tests.
  - the Wassermann reaction (WR)
  - the VDRL slide test
  - the RPR card test.

False-positive tests may be seen with chronic inflammatory diseases, yaws, narcotic abuse and pregnancy.

2 Specific tests:
  - the *Treponema pallidum* haemagglutination (TPHA) test
  - the fluorescent treponema antibody (FTA) test.

These two tests are specific for *T. pallidum* and become positive some 2 weeks after the initial infection. They remain positive forever once the patient has had the disease and do not produce biologically false-positive tests.

Effects on the fetus

The outcome for the fetus varies depending on the gestational stage at which infection is acquired:
1 Untreated early syphilis may result in neonatal death or stillbirth in 30%.
2 Congenital syphilis results in lasting neurological and skeletal damage.

Management

- *T. pallidum* is extremely sensitive to penicillin. Adequate treatment in early pregnancy protects the fetus. Even if the infection is discovered only in late pregnancy, treatment should still be given.
- Benzathine penicillin 2.4 MU i.m. in two doses (days 1 and 8)
- Pregnant women who are allergic to penicillin should be given erythromycin 500 mg orally every 6 hours for 15 days. As a result of lower efficacy and poor placental transfer of this drug, it is recommended that babies be examined and re-treated at birth with benzylpenicillin and the mother retreated with doxycycline after breastfeeding has ceased.
- The woman should be followed by the genitourinary physicians who should contact her sexual partners.

Herpes genitalis (see also Chapter 6)

Herpes simplex virus (HSV) is a large DNA virus that enters the body through a mucocutaneous surface, and then migrates along nerves.

Symptoms

- The first attack of herpes genitalis is usually acutely painful and may cause acute urinary retention.

• Vesicles break down to form shallow ulcers on the cervix, labia, perineum or perianal areas.
• There is inguinal lymphadenopathy.
• Recurrent attacks are less severe; many give warning symptoms of a tingling sensation.

Diagnosis
• The lesions are usually clinically obvious.
• Ulcers should be scraped and the scrapings sent for viral identification.

Effect on the newborn
• Herpes neonatorum may kill up to 50% of those who develop encephalitis but it is rare. A third of those remaining will have some residual neurological damage.
• The infection is acquired during the process of delivery or by ascending infection if the membranes have been ruptured for more than 4 hours.

Treatment
• Active infection in late pregnancy or early labour: consider caesarean section to avoid herpes neonatorum.
• Aciclovir may be used in pregnancy.
• Aciclovir is used widely for infants with herpes infection.

Vaginal streptococcal infections

Group B (β-haemolytic) streptococcal (GBS) infections may cause:
• Preterm rupture of the membranes and preterm labour
• Severe postpartum sepsis, particularly after caesarean section
• Overwhelming neonatal sepsis that may lead to death:
   — About 20% of women will carry group B streptococci in the vagina. About 2% of these women will give birth to an infected infant and about 30% of these could die from overwhelming sepsis.
   — Screening all pregnant women for the infection is not practical.
   — All women presenting with preterm rupture of the membranes should have a sample of the amniotic fluid sent to identify the organism. If present, the baby should be delivered immediately with penicillin cover.
   — A woman who is known to be a carrier for GBS should be given prophylactic antibiotics, eg intravenous benzylpenicillin or erythromycin during labour.

Group A streptococcal infections (puerperal fever) can be overwhelming and cause maternal death, most commonly during labour or in the early puerperium. The women are commonly relatively asymptomatic initially with a low-grade pyrexia and mild flu-like symptoms; within a few hours they may develop acute toxic shock and multiple organ failure, leading to death within a few hours or days. The diagnosis may only be made *post mortem*.

Listeriosis

Between 1% and 5% of pregnant women will carry *Listeria monocytogenes* in the rectum. The organism may in addition be acquired in pregnancy from eating unpasteurized cheese and cooked meats. It may produce the following symptoms:
• Maternal diarrhoea accompanied by a pyrexia
• Premature labour.

   Listeriosis septicaemia of the preterm infant acquired at birth may be rapidly fatal and may occur in the presence of few symptoms in the mother.

Treatment

Intravenous amoxicillin.

Infections that cross the placenta

The placenta acts as an efficient barrier against some infections in the mother. The following, however, are not uncommonly found in pregnant women and often cause serious consequences to the fetus:
• Syphilis (see pp. 77, 163)
• Rubella
• Cytomegalovirus (CMV)
• Toxoplasmosis
• Human immunodeficiency virus (HIV).
• Parvovirus B19.

Rubella

The widespread policy of immunizing schoolgirls and more recently all children means that German measles (rubella) is becoming rarer. All pregnant women are tested for the levels of rubella antibodies at the antenatal clinic; if they are seronegative, they are offered immunization in the puerperium.

Rubella rapidly crosses the placenta and may cause:

- learning difficulties and microcephaly
- cataract
- congenital heart disease
- deafness
- hepatosplenomegaly with thrombocytopenia if the mother is infected in the second half of the pregnancy.

Women suspected of having acquired rubella in early pregnancy should have a rubella-specific IgM test. If positive, then the following options are available:

- Termination of pregnancy: this applies particularly if the primary infection was less than 10 weeks' gestation because more than half of the babies will be affected.
- A chorionic villous sample: electron microscopy and modern immune methods may be able to determine if the virus has crossed the placenta. This test can be performed at 11–14 weeks' gestation.
- A fetal blood sample at 18–20 weeks' gestation (cordocentesis) to determine if the fetus is IgM positive for rubella. If negative, the patient can be reassured. If positive, it confirms that the fetus has been infected but does not guarantee that it is affected. Most would ask for a termination of pregnancy on these grounds.

Cytomegalovirus

CMV infection is now the most common perinatal infection in both the UK and the USA. The most serious manifestations associated with primary maternal infection include:

- stillbirth
- hepatosplenomegaly and jaundice
- thrombocytopenia
- microcephaly
- chorioretinitis.

CMV may be acquired:

- in childhood from other children's saliva, tears, urine or stool
- as an adult by sexual contact or blood transfusions
- in the perinatal period by direct transmission across the placenta.

By the time pregnancy occurs, about 75% of women will be immune to CMV. Of women who acquire CMV in pregnancy, some 5% have a seriously damaged infant. Unlike rubella, there is no immunization against the disease.

If the disease is suspected, it can be confirmed by looking for the IgM specific to CMV. Transplacental passage is not inevitable and the organism may be sought in the fetus by means of chorionic villous sampling (early) or fetal blood sample (late) (see rubella).

Toxoplasmosis

Toxoplasma gondii comes from parasites in cats' intestines. Human infection occurs as a result of eating poorly cooked meats that contain tissue cysts or that have been exposed to infected cat faeces. Infection readily crosses the placenta. In the mother, it may be asymptomatic, or produce a glandular fever-like illness. Transplacental infection may cause:

- microcephaly or hydrocephaly
- cerebral calcification leading to epilepsy and cerebral damage
- chorioretinitis.

The disease is diagnosed in the mother by finding an IgM specifically against toxoplasmosis. The mother can be treated by spiromycin to prevent further transplacental passage of the organism. Fetal infection may be diagnosed by fetal blood sampling and the search for specific IgM.

There is treatment available for the fetus through the mother but many women are offered a termination if their fetuses are infected.

HIV in pregnancy

- The fetus can be infected with HIV from the mother *in utero*, although it is thought that most transmissions occur at birth and through breast-feeding. Without intervention, the rate of mother-to-child transmission is 15–30%, rising to even higher rates with increasing duration of breastfeeding.

• The current policy in the UK has dramatically reduced the risk of mother-to-child HIV transmission to <1% (see Fig. 6.5) by:

— a routine offer and recommendation of antenatal testing of all pregnant women for HIV (women have to opt out of the test rather than opt in)

— prescribing antiretrovirals in the second and third trimesters to the pregnant woman and for 4 weeks to the neonate

— performing a caesarean section

— avoiding breastfeeding.

• Essential to the success of this policy is encouragement for all pregnant women to undergo HIV testing at antenatal booking. Consideration should be given to repeat the HIV test at a later stage if the woman is at risk of seroconverting during pregnancy. Rapid HIV testing should be offered to women who present to services late in their pregnancy or at labour.

• Factors that increase the risk of mother-to-child transmission include:

— high maternal HIV viral load and low CD4 count. Antiretroviral treatment is aimed at achieving undetectable HIV viral load during delivery. However, there have been reports of HIV transmission even when maternal plasma viral load is undetectable.

— the presence of concomitant sexually transmitted infections (STIs), especially genital ulcer disease. STIs increase maternal cervical HIV viral load and are also associated with preterm labour and chorioamnionitis.

— prematurity, especially gestation age <32 weeks; prelabour preterm rupture of membranes also increases risk.

— vaginal delivery: elective pre-labour caesarean section at 38 weeks is recommended. It is currently unclear whether caesarean section provides any additional protection if the maternal viral load is undetectable at <50 copies/ml on antiretroviral treatment around 38 weeks. BHIVA

(British HIV Association) guidelines offer the option of a planned vaginal delivery for such women if there is no other indication for a caesarean section.

— invasive procedures or monitoring during labour. It is also considered prudent to avoid invasive diagnostic antenatal procedures such as amniocentesis.

— breastfeeding: the risk of transmission increases with the duration of breastfeeding. It should be pointed out that, in resource-poor countries, a balance has to be made between the risk of preventing HIV transmission through stopping breastfeeding and the risk of gastroenteritis through imperfect bottlefeeding. If exclusive bottlefeeding cannot be achieved, breastfeeding is a preferred option to mixed feeding. In resource-rich countries formula feeding is recommended.

• There is no evidence that pregnancy has a detrimental effect on the health of an HIV-positive woman.

• Women who are HIV positive need preconception counselling about conceiving, especially if their partner is HIV uninfected. Care should be through a multidisciplinary approach including obstetricians, HIV physicians and paediatricians. Psychosocial problems are common and may require specialist input.

• Knowledge of the HIV status of newborn babies of high-risk women is essential in planning their immunization policy against other infections. Immunization with live attenuated vaccines should be avoided. With the use of DNA and RNA assays for HIV, much reassurance can be given within weeks of delivery if no neonatal virus is detectable.

Treatment with antiretrovirals during pregnancy

• The two aims of treatment in a pregnant woman are to treat the HIV infection as necessary for her own health and to prevent mother-to-child transmission of HIV. She is assessed both clinically and based on CD4 count and viral load results.

• If she meets the criteria for starting HIV treatment for her own health (see below), this should be done with HAART (highly active antiretroviral therapy) as soon as possible after the first trimester if there is no urgency.

• If the woman does not require treatment for herself, temporary treatment with HIV drugs is started in mid-second trimester, preferably before the fetus is viable, ie at 20–22 weeks. AZT monotherapy remains an option if the mother is ARV naïve and has a low viral load 6000–10 000 copies/ml. Delivery will be by elective prelabour caesarean section at 38 weeks if AZT alone is used and viral load is not undetectable. For women with higher viral loads and those with low viral loads of 6000–10 000 copies/ml, who prefer a normal vaginal delivery or may not have access to caesarean sections in the future, three drugs are used. There is some evidence, however, of an association between the use of HAART and premature delivery.

• Women who take three drugs and achieve an undetectable HIV viral load at 36 weeks can undergo a trial of normal vaginal delivery if there are no other contraindications. Those who opt for a caesarean section with an undetectable viral load should have this at 39 weeks. The mode of delivery needs to be discussed, planned and documented in the birth plan.

• Intrapartum AZT is given to mothers if HIV viral load is detectable at 36 weeks, 4 hours before caesarean section.

• The newborn is given AZT alone or as part of three-drug HAART for 4 weeks depending on maternal viral load at delivery.

• Women who conceive on HIV treatment should remain on treatment throughout pregnancy, although certain drugs may be switched because of safety concerns.

• The risk of health workers acquiring infection is small but delivery presents problems to the staff because the woman's blood and body products may contain live virus. In consequence, universal precautions should be taken.

• Knowledge of the HIV status of newborn babies of high-risk women is essential in planning their immunization policy against other infections. Immunization with live attenuated vaccines should be avoided.

Hepatitis B

Hepatitis B virus is transmitted by contaminated blood products and sexual intercourse. Transplacental rates of transmission are low among Europeans (<5%) but higher among Asians (40–90%). Rates of transmission are greater in women who are hepatitis B surface antigen (HBsA) positive.

The baby may be born apparently normal but develop hepatitis problems later. Rates may be reduced by both passive immunization with hepatitis B IgG and active immunization with hepatitis B vaccine.

Uterine conditions in pregnancy

Retroversion

Retroversion is the normal position of the uterus in 20% of women. If pregnancy occurs in a retroverted uterus:

• It usually comes upright as it enlarges.
• If tethered in the pouch of Douglas by old adhesions, it may enlarge by anterior sacculation.
• If the uterus is tethered it may grow and impact below the promontory of the sacrum. Growth can continue for a short time but soon there is:

— backache from pressure on the sacral peritoneum
— retention of urine from stretching of urethra by displacement of bladder into abdomen.

Unless this is relieved, the pregnancy will miscarry.

Management

1 Indwelling catheter and continuous drainage.
2 Uterus often slides up into the abdomen. Once up, it will not go back so no pessary is required.
3 Manual manipulation *per vaginum* under general anaesthesia before 16 weeks.

Pelvic tumours

Fibroids (see also Chapter 17)

Seen more commonly in the pregnancy age group among African and African–Caribbean women.

Diagnosis

Firm bosselated swellings detected, usually in early pregnancy. Later they soften and are difficult to locate. Ultrasound can usually detect fibroids (see p. 244).

Complications

1 Miscarriage (usually submucosal fibroids)
2 Pressure:
  - on pelvic wall veins (oedema of legs), thrombosis
  - on bladder (increased frequency)
  Effects in the baby include talipes.
3 Red degeneration:
  - Venous blood supply may be cut off and fibroid becomes stuffed with blood. Local pain and tenderness. May lead to premature labour.
  - If diagnosed correctly, analgesia and bed rest allow resolution.
  - If in doubt, do laparotomy to check. If red degeneration seen, leave alone. Myomectomy during pregnancy is contraindicated.
4 Malpresentation: oblique or transverse lie may persist because of position of fibroids.
5 Obstruction to labour:
  - Very rarely happens, because lower uterine fibroids usually ride up into the abdomen when lower segment is formed and stretched.
  - If cervical fibroids obstruct, caesarean section must be performed, but do not do myomectomy at the same time because of risk of heavy bleeding.
6 Dysfunction:
  - masses of fibrous tissue distort the smooth transmission of contractile impulses through the uterus
  - increased risk of PPH.

Ovarian cysts

In pregnancy:
- Corpus luteal cysts: 70%
- Benign mucous or serous cystadenoma: 20%
- Dermoid cyst: 5%
- Malignant tumour: 1%.

Diagnosis

Mobile mass alongside or displacing uterus in early pregnancy. Ultrasound can usually help diagnosis.

Complications

- Rupture of cyst
- Torsion of cyst
- Bleeding into cyst
- Obstruction in labour (rare).

Management

If any cyst >10 cm diameter is detected, it should be removed. Try to do this in the middle trimester of pregnancy. Excise because:
- it may be malignant
- It may undergo any of the above complications in labour or the puerperium.

Chapter 12

Normal labour

Labour is the expulsion of the fetus and placenta from the uterus and is traditionally divided into three stages, unequal in length (Fig. 12.1).

Stages

1 *The first stage, dilatation*: from the onset of labour until the cervix is fully dilated. More recently it has been divided into two phases:
  • The *latent phase* of effacement of the cervix: to 4 cm dilatation.
  • The *active phase* of active cervical dilatation: from 4 cm to full dilatation.
2 *The second stage, expulsive*: from full cervical dilatation to birth of the baby.
3 *The third stage, placental*: from birth of the baby to the delivery of the placenta.

Changes in pelvic organs during labour

• The cervix becomes effaced and dilates fully.
• The uterus and vagina become one elongated tube.
• The pelvic floor muscles are stretched backwards.
• The bladder becomes an abdominal organ and the urethra is lengthened.
• The bowel is compressed.

Lecture Notes: Obstetrics and Gynaecology, 3rd edition. By Diana Hamilton-Fairley. Published 2009 by Blackwell Publishing. ISBN: 978-1-4051-7801-3.

Uterine action

The fetus is propelled down the birth canal by the action of the myometrium. Normal uterine activity is fundally dominant, so waves of contraction pass down from each cornu to the lower uterine segment.

During labour, contractions increase in frequency and strength. Contractions are painful and this may be due to:
• hypoxia of the myometrium because of the duration of the contraction
• compression of the nerve endings in the myometrium
• cervical stretch and dilatation.

The patterns of propagation of the uterine activity start at each cornu and travel downwards. Labour starts with contractions about one in every 20 minutes increasing to one in every 2–3 minutes. The upper uterine segment contracts and retracts so that the lower segment and, later, the cervix are pulled over the baby's head rather like putting on a tight polo-neck sweater.

Figure 12.2 illustrates the intrauterine pressures that are achieved during normal labour.

Mechanism of labour

In humans, the mechanism for the onset of labour is unknown. The following facts are accepted:

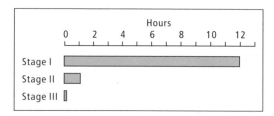

Figure 12.1 Average length of stages of labour in a nullipara.

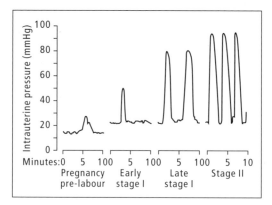

Figure 12.2 Intrauterine pressure patterns.

- Oestrogens increase uterine muscle activity whereas progesterone suppresses it.
- In late pregnancy the fetal adrenal glands produce more dehydroepiandrosterone sulphate (DHEAS), which is converted by the placenta into oestrogen. This encourages uterine contractions.
- The decidua releases prostaglandins (PGs), mainly PGE_2 and $PGF_{2\alpha}$. Such PGs cause minor uterine contractions, which result in further hypoxia of the decidua and further PG production.
- The final common pathway for a contraction is an increase in the cytosol-free calcium which causes a joining together of actin and myosin. This is common to all involuntary muscle contractions.
- Oxytocin, released from the posterior pituitary, cannot be detected in the blood in early normal labour. The release of oxytocin is dependent upon a monosynaptic reflex, initiated when the presenting part presses on the pelvic floor.

The uterus in the first stage

1 Uterine muscle fibres contract and retract, so that they do not return to their original length after contraction but remain shorter.
2 There is a heaping up and thickening of the upper uterine segment while the lower uterine segment becomes thinner and stretched.
3 The cervix is pulled up and the canal is effaced so that its length diminishes.
4 The cervix is pulled up and open and so the os is dilated.

These changes often start with the painless Braxton Hicks' contractions of late pregnancy, so that by the beginning of labour the cervix is often already partially effaced and a little dilated, particularly in multiparous women.

The uterus in the second stage

1 A diminution in the transverse diameters because of:
- pulling up of the lower segment
- straightening out of the fetus.
2 The fetal head is forced into the upper vagina, which now forms a continuous tube with the uterus and a fully effaced cervix.
3 As well as uterine contractions, expulsive efforts are made by the mother using:
- the abdominal wall muscles
- the fixed diaphragm, thus raising intra-abdominal pressure.
4 Voluntary efforts are not essential; paraplegic women and those with epidural analgesia have normal deliveries. Pushing is instinctive, and very satisfying to the woman who then assists at her own delivery.

The uterus in the third stage

1 The uterine muscles contract so constricting the blood vessels passing between the fibres, and thus preventing excessive bleeding (Fig. 12.3).
2 The placenta separates at the delivery of the fetus when the uterus contracts sharply in size. Haemostasis is mostly mechanical immediately after

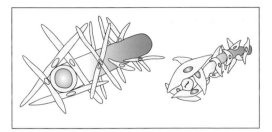

Figure 12.3 Uterine blood vessels become constricted when the surrounding muscle fibres contract.

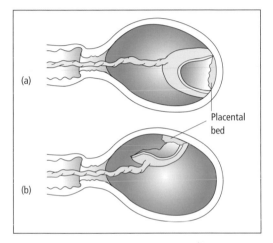

Placental bed

Figure 12.4 (a) The more common mechanism of placental separation in which the whole organ separates from its bed and balloons inside out into the uterine cavity. (b) Less commonly, the placenta separates at one side of the disc and is peeled off as the uterine muscle contracts and makes the placental bed much smaller in area.

delivery, with muscle fibres kinking blood vessels. During pregnancy and most of the labour, the placental bed and the placenta are roughly the same size. With the fetus removed, the area of the placental bed is reduced to about half that of the placenta (Fig. 12.4). The placenta is therefore sheared off and finally expelled from the uterus by contractions passing down into the lower segment.

The signs of descent of the placenta in the uterus are:
- the uterus becomes hard
- the umbilical cord lengthens
- there is a show of blood.

Management of normal labour

Diagnosis of labour

The onset of labour is defined as regular painful uterine contractions that cause cervical change. By definition it is often a retrospective diagnosis.

Admission

1 Of women in the UK 97% deliver in the hospital or midwifery-led maternity unit.
2 Women should be advised to come into hospital when:
- uterine contractions are occurring every 5–10 min
- their membranes rupture and amniotic fluid is released.
3 Assuming that the woman had full antenatal care, on admission and her records are available:
- a short history of labour is taken.
- a brief examination is performed including the following:
  — check the blood pressure
  — determine the lie and presentation of the fetus
  — determine the degree of engagement of the presenting part
  — perform a vaginal examination to assess the degree of effacement and dilatation of the cervix
  — perform a speculum examination only if the woman reports that her membranes may have ruptured or she is bleeding
- the woman is offered a warm bath.

First stage of labour

Progress in labour is monitored by descent of the fetal head together with dilatation of the cervix. As little or nothing is known about the rate of cervical dilatation before admission to the labour ward, the partogram is started on admission.

The partogram (Fig. 12.5), used by most maternity units, is an easy, graphic method of assessing the progress of labour and helps facilitate handover

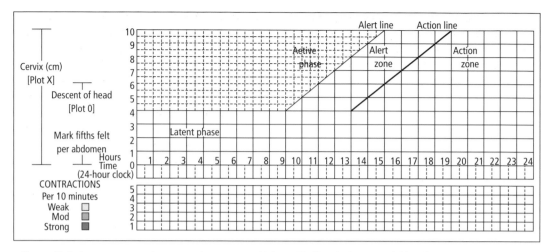

Figure 12.5 A partogram used to assess the progress of labour. The lines in the cervical dilated section are the expected patterns of cervical dilatation in labour, showing a slow latent phase and faster active phase. If dilatation crosses the action line the patient should be reviewed and/or an artificial rupture of the membranes and Syntocinon infusion started to accelerate labour.

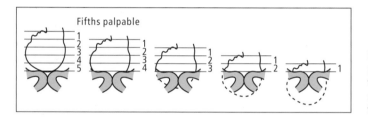

Figure 12.6 The expected normal progress and descent of fetal head through pelvis. Engagement, the maximum head diameter passing through the inlet of the pelvis.

between midwives. It contains the following information:

- High-risk factors: obstetric, paediatric or anaesthetic.
- A record of the fetal heart rate: higher-risk women have continuous electronic fetal heart rate monitoring (EFM) by the cardiotocograph (CTG). Low-risk women usually have the fetal heart rate measured with Pinard's stethoscope every 30 min, immediately after contractions. These records are plotted on the partogram.
- The cervicogram: graphic record of the rate of cervical dilatation always marked by a cross.
- Descent of fetal head marked by a circle.
- Frequency, duration and strength of uterine contractions are recorded.
- If membranes are ruptured, the amniotic fluid colour is recorded.
- The volume of maternal urine that is produced, tested for ketones and protein.

- A record of the drugs given, in particular analgesics.
- Maternal blood pressure, pulse and temperature.

After the first examination the following should be plotted:

- The amount of the fetal head that can be palpated per abdomen in terms of fifths of the head descent. Figure 12.6 illustrates the system of fifths.
- The cervical dilatation (0.5 cm/h beyond 4 cm in women in their first labour, >1 cm/h in subsequent labours).
- A line of expected cervical dilatation should then also be plotted. The World Health Organization (WHO) has produced an international partogram with two parallel straight lines plotted at 1 cm/h. In normal labour progress should follow a line that is parallel or steeper than the first line on the partogram (see Chapter 13).

The level of descent of the presenting part should be checked and plotted every hour by abdominal palpation, whereas vaginal examinations may be performed every 3–4 h. As long as the rate of cervical dilatation stays on or to the left of the nomogram, labour progress is considered to be normal.

Care of the patient

• The woman should not be left alone during labour. Ideally there should be a midwife present with her throughout. In addition, many women choose to have their partner, companion or relative present. Good support both emotionally and physically from a known midwife or trusted companion, whether the partner or other person, has been shown to increase the chances of a woman having a normal delivery.

• Analgesia should be given sufficient for the woman's need (see p. 174).

• She should be encouraged to pass urine frequently. If the woman cannot void and the bladder becomes palpable in the abdomen, she should be catheterized.

• Light snacks, soup or cool fluids are offered.

Second stage of labour

1 During the expulsive stage, the woman is encouraged to push with uterine contractions. If she is sitting propped up, this is done by taking a deep breath and holding it, putting her chin on her chest and pulling on the backs of her knees. Women usually achieve two or three expulsive pushes during each uterine contraction. Many women adopt different positions in labour and this must be allowed because there is a great deal of individual variation. Birthing stools, birthing balls and water in a birthing pool are all available and can help the woman to push effectively.

2 Monitoring progress in the second stage of labour is by vaginal assessment of the lowest part of the presenting pole related to the ischial spines. This applies until the presenting part becomes visible. Normally no vaginal assessment is necessary unless the vertex (crown of the head) is not visible after 1 hour of pushing.

3 The fetal heart should be listened to with a Pinard stethoscope or portable Doppler ultrasonography after every contraction for 1 minute to ensure that there are no late decelerations.

4 Inhalational analgesia should be offered if the woman needs it. With organized pushing, many women do not require pain relief.

5 Episiotomies are no longer performed routinely in normally progressing labours but are indicated for the following reasons:

  • fetal distress (see Chapter 13)
  • the presence of a rigid perineum which, in the opinion of the midwife, is delaying delivery
  • if an experienced midwife believes that there is going to be a major perineal tear.

Minor tears (primary and some secondary) often do not need suturing and heal well.

If an episiotomy is to be performed, local anaesthetic (lidocaine 1% plain) is injected into the subcutaneous tissues of the vagina and perineum as the head distends the perineum. Just before crowning, a right mediolateral episiotomy is usually performed. With slow extension of the head the episiotomy does not extend.

6 When the head is delivered, it is allowed to rotate (restitute) and then lateral traction is applied in the direction of the mother's anus which allows the birth of the fetal anterior shoulder.

7 Now give 5 IU Syntocinon or 0.5, mg Syntometrine i.m. to aid delivery of the placenta.

8 The baby's head is raised towards the mother's abdomen so that the posterior shoulder passes over the perineum and the rest of the baby usually then slips out.

9 The baby should be delivered on to the mother's abdomen and covered with a clean dry towel to let the parents see the baby immediately and ensure early skin-to-skin contact and keep the baby warm. A note should be taken of the Apgar score (see Table 15.1, Chapter 15) at 1 and 10 min.

10 The umbilical cord is clamped twice, and divided between the clamps. In developed countries, hospital units use disposable plastic umbilical clamps, although Spencer Wells forceps suffice. In the developing world sterile string may be used. There is no need to hurry to clamp the cord unless the baby requires active resuscitation. There is

some evidence to suggest that babies regain their birth weight and suckle better if the cord is allowed to stop pulsating before it is clamped.

Third stage of labour

1 Syntometrine has been given with the delivery of the anterior shoulder. Signs of placental separation should be awaited before applying controlled cord traction.

2 The operator's left hand is placed above the symphysis pubis and guards the front wall of the uterus to prevent uterine inversion.

3 The umbilical cord is grasped in the operator's right hand and steady traction is applied until the placenta is delivered down into the vagina and on into a kidney dish.

4 The membranes usually follow the placenta and can be removed by gentle rotation of the placenta, helping them to peel off the uterus.

5 The placenta and membranes are checked for completeness.

6 Blood loss should be estimated; it is usually between 100 and 300 ml.

7 Any tear or episiotomy should be carefully repaired under local anaesthetic with absorbable sutures such as Vicryl/Dexon (Fig. 12.7). Massaging the perineum with almond oil, before delivery, has been shown to reduce the risk of tearing.

Pain relief in labour

- Labour is usually painful. Relief of pain is better given before the woman feels the pain of the contractions.
- Careful timing of analgesia is as important as correct dosage.

Drug analgesia

Nitrous oxide

This is self-administered, pre-mixed with O_2 (50% of each), in Entonox machines. Inhalation should start as each contraction is felt and before the woman feels pain (Fig. 12.8) because it takes some seconds to work.

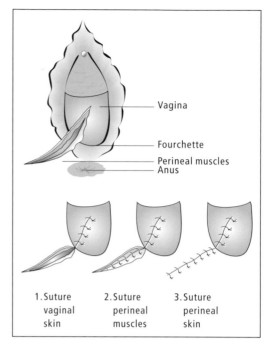

Figure 12.7 Repair of an episiotomy.

Pethidine

Pethidine has been used for many years as an analgesic in labour. Many units have now withdrawn it because of evidence that it is a poor analgesic and has a prolonged depressant effect on neonatal respiratory effort:

- Synthetic analgesic and antispasmodic
- Dose:
  — 50–150 mg i.m.
  — 50–100 mg i.v. (slowly, because it can cause nausea)
- Use in first stage: try to avoid giving within 2 hours of expected delivery if possible because of depression of neonatal respiration
- Can cause drop of maternal blood pressure
- Causes nausea in 20%; give antiemetic.

Morphine

- An alkaloid of opium. Stronger analgesic with no antispasmodic action. Used for the pains of occipitoposterior positions and long labours.

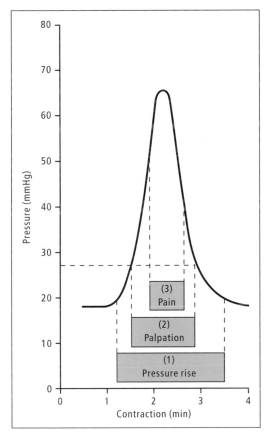

Figure 12.8 Pressure recording of contraction in late labour: (1) tocograph pressure readings show contraction for 2.5 min; (2) clinical abdominal palpation diagnosis shows it for 1.5 minute; (3) pain is felt by the woman for 45 s.

- Dose: 10 mg i.m.
- Morphine depresses the neonatal respiratory centre, and should be avoided for 2 hours before delivery if possible.
- May cause maternal vomiting (about 15%) so give antiemetic (eg prochlorperazine 3 mg sub-buccally/metoclopramide 10 mg i.m. or i.v.).

Diamorphine (heroin)

- Very powerful opiate. Good for anxious mother or long labour.
- Dose: 5–10 mg i.m.
- Depresses neonatal respiratory centre if given within 3–4 hours.

Note: barbiturates, tranquillizers and sedatives given in labour are *not* analgesics. They often potentiate analgesics and help progress by their own properties.

Non-drug analgesia

Increasing numbers of women are turning to non-pharmacological methods of pain relief. Pain is such a subjective symptom that anything that helps a woman and does not put her or her fetus at increased risk should be explored. Maybe these methods cause the release of endorphins and so postpone the need for more formal analgesia; this reduces the total dose, giving the woman a greater sense of self-participation.

Transcutaneous electrical nerve stimulation (TENS)

Small pulses of electrical vibration to the muscles of the back, from a portable battery-driven pack, provide distraction therapy. Some find it helpful in the early stages of labour. Even though it might not work for full labour, it could postpone the need for a stronger, more depressant analgesia and so its use should be encouraged if women want to try it. However, labour ward staff must know how to work the machines and be sympathetic to their use.

Water

Immersion in warm water so that the woman becomes weightless reduces the sensation of pain and many women find passing the first stage of labour in a birth pool or large bath very helpful and soothing. Some women choose to stay in the water for second stage and delivery. In this situation the baby is monitored using a special Doppler/Sonicaid that is waterproof. When the baby is born it is vital that the water is at 37°C and the baby brought to the surface quickly so that it does not take its first breath under water. The main risks for the infant are of drowning and infection and, although both of these are rare, they can be fatal.

Relaxation

The woman should take training in how to relax in pregnancy. The method works best if there is a sympathetic attendant to guide in labour (eg partner). It is safe for mother and fetus.

Hypnosis

If both woman and attendant are trained, this can give good pain relief. It is expensive on the attendant's time and works only for susceptible women. If it works, it is safe for the fetus.

Acupuncture

Some women opt for acupuncture in labour. The effects are very variable from one person to another and the need for several needles in various points of the body limits mobilization which many women find unacceptable.

Anaesthesia

Depression of the central or peripheral nervous system to prevent transmission and reception of painful impulses.

Local

Pudendal

- Block pudendal nerve with xylocaine 0.5 or 1% as its two or three branches circumnavigate the ischial spine—given through either vagina or perineal skin. Numbs the area on the right only as shown in Fig. 12.9, and therefore needs a field block as well.
- Used for outlet manipulations in the second stage of labour, eg easy forceps delivery.

Field block

A local infiltration of the nerve endings in the vulva and labia:
- before episiotomy or its repair
- as an adjunct to pudendal block.

Proper analgesia and anaesthesia in labour work best when the woman and her partner have been

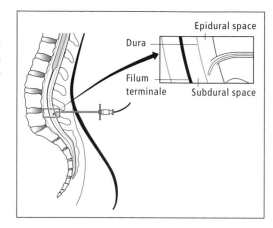

Figure 12.9 An epidural block: the outer cannula is removed and the flexible plastic catheter remains in peridural space.

instructed antenatally and have had a chance to learn about the methods available. She should talk to other women who have benefited from analgesia. All this is then applied by sympathetic attendants who look to the needs of the individual woman and tailor the therapy to her needs, preferably preventing pain being felt rather than trying to remove it after it has arrived

Regional

Nerve roots are blocked at their outflow.

Spinal block

This is not used in normal labour. It is now commonly used for caesarean section, emergency and elective because the onset of a good block is rapid and reliable. An epidural catheter can be sited at the same time for postoperative pain relief.
- Heavy bupivacaine into subarachnoid space.
- Give at L3–4, put woman in head-up position.
- Blocks L2–S1.
- Used once only, usually for surgical delivery (eg caesarean section).
- Good anaesthetic used increasingly in UK.

Epidural block

This is the most commonly used analgesia in labour—40% of all labours and 55% of first labours.

It is particularly useful for women who are experiencing a prolonged labour as it can allow them some rest.

● Bupivacaine (Marcain) 1% or Marcain 0.25–0.5% through a cannula inserted into peridural fat. Affects nerve roots L2–S4.

● Pain relief rapid, lasting 2–3 hours.

● Repeated doses can be given, so used for pain relief in labour.

● Requires expert anaesthetist (Fig. 12.10).

● Loss of sensation from the uterus means that the woman needs help in the second stage to recognize uterine contractions.

● Using a constant infusion of bupivacaine with fentanyl reduces the density of the block and allows some mobilization for the woman (walking epidural).

It can be topped up easily for operative delivery.

Complications

● A serious complication of the epidural block is puncture of the dura and so unwittingly performing a spinal anaesthetic with a big needle. This could lead to nerve blockage and stopping respiration if the anaesthetic agent flows up into the cervico-/thoracic region. Such a complication is watched for carefully by an experienced anaesthetist; it occurs in 1 : 500 cases. It is resolved by injecting some blood over the puncture.

● A rarer complication is infection that might enter through the skin to the peridural area.

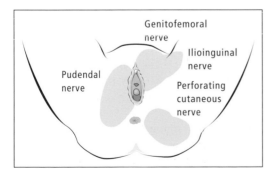

Figure 12.10 The sensory nerve supply of the skin of the perineum. Although the pudendal nerve principally supplies this area, other nerves are involved and need consideration in anaesthetizing the perineum locally.

Caudal block

● Localized epidural through sacral hiatus.

● Gives good anaesthesia for operative deliveries but only 80% effective.

General

This is avoided if at all possible and is used only in an emergency when a spinal anaesthetic cannot be achieved in a short enough time frame or if the woman has a contraindication for a combined spinal/epidural (CSE). It is never used in normal labour. Total anaesthesia induced by injection (eg propofol) and followed by inhalation (eg isoflurane or nitrous oxide) results in an unconscious patient completely under the anaesthetist's control.

In labour one of the risks is regurgitation of acid stomach contents and their inhalation into the lungs producing aspiration pneumonia (Mendelson's syndrome). To avoid this:

● have as empty a stomach as possible

● if really necessary, ensure that stomach is empty—pass a tube

● reduce acidity of stomach contents—give sodium citrate (30 ml) or H_2-receptor blocker, eg ranitidine.

● Once induced, pass cuffed endotracheal tube.

● Tilt head up for intubation and use cricoid pressure.

● Only skilled senior anaesthetists deal with women in labour.

General anaesthesia is useful for operations such as an emergency caesarean section when speed is essential.

The fetus during labour

During labour the fetus descends down the birth canal and is then delivered. The process is conventionally broken down into the series of mechanisms detailed below, but these merge with each other and are inseparable.

Flexion

Uterine activity is fundally dominant; the line of force is down the fetal spine and causes flexion of the fetal head. The head then engages when the presenting diameter passes through the pelvic brim. In most cases this is in the right occipitotransverse position.

Descent

Further uterine activity causes the fetal head to descend through the pelvic brim to the midcavity.

Internal rotation

Due to the angle of inclination between the lumbar spine and the pelvis (about 135°), the fetal head engages in the pelvis with one parietal eminence lower than the other (asynclitism). The leading parietal eminence is pushed into the pelvic floor with uterine contractions. When the uterus relaxes, the reaction from the pelvic floor muscles causes the fetal head to rotate until the head is no longer asynclitic. The head rotates from the right occipitotransverse position at engagement to become direct occipitoanterior (Fig. 12.11).

Further flexion

Further descent through the pelvis causes the chin to be forced tightly up against the fetal chest. The fetal occiput comes to lie behind the maternal symphysis pubis and the chin comes down to the lower part of the birth canal.

Extension

Further descent pushes the fetal head forward and gradual extension of the fetal head occurs, distending the perineum. With more extension, the widest diameter passes through the vulval introitus (crowning) and the head is born by extension at the fetal neck.

Restitution and internal rotation

As the head is born, the shoulders enter the maximum diameter (the transverse diameter) of the maternal pelvic inlet. As they descend through the canal, one shoulder leads because of the angle of inclination. This causes the shoulders to rotate (just as the head did in internal rotation) and, as they do so, the head (outside the body now) rotates 90°. The shoulders now lie in the anteroposterior diameter behind the maternal symphysis pubis; the head rotates to its usual alignment with the shoulders.

Delivery of the body

By gentle lateral flexion of the fetal head, the anterior shoulder is helped to slip under the pubis and is born. The posterior shoulder and the rest of the body follow, usually very easily.

During each uterine contraction, the maternal blood supply to the intervillous space is severely reduced and may be cut off. This reduces the fetal O_2 supply and allows less time for exchange of

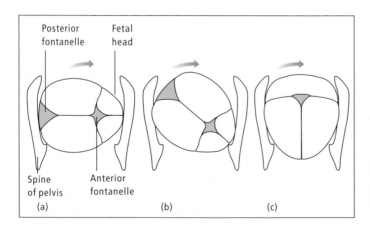

Figure 12.11 Internal rotation of the fetus: (a) inlet: right occipitotransverse position; (b) midcavity: right occipitoanterior position; (c) outlet: direct occipitoanterior position.

waste products from the fetus to the mother. Most normal fetuses can stand intermittent hypoxic ischaemia and do not require continuous monitoring during the second stage.

Monitoring the fetus during labour

There has been much recent controversy about the value of EFM in labour. There is probably little value in continuous EFM in low-risk pregnancies. Recent evidence has shown that women who have reached term with a baby that is well grown and no previous or pregnancy-acquired complications can be safely monitored intermittently using either a Pinard stethoscope or a hand-held Doppler machine. In the first stage this should be performed every 30 minutes for the duration of a contraction and 1 minute beyond to detect early, late or variable decelerations. The mother's pulse rate should be measured and recorded around the same time in order to confirm that it is the fetal heart being heard and not the aortic/uterine blood flow of the mother. If a deceleration is heard the woman is no longer low risk and should be transferred from home or a midwifery/GP maternity unit to an obstetric unit where EFM can take place and in case an operative delivery is required.

Home deliveries

Until the 20th century, in the UK the place of birth was most usually the home. Hospital deliveries started in the mid-eighteenth century for charitable reasons to help single mothers and poor women with unsuitable conditions at home. It grew gradually from 2% in 1900 to 98% in 1990.

Home deliveries had reduced to about 1% by 1986, but increased slightly to a figure of 2% in 2001; unfortunately there has been little increase since then, although the rate can vary around the UK from 0% to 20% (Fig. 12.12).

The drift to hospitalization occurred for the following reasons:

• As part of the fashion of using a hospital for more medical management.

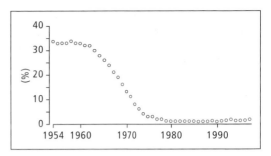

Figure 12.12 Percentage of home deliveries (England and Wales) 1954–93.

• For safety: in the isolation of the home, it would be difficult to care for:
  — PPH
  — delayed onset of baby breathing
  — shoulder dystocia.

Against this, the advantages of home delivery are:

• familiar surroundings for the woman
• more relaxation because of confidence at home
• the woman would probably know the midwife who was delivering her
• that more family members could attend at the birth and afterwards.

The slight increase in home deliveries means that a community service must be kept going. Two midwives attend each home delivery and these are usually more senior than some of those working in the hospitals. A general practitioner can be called in an emergency. If the woman has to be transferred to hospital, it is necessary to have the use of an ambulance with paramedics skilled in resuscitation.

The future of the hospital/domiciliary debate could be helped by the following:

• Increasing the availability of midwifery practices that look after women during the antenatal, intrapartum and postnatal period. This has been shown to increase the number of normal deliveries, increase the breastfeeding rate, increase the smoking cessation rate and reduce anxiety among women and their families. In the UK each midwife has a caseload of 36 women per year to look after throughout. The midwives find the continuity of care, the autonomy of practice and the relationships they build with the mothers very rewarding, so the service is satisfying to provider and receiver. The midwives are usually more confident about carrying out a delivery in the home and it is these midwives who achieve up to 20% of deliveries at home.

• The use of a midwifery-led birthing unit outside the hospital, or away from the main delivery suite. If delivery is normal and all goes well, they can return home a few hours later and so seem to have never really entered the hospital.

• Use of formal DOMINO (domestic in and out) services.

• Reduce the regimentation of hospital.

• Reduce the noise of the wards.

• Provide clean wards, enough linen and bathrooms.

• Get the woman back home early on day 1 or 2.

Chapter 13

Abnormal labour

Dysfunctional uterine action

Prolonged labour is more common in primigravidae and may be due to primary or secondary myometrial dysfunction or to malpresentation of the fetus, eg occipitoposterior position. The progress of labour should be monitored on a partogram. Figure 12.5 (p. 172) illustrates the normal rate of cervical dilatation from the start of labour. During the first 8 hours in primiparous women there is minimal change in the cervical dilatation but effacement (shortening and softening) occurs—the latent phase. Effacement is the taking up of the cervix, merging with the lower segment; eventually there is no length to the cervical canal.

Three abnormalities of labour may be recognized.

Prolonged latent phase (PLP)

This is a rare abnormality in which the cervix fails to dilate and or shorten despite many hours of regular, strong, painful contractions and occurs almost exclusively in primigravidae. The cervix in multigravidae who have previously laboured is usually partially effaced and dilated before labour

commences. Figure 13.1 illustrates this together with the possible outcome. The following are aetiological factors:

- An incorrect diagnosis of labour
- An abnormal or high presenting part
- Premature rupture of the membranes
- Idiopathic: cervical dystocia:
  — primary: failure of a ground substance of the cervix to soften in late pregnancy
  — secondary: previous surgery on the cervix causing fibrosis.

Management

- Women who present with regular uterine activity should be assessed by vaginal examination; if the cervix is long and closed, they may be in early labour or not in labour. The uterus should be carefully palpated.
- The woman should be allowed to walk around or to sit comfortably. She should be re-examined again 4 hours later if the contractions persist:
  — If labour has ceased the woman should go home.
  — If labour continues and pain relief is required, then it should be given.
  — The first line represents the expected progress of a normal labour. If cervical dilatation falls below the first/alert line and reaches/crosses the second/action line an artificial rupture of the membranes (ARM) should be performed if they

Lecture Notes: Obstetrics and Gynaecology, 3rd edition. By Diana Hamilton-Fairley. Published 2009 by Blackwell Publishing. ISBN: 978-1-4051-7801-3.

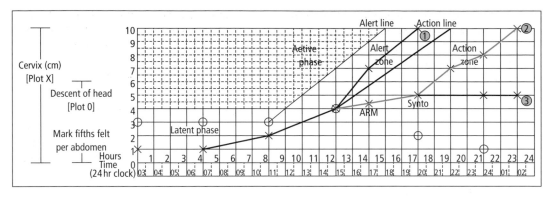

Figure 13.1 Prolonged latent phase in labour and possible outcomes: 1 and 2, vaginal delivery; 3, caesarean section. ARM, artificial rupture of membranes; Synto, Syntocinon infusion.

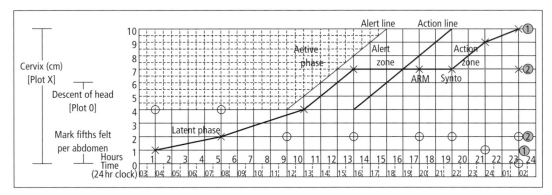

Figure 13.2 Secondary arrest of cervical dilatation and outcomes: 1, vaginal delivery; 2, caesarean section. ARM, artificial rupture of membranes; Synto, Syntocinon infusion.

have not ruptured spontaneously. If progress after 2 hours is not parallel to the action line Syntocinon should be started to make the contractions stronger and more frequent. Labour should then follow the action line; if it does not a caesarean section is indicated.

— The level of descent of the presenting part should be checked and plotted every hour, while vaginal examinations may be performed every 3–4 hours. As long as the rate of cervical dilatation stays on or to the left of the nomogram, labour progress is considered to be normal. If the cervix continues to efface but not dilate and progress falls more than 2 hours to the right of the partogram, the membranes should be ruptured (ARM) and labour stimulated by Syntocinon.

— In 85% of cases, labour will progress rapidly and will reach a normal active phase.

— In 15% of cases, adequate uterine activity fails to cause cervical dilatation. If, after 4–8 hours of Syntocinon, the cervix is not further dilated, a caesarean section should be performed.

Secondary arrest of cervical dilatation

The woman enters the active phase of labour, reaches 5–7 cm dilatation and then the cervix stops dilating (Fig. 13.2). Uterine contractions have become less frequent and may even stop:

• The fetal head engages in the occipitotransverse position and, if it is well flexed and asynclitic, will undergo rotation in the midcavity to the direct occipitoanterior position. Poor flexion leads to failure of rotation in the midcavity; this leads to persistent occipitotransverse position.

• Intravenous Syntocinon leads to regular, coordinated uterine contractions that initially cause the fetal head to flex. In most cases (85%) this allows the head to rotate so that a spontaneous vaginal delivery will occur.

• If Syntocinon administration over 4 hours (multigravida) or 8 hours (primigravida) fails to lead to further cervical dilatation, a caesarean section should be carried out for relative cephalopelvic disproportion (CPD). This occurs in about 15% of cases.

• This is a benign condition as far as the fetus is concerned and very rarely leads to fetal distress.

Primary dysfunctional labour

This is defined as slow progress after the onset of established labour and is the most worrying of the abnormalities of labour because it can lead to:

• fetal distress in a well-grown or a large baby
• prolonged labour leading to an increase in maternal fear and anxiety
• incoordinate uterine activity which increases maternal pain
• maternal dehydration which leads to maternal acidosis.

The release of catecholamines stimulates uterine activity to arise from the lower segment. This means that the fundus and the lower uterine segment contract against each other, and the cervix fails to dilate or dilates very slowly.

Maternal dehydration and acidosis lead to hydrogen ions competing with calcium (the final common pathway for smooth muscle contraction) and further dysfunctional uterine activity occurs.

Predisposing factors to dysfunctional labour are:
• first labour at term
• induction of labour
• a malpresentation such as a brow
• occipitoposterior position
• relative CPD: the fetus is only just small enough to pass through the pelvis but, if all goes well, it will succeed; if there is poor flexion or rotation, delay occurs
• macrosomia.

Once diagnosed, the dysfunction is treated with Syntocinon. In very few cases the rate of cervical dilatation returns to normal, but often it can be increased. The outcome is:
• spontaneous vaginal delivery (15%)
• caesarean section for fetal distress (50%)
• a vaginal instrumental delivery (35%). Care should be taken because, even if full dilatation of the cervix is obtained, the fetus may still be high in midcavity. This could mean a difficult, rotation forceps delivery.

Induction of labour

Definition

A planned initiation of labour.

Incidence

Varies with the population and the type of obstetric cases seen; in the UK between 5% and 25%.

Indications

• Maternal disease:
 — existing before pregnancy, eg diabetes
 — occurring in pregnancy, eg pre-eclampsia.
• Fetal disease, eg rhesus (Rh) disease.
• Fetuses at risk from reduced placental perfusion, being small for gestational age (SGA).

In the UK the following are the most common indications:
• Post-maturity (or more strictly post-dates), T^{+10-14}
• SGA
• Maternal disease
• Rh incompatibility
• Fetal death or abnormality.

In addition, there are several softer indications that obstetricians commonly employ for which there is little or no scientific basis:
• Poor past obstetric history
• Recurrent unexplained antepartum haemorrhage (APH)
• Maternal request: these women often have a fear of labour that needs psychological assistance

before delivery to discover and treat the reason for this fear. The women who accept this route often have a successful vaginal delivery if properly supported. It should never be forgotten that there are increased risks for both mother and baby if an elective caesarean section is undertaken. It is therefore important to avoid any intervention unless there is a clear medical indication that a vaginal delivery would carry greater risks to the mother, baby or both.

Before undertaking an induction the woman should be examined vaginally to determine Bishop's score (Table 13.1) and a membrane sweep performed. This can be done if the cervix admits a finger (>1 cm dilated). A circular motion round the edge of the internal os releases prostaglandins. Seventy per cent of women at term will go into spontaneous labour within 48 hours, so avoiding an induction. Bishop's score is a weighted means of assessing how likely it is that the woman will go into labour. Women with Bishop's score >6 are considered favourable and failed induction rates are usually less than 1%.

The most common method of induction of labour in the UK is using prostaglandins followed by ARM, or the latter alone. The usual system is:

1 Give prostaglandin (PG) in either vaginal pessaries (PGE$_2$, 2 mg) or as a gel (1 or 2 mg PGE$_2$) or orally (200 µg). In up to 40%, this will start labour on its own and no further action is required.

2 If not, 6 hours later, repeat the PG and wait 4–6 hours.

3 If not in established labour (>4 cm) rupture membranes.

4 Administer Syntocinon if uterine contractions do not follow within 2–4 hours or if labour becomes prolonged and abnormal, so that the rate of

cervical dilatation is to the right of the cervical partogram.

Prostaglandins

A ubiquitous group of fatty acids found in many body fluids first described in seminal plasma, hence their name. PGs E and F stimulate uterine activity and are involved in the initiation of normal labour.

Mode of action

This is directly on the muscle cells. A secondary effect is that a uterus primed with PGs will respond much better to intravenous Syntocinon.

Route

• Intravaginal: putting either a gel or a pessary into the vagina—most common method for induction of labour. A dose of PGE$_2$ in a 2 mg pessary or a 1 or 2 mg gel is placed high in the vagina. If labour is not established and the cervix is not dilating some 6 hours later, the PGE$_2$ may be repeated. Four hours after this it is usual to do an ARM and then to add Syntocinon if necessary.

• Extra-amniotic: a fine catheter passed through the cervix comes to lie between the membranes and the uterine sidewall. PGs are then injected through the catheter. This is sometimes used for late therapeutic abortions.

• The oral route: this is not commonly used because of the side effects of gastrointestinal colic and diarrhoea.

• Intra-amniotic: by direct injection of PG into the amniotic sac; may be used for late therapeutic abortions but is not used to induce labour.

Artificial rupture of membranes

Figure 13.3 illustrates rupture of the forewaters in order to induce or accelerate labour. This is carried out with an amnihook.

The following conditions should exist before ARM is carried out:

• The fetal head or presenting part should be firmly engaged.

Table 13.1 Bishop's score

Cervix	0	1	2
Dilatation (cm)	0	1–2	3–4
Consistency	Firm	Medium	Soft
Length (cm)	>2	1–2	<1
Position	Posterior	Mid	Anterior
Station of head above ischial spines (cm)	3	2	1

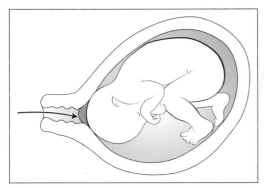

Figure 13.3 Artificial rupture of membranes: rupture of the forewaters (arrowed).

• The woman should be informed of the procedure and the reasons for it; oral consent should be obtained.

Syntocinon

This is an artificially produced oxytocic agent that mimics the activity of the normally released oxytocin. In normal labour, oxytocin is not detectable until the cervix has reached 7 cm dilatation.

Nowadays labour is not commonly induced with oxytocin alone; it is used:
• when PG pessaries and ARM fail to result in uterine activity and active dilatation of the cervix
• to augment abnormal labour when the rate of cervical dilatation has fallen to the right of the cervical partogram.

Success of induction of labour
Even with an unfavourable cervix the use of PGs, ARM and Syntocinon should result in a failed induction rate of no more than 5%.

Management of women who have a failed induction depends upon the obstetrician's opinion, which may be either of the following:
• The need for induction indicated a need for delivery and therefore failure of induction should lead to a caesarean section.
• The indications for induction were borderline and it is therefore reasonable to stop the induction process and attempt it again the next day. This can be carried out only if the membranes have not

been ruptured. It is not to be encouraged because it leads to the woman's loss of confidence in the method.

Risks of induction
• Uterine hyperstimulation may lead to fetal distress and so to a caesarean section unless reversed with the use of a tocolytic.
• Prolonged rupture of the membranes may increase the risk of intrauterine infection.
• Prolonged labour may lead to a caesarean section.
• Women whose labours are induced have a higher incidence of caesarean section (a risk factor of times three). Often this is due to the reason for the induction, eg an SGA fetus, but in many cases it results from prolonged labour.

Preterm labour

Definition

Labour occurring at <37 completed weeks' gestation.

Incidence

• Six per cent of deliveries occur before 37 weeks' gestation.
• Two per cent of deliveries occur before 34 weeks' gestation.

Prognosis

This depends upon the following:
• The availability of a neonatal intensive care unit (NICU). All infants born at <30 weeks' gestation should be transferred to a hospital that contains a NICU (level 3) if time and maternal/fetal condition allow.
• The gestational age and birth weight. The perinatal team at a typical obstetric and neonatal combined unit usually achieves a 50% survival rate at 26 weeks' gestation.
• The condition of the baby at birth. Asphyxiated infants are more likely to die later from respiratory distress syndrome (RDS).

- Immediate neonatal management.
- The use of antenatal steroids to improve the maturity of the fetal lungs and reduce the risk of intraventricular haemorrhage (IVH) in fetuses <37 weeks' gestation.

Diagnosis

Half the women who present with painful contractions before 37 weeks' gestation will stop spontaneously. Conversely, preterm labour may be insidious. The following plan is therefore recommended:

1 Look for a cause for preterm labour (Box 13.1).

2 A speculum examination should be performed to view the cervix, confirm rupture of membranes and take a high vaginal swab.

3 The fetal heart rate and uterine activity should be electronically recorded continuously.

4 Repeat the vaginal examination 2 hours later if there are more than two contractions every 10 min. Change in cervical effacement or dilatation confirms preterm labour.

5 Check fibronectin levels in cervical fluid; presence of fibronectin identifies a group of women at high risk of establishing preterm labour. If the fibronectin is negative it is highly unlikely that labour will proceed and the woman can be reassured.

Box 13.1 Risk factors and causes of preterm labour

Risk factors
Previous preterm labour
Multiple pregnancy
Polyhydramnios
Antepartum haemorrhage
Uterine abnormalities
Causes of preterm labour
Premature rupture of the membranes
Maternal pyrexia (urinary tract infection and other infections)
Fetal death
Bacterial vaginosis
Cervical incompetence

Principles of management of ongoing labour (intact membranes)

1 Full electronic monitoring is mandatory in preterm babies and those who are SGA because they may run into danger during labour through recurrent episodes of hypoxia during contractions.

2 Arrange *in utero* transfer if neonatal intensive care facilities are not available.

3 Give tocolytics for 48 hours to allow steroid therapy to mature fetal lungs and reduce risk of intracerebral haemorrhage.

Tocolysis

There is no convincing statistical evidence that tocolytic agents such as β agonists, ritodrine, calcium channel blockers (nifedipine), oxytocin antagonists (atosiban), non-steroidal anti-inflammatory drugs (NSAIDs, eg indometacin) or uterine muscle action inhibitors (progesterone) usefully prolong pregnancy by more than 1 week. However, at <4 cm dilatation they may delay delivery for 24–48 hours in order to allow time for steroids to act or for the woman to be transferred to a delivery site with a neonatal intensive unit.

Contraindications to tocolysis
Absolute
- Thyroid disease
- Cardiac disease
- Severe hypertension (>160/110 mmHg)
- Sickle cell disease
- Chorioamnionitis
- Intrauterine death.

Relative
- Advanced labour, >4 cm cervical dilatation.
- APH
- Maternal diabetes mellitus.

Side effects
These include:
- Tachycardia: treatment should be stopped if the maternal pulse rate exceeds 120/min.
- Hyperglycaemia: β agonists are diabetogenic as are steroids. As steroids are usually given at the

same time as tocolytics, the maternal blood glucose should be checked 2-hourly and a sliding scale of insulin started if the blood sugar exceeds 9 mmol/l.

• Pulmonary oedema: this is caused by fluid overload and tachycardia. It can be avoided by giving the tocolytic through a syringe pump to reduce the volume of colloid given, as well as ensuring that the woman does not have a prolonged tachycardia of >120/min.

A new tocolytic—Atosiban—has been introduced. This is an oxytocin antagonist. Other agents that have been used include NSAIDs (indometacin) and glyceryl trinitrate (GTN). NSAIDs may cause oligohydramnios and closure of the patent ductus arteriosus in the fetus if used for more than 48 hours.

Steroid therapy

Maternal steroids have been shown to reduce the incidence and severity of RDS between 26 and 36 weeks' gestation. They also reduce the risk of intracerebral haemorrhage in babies <34 weeks. They are recommended for all anticipated deliveries at less than 36 weeks.

Conduct of a preterm delivery

• The fetal heart should be electronically monitored.
• A senior obstetrician should be present.
• A neonatal paediatrician should be present.
• Forceps may be used carefully.
• Ventouse delivery is contraindicated because of the increased risk of bleeding under the scalp (cephalohaematoma).

Preterm premature rupture of membranes

PROM refers to rupture of the membranes before the onset of labour. At less than 37 completed weeks' gestation this is referred to as preterm premature rupture of the membranes (PPROM).

Problems

Risks of preterm delivery versus risk of intrauterine infection.

Confirm the diagnosis

• Avoid vaginal digital examinations
• Perform a sterile speculum examination
• If amniotic fluid is seen coming through the cervix, membranes have ruptured
• The smell of amniotic fluid is characteristic
• A positive nitrazine stick test (pH change) is of imprecise help.

Management

PPROM after 34 weeks' gestation
Management is controversial and follows one of two lines:
1 Immediate delivery to avoid intrauterine infection. Perinatal mortality because of immaturity is almost identical to that at term. However, these babies do have an increased morbidity.
2 Perform an amniocentesis to exclude an infection and, if not present, manage the woman conservatively:
  — give steroids
  — give erythromycin until delivery.

PPROM at <34 weeks' gestation
Care must be individualized but the following lines of management are reasonable:
• *In utero* transfer to a hospital with an NICU for all women <34 weeks' gestation.
• Admit for up to 1 week or more as most likely to deliver during this time.
• Conservative management in the absence of labour/chorioamnionitis after 7 days.
• Give steroids.
• Give erythromycin for 10 days or until 36 weeks.
• Monitor infection markers twice a week—white blood cell count (WBC) and C-reactive protein (CRP).
• Indications for augmentation of labour with Syntocinon are:

— evidence of chorioamnionitis (pus-coloured liquor, raised WBC and CRP)

— maturity (>37 weeks)

— spontaneous onset of labour.

• Perform an amniocentesis. If the amniotic fluid shows organisms, this suggests intrauterine infection and the woman should be delivered.

Chorioamnionitis

This is usually diagnosed by one or more of the following:
• Maternal temperature and tachycardia
• Tender uterus
• A foul-smelling vaginal discharge
• Fetal tachycardia
• Rise in maternal WCC and or CRP
• Organisms in amniotic fluid.

Management

• Obtain high vaginal swab, a mid-stream urine (MSU) sample and blood culture.
• Induce labour. Caesarean section is preferably avoided because of the risk of maternal infection, but it is indicated in the following circumstances:
— fetal distress
— preterm breech or other abnormal lie
— a failed induction.
• Start intravenous broad-spectrum antibiotics such as erythromycin for both mother and baby.

Monitoring the fetus during labour

There is a high risk of hypoxia in the following circumstances, so continuous electronic fetal monitoring (EFM) is recommended:
• Preterm infants (<37 weeks' completed gestation)
• Fetuses that are or are suspected to be SGA
• Multiple pregnancies
• Breech presentations
• Women with epidural analgesia
• Women with Syntocinon augmentation of labour
• Women who have been induced
• Women who are hypertensive

• Women with major medical disorders, including diabetes
• Women who develop meconium staining of the amniotic fluid during labour
• Women who undergo a trial of uterine scar (vaginal birth after caesarean section — VBAC)
• If a fetal heart abnormality is recorded with the Pinard stethoscope/Sonicaid.

Continuous electronic fetal heart rate monitoring

In all modern labour wards, this is performed with one of the following:
• An external fetal heart rate monitor with Doppler ultrasound echoing off movements of the fetal cardiac walls or the cardiac valves.
• An electrode attached to the fetal scalp (Fig. 13.4) showing the fetal heart rate derived from the fetal ECG. These should not be used if the mother has a viral illness that could be transmitted to the baby.

Either of these provides the fetal heart rate and this is recorded on a continuous trace. In normal

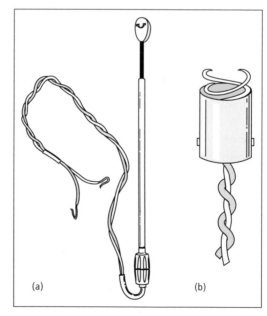

(a)   (b)

Figure 13.4 Fetal scalp electrodes for (a) clipping onto or (b) screwing into the skin of the fetal presenting part thus providing electrical continuity.

labour at term, this should be between 110 and 160 beats/min. EFM is used as a screening test to detect those babies who are developing metabolic acidosis. The diagnostic test is to perform a fetal scalp sample and measure the scalp pH.

The trace should have the woman's name, date of birth and hospital number recorded at the start, with the date and time of commencement. The reason for starting EFM should be documented in the notes and on the recording paper. The fetal and maternal heart rate should be recorded clearly in the notes every 30 min during active labour. The note should be signed, timed and dated recording:
- baseline rate
- variability
- accelerations
- decelerations.

This should be followed by a statement of whether the professional considers the trace to be normal (all four elements are within acceptable limits—reassuring), suspicious (one element is outside the acceptable range—non-reassuring) or pathological (two or more elements are non-reassuring or one feature is abnormal) (Tables 13.2 and 13.3). To reduce errors a systematic way of recording the elements of the trace has been introduced (see cardiotocograph Chapter 9).

Speed of heart rate

- A *fetal tachycardia*: Fig. 13.5 demonstrates a fetal tachycardia of about 170 beats/min. The causes of this might be:
  — a maternal tachycardia due to pyrexia, pain, fear or dehydration
  — fetal hypoxia.
  Management is to exclude or correct a maternal cause and, if the tachycardia persists, a fetal blood sample should be performed.
- A *baseline bradycardia*: baseline bradycardias are uncommon and provided that they are in the 110–120 beats/min range and there is baseline variability they are not of serious significance (Fig. 13.6). Bradycardias <110 beats/min in labour are often due to congenital heart block.

Table 13.2 Definition of normal, suspicious and pathological FHR (fetal heart rate) traces

Category	Definition
Normal	An FHR trace in which all four features are classified as reassuring
Suspicious	An FHR trace with one feature classified as non-reassuring and the remaining features classified as reassuring
Pathological	An FHR trace with two or more features classified as non-reassuring or one or more classified as abnormal

Table 13.3 Classification of FHR trace features

Feature	Reassuring	Non-reassuring 1	Non-reassuring 2	Abnormal
Baseline (beats/min)	110–160	100–109	161–180	<100/>181
Variability (beats/min)	≥5	<5 for 40–90 minutes		Sinusoidal pattern ≥10 min <5 for 90 min
Decelerations	None	Typical variable decelerations with over 50% of contractions, occurring for >90 min	Single prolonged deceleration for up to 3 min	Either atypical variable decelerations with >50% of contractions or late decelerations, both for >30 min
Accelerations	Present	The absence of accelerations with otherwise normal trace is of uncertain significance		

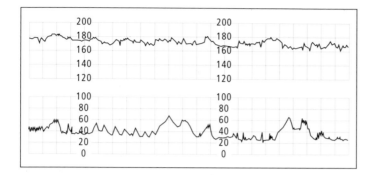

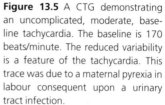

Figure 13.5 A CTG demonstrating an uncomplicated, moderate, baseline tachycardia. The baseline is 170 beats/minute. The reduced variability is a feature of the tachycardia. This trace was due to a maternal pyrexia in labour consequent upon a urinary tract infection.

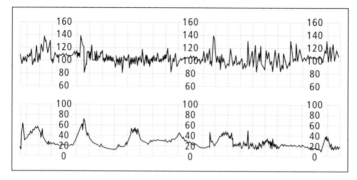

Figure 13.6 A CTG demonstrating a moderate baseline bradycardia. The baseline is 100 beats/minute. No cause for this was found.

Baseline variability

Terminology in this area is difficult because of the way in which the machinery records the heart rate. Most external Doppler machines group average beats, and so the term 'beat-to-beat variation' should be reserved for fetal heart rate traces that are obtained by fetal scalp electrodes where true beat-to-beat measurements are made.

The variation in fetal heart rate from one beat to the next (baseline variability) is caused by the balance between the parasympathetic and sympathetic nervous systems. In normal labour this varies by 5–15 beats either side of the baseline.

The following are the major variations of baseline variability:

• *Loss of baseline variability*: this is illustrated in Fig. 13.7 and may be caused by:

— administration of drugs to the mother including pethidine, diazepam and many antihypertensive agents, especially β blockers

— fetal sleep, especially in early labour

— fetal hypoxia: in the absence of maternal drugs, prolonged loss of baseline vari-

ability should lead to a fetal blood sample (> 40 mins).

• *Increased baseline variability* (sinusoidal rhythm): this is illustrated in Fig. 13.8 and usually is of serious significance. The causes of it are as follows:

— fetal asphyxia

— fetal anaemia, eg due to Rh incompatibility.

Intermittent variations

• *Accelerations* (see Fig. 9.7) are intermittent periods in which the fetal heart rate is raised quite markedly above the baseline. They are a sign of fetal health.

• *Decelerations*: intermittent changes in the baseline, falling into four categories:

— Early decelerations: the maximum descent occurs at the peak of the contraction with immediate recovery to baseline. These are illustrated in Fig. 13.9 and result from vagal stimulation after head compression as the fetus descends the birth canal. They usually have no significance and do not require a fetal blood sample unless the fetus is preterm.

— Late decelerations: these are illustrated in Fig. 13.10. They differ from early decelerations

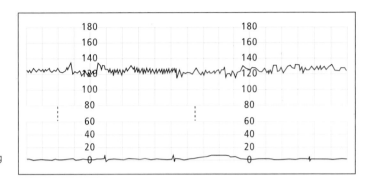

Figure 13.7 A CTG demonstrating loss of baseline variability.

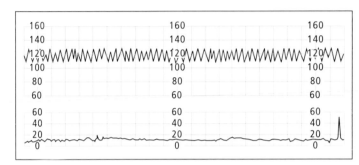

Figure 13.8 A CTG demonstrating minor sinusoidal rhythm. The baseline is 110 beats/minute.

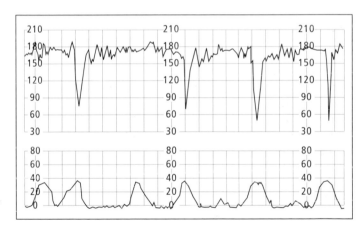

Figure 13.9 Type I or early deceleration.

in that they are U shaped, start more than 30 seconds after the contraction has started and continue after the contraction has finished. They are thought to be metabolic in nature and always warrant a fetal blood sample.

— Variable decelerations: these are also of two types: isolated and variable decelerations:

Isolated variable decelerations (Fig. 13.11): commonly seen in labour after the use of a bedpan or an epidural top-up. They may also result from umbilical cord compression and will usually disappear if the woman is turned on her side. Provided that the fetal heart rate trace returns to normal the baby is not asphyxiated and fetal blood sampling is not required.

Recurrent variable decelerations (Fig. 13.12): the important features to note are that the decelerations vary both in shape and in their relationship to the uterine contraction. The

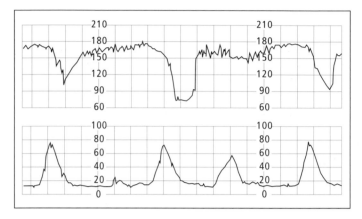

Figure 13.10 Late deceleration.

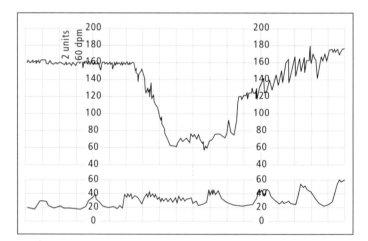

Figure 13.11 Oxytocin-induced prolonged deceleration.

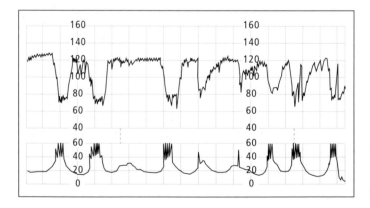

Figure 13.12 Variable decelerations.

most common cause of these is cord compression. The cord is either compressed between the presenting part and the pelvic side walls or around the fetal neck or a limb. Usually these decelerations do not indicate a fetal blood sample but, if associated with meconium or a change in the baseline heart rate, one should be performed.

Passage of meconium

Stimulation of the vagus *in utero* causes the fetal gut to contract and the anal sphincter to relax so that meconium (fetal stool) is passed into the amniotic fluid. Meconium is made up of swallowed cells in late pregnancy and alimentary tract cells, all of which are stained with bile.

With a normal fetal heart rate trace, the fetus is unlikely to be hypoxic, but if the fetal heart rate trace is abnormal when meconium is passed, a fetal blood sample (FBS) should be performed.

Fetal blood sample

Fetal blood sampling is a diagnostic test for fetal acidosis. A bead of blood is taken from the fetal scalp and the pH and base deficit can be measured. During a uterine contraction the following happens:
- Maternal blood flow to the intervillous space is vastly reduced or may even cease.
- Passage of O_2 from the mother to the fetus is reduced and thus the fetus may become hypoxic.
- The fetus withstands these periods of hypoxia by employing anaerobic metabolism. To do this, the fetus must mobilize glycogen from liver and muscle stores to produce glucose as an energy source.
- Anaerobic metabolism results in the production of large amounts of lactic acid and an increase in the arterial CO_2. In normal circumstances, the rise in arterial CO_2 is buffered, mostly by fetal bicarbonate.
- Between contractions the lactic acid and the buffered CO_2 are passed back to the mother who excretes them.
- If glycogen stores are poor (the preterm or those with SGA), other sources of energy are required for anaerobic metabolism. These produce more CO_2 and more lactic acid, and thus fetal buffering systems become overloaded. This results in a gradual fall of pH; the fetus demonstrates a metabolic acidosis.

If uterine activity is too frequent or sustained, blood flow to the fetus may be impaired for a long space of time and this, again, will result in a metabolic acidosis with an increasing base deficit.

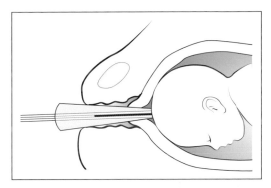

Figure 13.13 Fetal blood samples can be taken from the scalp through an amnioscope.

Figure 13.13 illustrates the mechanism by which the FBS is acquired. The fetal scalp is punctured with a 2 mm guarded blade and the blood is aspirated into a capillary tube.

The pH results are interpreted as follows:
- pH >7.25: normal
- pH 7.20–7.25: pre-asphyxia
- pH <7.20: asphyxia
- Base deficit <6.0 mmol/l: normal
- Base deficit 6.1–7.9 mmol/l: pre-asphyxia
- Base deficit >8.0 mmol/l: asphyxia.

In obstetric practice it is common to use the term 'asphyxia' but what is truly meant is a metabolic acidosis. If a fetus has a pH <7.20 and a base deficit >8.0 mmol/l he or she should be considered for delivery by the most appropriate route. Fetuses that demonstrate pre-asphyxia and are in the second stage may be allowed normal delivery, but only if this is imminent.

The scalp pH reflects the state of the fetus only at the time of the sample; the base deficit reflects a slower change, and is therefore a longer predictor. If the fetal heart rate trace continues to be abnormal, the FBS should be repeated hourly or the baby delivered.

Fetal blood sampling is contraindicated in babies of mothers with HIV or high infectivity for hepatitis B.

Cephalopelvic disproportion

Classically, cephalopelvic disproportion (CPD) is classified as follows:

• *Absolute*: there is no possibility of a normal vaginal delivery even if the mechanisms of labour are completely correct. In the western world, this condition is extremely rare; it may result from the following:

— fetal hydrocephalus

— congenitally abnormal pelvis (such as Robert's or Naegele's pelvis) in which one or both sacral ala are missing, leading to a narrowing of the pelvic inlet

— a pelvis that has been damaged usually due to a severe roll-over road traffic accident in youth

— a pelvis that has been grossly distorted from osteomalacia.

• *Relative CPD*: this means that the baby is large but would pass through the pelvis if the mechanisms of labour functioned correctly. If, however, the head is deflexed or fails to rotate in the midcavity, then prolonged, abnormal labour will occur.

The above definitions do not include estimates of the weight of the baby or radiological measurements of the pelvis. CPD can only truly be diagnosed after a trial of labour. This means awaiting the onset of spontaneous labour and, if that labour becomes prolonged and abnormal, stimulating with Syntocinon as described above.

CPD may be suspected antenatally in women who are less than 5 feet 2 inches (1.58 m) in height. These women tend to have a small gynaecoid pelvis but they often also have small babies. In a cephalic presentation there is now little evidence that X-ray pelvimetry or a CT scan helps in management. These women should have a trial of labour and in many cases will deliver vaginally.

All women with a high head at term should have an obvious cause excluded by an ultrasound examination. This will diagnose placenta praevia, uterine fibroids or an ovarian cyst as the cause. In the absence of these findings, one should suspect that the cause is CPD.

Head-fitting tests and X-ray pelvimetry have been shown to be of no value in determining the outcome of labour in women who have had a previous caesarean section or are thought to have a large baby and a cephalic presentation. The correct management is the proper use of a trial of labour.

Malpresentations and malpositions

Breech presentation

Incidence

At term 2–3%; more in preterm deliveries.

Aetiology

• The ratio of amniotic fluid volume to fetal size may be high, allowing freer movement (eg polyhydramnios and before 32 weeks).

• Extended legs of the fetus can splint and prevent flexion of the fetal trunk so stopping further turning and causing the fetus to stay as a breech presentation.

• Fetuses in multiple pregnancies may interfere with each other's movements.

• Something might be filling the lower segment (eg placenta praevia or fibroids).

• Fetal malformations may prevent cephalic presentation (eg hydrocephaly).

Types (Fig. 13.14)

Flexed or extended knee joints:

• Neither knee joint flexed so that both legs are extended: a frank breech or extended breech. This is the most common presentation.

• Fully flexed fetus with both knees flexed: a flexed breech.

• One leg flexed and the other leg extended: an incomplete breech.

• Both hips extended; a footling. Often occurs with very small babies.

On vaginal examination, the breech presentation in labour is described according to the relation of the fetal sacrum to the maternal pelvis (Fig. 13.15).

Diagnosis

Abdominal examination

No head is felt at the lower end and a hard, rounded knob is ballottable at the upper end of the uterus.

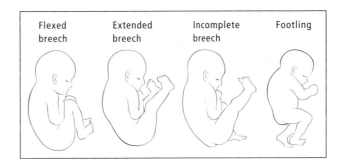

Figure 13.14 Types of breech presentation.

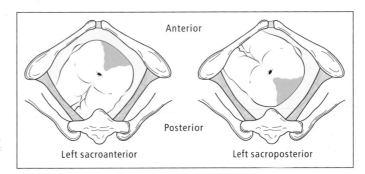

Figure 13.15 Using the fetal sacrum as the denominator, the position of the breech presentation is described.

Vaginal examination

Confirms that there is no head in the pelvis.

Investigations

Ultrasound scan confirms the situation.

Management of a breech presentation in pregnancy

• From about 37 weeks onwards external cephalic version (ECV) is worth trying without general anaesthesia. If the mother is Rh negative, anti-D-immunoglobulin should be given after the first attempt.

— listen to the fetal heart immediately before and after the procedure.

Administer subcutaneous salbutamol or ritodrine as a uterine relaxant.

The operator then disengages the breech from the pelvis and pushing the head and the breech in opposite directions slowly rotates the baby through 180° to lie cephalically.

— if it works, the woman should be seen weekly to ensure the fetus stays as a cephalic presentation

— if it fails, the woman should be counselled about the route of delivery.

— The reasons for failure of ECV:

— breech too deeply engaged in pelvis

— too tense a uterus

— too tense an abdominal wall

— fetal abnormality: request an ultrasound

— undiagnosed twins: request an ultrasound.

— Contraindications to doing ECV:

— previous uterine scar from caesarean section (relative)

— hypertension in the mother

— planned delivery by caesarean section anyway

— ruptured membranes

— multiple pregnancy

— antepartum haemorrhage.

• If ECV does not succeed then the woman should be advised about the pros and cons of vaginal breech delivery compared with caesarean section (Box 13.2).

• An ultrasound scan of the fetus will establish its estimated weight. In a breech delivery the head (the largest and hardest part of the fetus) is coming last and it is too late to wait and see if

---

Box 13.2 The pros and cons of vaginal breech delivery

Requires
Pelvic inlet >11 cm (AP)
Pelvic outlet >11 cm (transverse)
Well-curved sacrum
Estimated fetal weight <3.5 kg

Pro	*Con*
↓ Maternal morbidity	↑ Risk of fetal intrapartum hypoxia × 3
↓ Maternal mortality (rare)	↑ Risk of head entrapment
	↑ Risk of intracranial damage
	May lead to emergency caesarean section done in less favourable circumstances

---

this fits the pelvis; most obstetricians would advise a caesarean section for babies >3.5 kg, although the estimated fetal weight can be incorrect by as much as 300 g.

- It is wise to deliver most breech presentations by 41 weeks. If the woman has not gone into spontaneous labour before this time, induce or do an elective caesarean section.

- If there is any other variation from normal, many obstetricians will deliver a breech-presenting baby by elective caesarean section at 38–39 weeks.

A recent randomized trial of vaginal versus elective caesarean section for breech presentation has suggested that the latter may be safer for the infant if an ECV fails. This is truer for developed countries than for developing countries where the perinatal morbidity and mortality for cephalic vaginal deliveries are higher and the risks of caesarean section for the mother are also higher.

Management of a breech presentation in labour

First stage

- Increased risk of early rupture of the membranes. When they do, a vaginal examination should exclude a prolapse of the cord.

- An epidural anaesthetic is a good method of pain relief as the normal delivery can rapidly be changed to a surgical one if necessary (but is not mandatory).

Second stage

- Delivery is by the most senior obstetrician or midwife available with an anaesthetist and a paediatrician close to the labour ward.

- A propped-up dorsal position of the mother is the easiest to manage. The labour bed should be capable of breaking in the middle for delivery of the baby's body, so that the mother can assume a semi-lithotomy position.

- The buttocks progress down the birth canal and the baby is rotated to sacroanterior.

- The baby will often progress as far as the umbilicus with the mother's own expulsive efforts. The legs are assisted down, especially if extended by flexing the knees.

- Commonly, the arms are flexed across the chest, so they deliver readily with the next contraction.

- If the arms are extended the body can be rotated to facilitate their delivery, which may require flexion of the elbows across the front of the baby.

- After delivery of the body, it is allowed to hang down to keep the head flexed until the suboccipital region appears under the maternal pubis.

- The head is delivered slowly by placing one finger in the baby's mouth or gently flexing the head with forceps, the blades applied to either side of the fetal head from the front of the body, which is held up by an assistant. The face is delivered over the mother's perineum and the nose and mouth are cleared of mucus and liquor, allowing the baby to breathe. The rest of the head is slowly delivered, not allowing any sudden decompression that could result in pressure alterations inside the skull and so cause intracerebral venous bleeding.

Third stage

- Syntometrine is given with the delivery of the head for there is an increased risk of PPH.

- The placenta is delivered as described in normal labour.

Caesarean section

This should be done if vaginal delivery is considered too hazardous because of:

- multiple pregnancy if the first twin is a breech
- other complications, eg pre-eclampsia or diabetes
- non-descent of buttocks in labour
- failure of progress in labour.

Risks to the fetus of breech delivery

Perinatal mortality in all breech deliveries is two or three times that of cephalic presentations but this is made up mainly of preterm births (26–30 weeks). Mature breech deliveries (36+ weeks) in reputable centres have no higher risk than mature cephalic deliveries. Hence the reasons for mortality are:

- prematurity
- intracranial damage: subdural and intracranial haemorrhage often after too rapid delivery of the head
- rarely hypoxia; this may be:
  — before delivery (prolapsed cord)
  — at the time of delivery (too slow delivery of the head).

Shoulder presentation (transverse lie)
(Fig. 9.21)

Incidence

Accounts for 0.3% of all deliveries.

Aetiology

As for other malpresentation but most commonly the following:

- Polyhydramnios causing an increased ratio of fluid to fetus
- Something preventing the engagement of the head in the pelvis:
  — placenta praevia
  — fibroids
  — contracted pelvis
- Abnormal shape of uterus (subseptate or arcuate uterus)
- Second twin
- Grand multiparity (5+).

Diagnosis

- Abdominal examination: the head is in one flank and the buttocks in the other. Commonly, the fetus can be rotated to a cephalic presentation quite readily but reverts back to a transverse position.
- Vaginal examination: the pelvis is empty of presenting parts.
- Investigation: ultrasound scan confirms diagnosis.

Management of transverse lie in pregnancy and labour

1 Before 36 weeks, the woman is referred back to the following week's clinic. The position is usually self-curing.

2 Past 37 weeks in a multiparous patient, and after 38 weeks in a primiparous one, admission to hospital should be advised, where ECV is attempted each day.

3 Should the woman go to term with the fetus still in a transverse position, management may be by either of the following:

- A *stabilizing induction*: ECV is done in the labour ward. The fetal head is held over the brim of the mother's pelvis and high membrane rupture is performed. Amniotic fluid escapes and the head often sinks into the pelvis. Labour follows in the normal fashion.
- An *elective caesarean* section: in the western world this may be the safer line of treatment for the fetus because it cuts down the risks of prolapsed cord during labour, but it does leave the mother with a scarred uterus for future pregnancies and an increased risk of postpartum problems.

4 Occasionally a woman is admitted in mid or late labour with a transverse lie. This would lead to an impacted shoulder presentation, the folded fetus having been driven a varying amount down the pelvis, depending on how far labour has gone. Treatment must be by immediate caesarean section, even if the fetus is dead, because of the risk of uterine rupture.

Occipitoposterior positions

The fetal head usually engages in the pelvic brim in the occipitotransverse position (long axis of head fitting into maximum diameter of bean-shaped pelvic brim). When labour starts, the head is driven down the birth canal and rotates:

- 80% rotate forward through 90° to an occipito-anterior position.
- 15% undergo long internal rotation through 270° to become occipitoanterior, having gone through directly occipitoposterior on the way.
- 3% rotate back 90° to a directly occipitoposterior position; these may deliver face to pubis.
- 2% stay in the transverse and descend in this position; a minority of these might rotate on the perineum but most end up in transverse arrest.

Aetiology

Pelvis

Flat sacrum with loss of pelvic curve and so loss of room for rotation.

Uterus

Poor or disorganized uterine contractions do not push the fetal head down and so there is no impetus to rotate.

Head

Poor flexion so that larger diameters present (sub-occipitofrontal >10.5 cm).

Analgesia

Epidural analgesia causes pelvic floor relaxation. This allows the gutter of the levator ani muscles to become lax, so not directing the occiput anteriorly. This is associated with lack of fetal head rotation.

Diagnosis

Pregnancy

Occasionally, by abdominal palpation when in a cephalic presentation, the back cannot be felt in the flank but fetal limbs can be felt all over the front of the uterus. The head is often not engaged after the time that it would be expected to be.

Labour

- Abdominal palpation as above
- Vaginal examination feeling the sutures and fontanelles. Both anterior and posterior fontanelles

can be felt (deflexion) and the triangular-shaped posterior fontanelle is in the posterior quadrant of the pelvis.

Management in pregnancy

Leave alone.

Management in labour

Laissez-faire. Await events for many will rotate spontaneously. Prepare for a longer labour because:

- pelvis may be minimally contracted or sacrum slightly flattened
- incoordinate uterine contractions
- deflexed fetal head.

    Therefore:
- Watch progress by both:
    — abdominal assessment of engagement and descent of fetal head
    — vaginal assessment:
        — head in relation to ischial spines
        — rotation of head
        — dilatation of cervix which is often poorly applied to the head
        — check no prolapse of cord by vaginal examination straight after membranes rupture
- Women often wish to push before the cervix is fully dilated. If the occiput is posterior there is extra pressure on the sacrum and rectum. Frequent vaginal examinations are needed to make accurate assessments of the real dilatation of the cervix and the progress of labour.
- Watch maternal condition. Especially remember that:
    — labour will be long, so maintain morale
    — pain relief should be thorough—epidural anaesthesia is good in this situation; if such regional anaesthesia is unavailable many would use morphine or diamorphine for this problem; no food and little fluids by mouth (general anaesthetic may be needed); give intravenous fluids.
- If head stays directly occipitoposterior (OP), delivery may occur spontaneously but, as larger diameters are passing through the birth canal, the

mother will have to work harder and an episiotomy may be required. Face-to-pubis delivery will occur.
- If head stays in occipitotransverse (OT) position it will not deliver spontaneously. It must be rotated to deliver and this will require good analgesia, usually an epidural. A rotational delivery is contraindicated if there is fetal distress and a caesarean section should be performed. Rotation and delivery may be by:
  — manual rotation to the occipitoanterior (OA) position and subsequent forceps delivery
  — Kielland's straight forceps rotation and subsequent delivery; these forceps have no pelvic curve
  — vacuum extraction: this applies only a linear pull on the fetal head so that any rotation can occur as determined by the pelvic muscles and bones.
- Give intravenous Syntometrine with the crowning of the head because the risks of PPH are greatly increased. Deliver the placenta promptly after the baby is born.
- Be prepared to repair the episiotomy quickly and it is important to check that the anal sphincter and rectal mucosa are intact because there is an increased risk of injury when the baby is born occipitoposterior or after rotation.
- If the head does not rotate a caesarean section is indicated. This can be difficult because the head is so low in the vagina.

Complications

Mother

After surgical delivery and an episiotomy, vaginal and vulval oedema and haematomata are more frequent.

Damage to the anal sphincter and rectum are more common and should be repaired by a senior member of staff who has been trained in this. After rotational deliveries lateral wall tears of the vagina are also more common and should be checked carefully.

Baby

As a result of the longer labour and high incidence of operative delivery, perinatal mortality and mor-

bidity are increased. The mortality is due to hypoxia and birth trauma. The morbidity is from these and the results of intracranial haemorrhage.

Face presentation

As the fetal head gets driven down the birth canal, the front of the head can become extended (Fig. 13.16). Distinguish from face-to-pubis delivery.

Incidence

This is some 0.3% of all deliveries.

Aetiology

- Lax uterus, multiple pregnancy, polyhydramnios
- Deflexed fetal head
- Shape of fetal head:
  — dolichocephalic (long head)
  — anencephalic (no cranium).

Mechanism
Head descends with face leading. Chin (mentum) used as denominator to determine rotation.

Eighty per cent engage in mentotransverse (submentobregmatic diameter—10 cm). With descent, most rotate to mentoanterior on the pelvic floor, the fetal chin coming behind the maternal pubis. After further descent, the chin can escape from under the lower back of the pubis and the head is then delivered over the vulva by flexion.

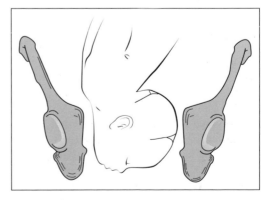

Figure 13.16 Face presentation: well engaged in the mentolateral position.

Up to this point, the mechanisms of flexion/extension of the fetal head are the reverse of those with a vertex presentation. After delivery of the head, however, the external rotations are the same, allowing the fetal shoulders to negotiate the pelvis.

A few face presentations rotate from the transverse to mentoposterior, so that the fetal chin is in the curve of the mother's sacrum; the fetal occiput and back are crushed into each other behind the pubic bone. Further descent is unlikely because the head cannot extend further and so cannot negotiate the forward curve of the birth canal, and caesarean section is needed.

Diagnosis

Rarely made before labour and of little significance if it is.

Abdomen

- Longitudinal lie with body nearer to midaxis of uterus.
- More head felt on the same side as the back.

Vaginal examination

- Do not expect the face to feel like the newborn baby's face. Oedema always obscures facial parts.
- Supraorbital ridges lead to the bridge of the nose.
- Mouth has hard gums in it and may suck on the examining finger.

Management

In pregnancy
- Await events.
- Membranes may rupture early (examine vaginally to exclude prolapsed cord).
- Check that pelvis is adequate and that fetus is not oversized. If either, consider caesarean section because face presentation in labour has a higher risk.
- Check with ultrasound that the fetus is not anencephalic because this might alter management.

In labour
- If anterior rotation to mentoanterior, a longer labour but spontaneous delivery will probably occur (90%).
- If head stays in mentotransverse, either manual rotation to mentoanterior and forceps extraction, or Kielland's forceps rotation and extraction or deliver by caesarean section.
- If face rotates posteriorly, this is impossible to deliver vaginally, so perform a caesarean section.

Results

Mother
Higher morbidity associated with operative delivery.

Baby
Higher mortality:
- Abnormalities incompatible with life (anencephaly)
- In the normal, hypoxia and cerebral congestion.

Brow presentation

A very poorly flexed head may present the largest diameter of the skull: mentovertex (13 cm) (Fig. 13.17).

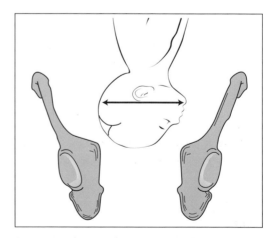

Figure 13.17 Brow presentation with mentovertex diameter presenting.

Incidence

Some 0.1% of all deliveries.

Diagnosis
Rarely made before labour and of little significance if it is.

Abdomen

- Head feels big.
- Not well engaged.
- Groove between occiput and back. Head felt on both sides of fetus.

Vaginal examination

- Anterior fontanelle presents.
- Supraorbital ridges and base of nose can be felt at edge of field.

Management

In pregnancy
- Await events. No point in trying to convert to more favourable presentation.
- Membranes may rupture early (examine vaginally to exclude prolapsed cord).

In labour
- If diagnosed early, await events for some convert spontaneously to face (by further extension) or vertex (by flexion).
- If presentation persists, it will be impossible to deliver vaginally, so deliver by caesarean section.
- If fetus is dead or there is hydrocephaly, the destructive operation of perforation of head and vaginal extraction is possible provided that the operator is skilled in these arts, but in the western world these are diminishing in number.

Results

Mother
Higher morbidity associated with operative delivery.

Baby
As a result of wider use of caesarean section, morbidity and mortality rates are low.

Surgical delivery

Before undertaking a surgical vaginal delivery the following five conditions should be met:

1 Adequate analgesia (epidural or pudendal block with infiltration of the perineum with lidocaine).
2 The fetal head should not be more than 1/5th palpable in the abdomen.
3 Full dilatation.
4 Presenting part at the spines or below with accurate knowledge of position of fetal head (OA/OT/OP).
5 Empty bladder via catheter.

Vacuum extractor

This instrument is used to get a purchase on the smooth fetal head, allowing traction to be applied (Fig. 13.18). The suction raises an edged dome of the soft tissues of the scalp and the pull is on the overhang of this edge.

Usage

Used widely in Europe and the UK, least in the USA; 5–10% of UK deliveries.

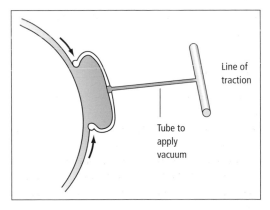

Figure 13.18 Vacuum cap on fetal head sucks up a chignon of subcutaneous tissues to give a button on which to pull. The tractive efforts are mostly on the overhang (arrowed).

Very useful in countries with developing health services (eg Africa) because it can be used by less experienced operators than forceps.

Indications

- Delay in second stage:
  — often with OP or OT position; commonly in association with an epidural
  — mother is too tired.
- Compound presentations—after replacing a presenting hand.
- High head of second twin.

(Less use in fetal distress for forceps are swifter but, if the operator is inexperienced, the vacuum extractor is safer.)

Contraindications

- Malpositions (face particularly)
- Breech presentation
- Premature infants (<36 weeks)
- Mother has HIV or high infectivity hepatitis B.

Methods

This is best learned by watching and helping in the labour ward. Here only essentials are given:
- Apply largest vacuum cap that slips through cervix—60 mm if possible.
- Hold cap flat against fetal head just anterior to the occiput and start to build up vacuum.
- With just enough vacuum to hold cap on head, check around the whole perimeter that maternal soft tissues have not been sucked under the cap's rim.
- Increase vacuum to the yellow line; check full circumference of cap to ensure correctly positioned and no inclusion of maternal tissues; increase vacuum to the green line.
- Pull on handle, apply traction to fetal head in a straight line (Fig. 13.19).
- Press cap onto head at right angles to line of traction with fingers of other hand.
- Remove cap by reducing vacuum suction.

Use modern Ventouse systems made of softer rubber with hand-held disposable caps which cause

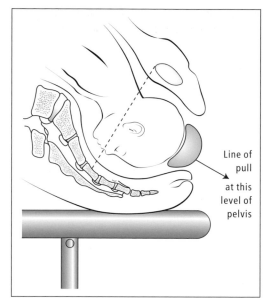

Figure 13.19 Line of traction with vacuum extractor.

fewer fetal abrasions. The old metal and Silastic cups have fallen out of use in the UK but are still in use in some parts of the world.

Complications

Maternal
- Cervical damage
- Vaginal wall damage; reduced if application of cap checked so as not to suck in walls when vacuum is being established
- Possible urinary retention later.

Fetal
- Skin abrasions (usually minor)
- Cephalohaematoma/subgaleal haemorrhage which may cause massive blood loss with hypotension and tachycardia, and collapse. This is fortunately rare but can be a cause of serious morbidity (59/10 000) and mortality.

Forceps

The function of forceps is to get purchase on a rounded object (the fetal head) and to apply traction. This is usually needed to hasten delivery, but it can control the speed of descent, eg slow down the aftercoming head in breech delivery.

Usage

Depends on availability of obstetricians. In the UK 5.10% of all deliveries.

Mechanism

There are many types of forceps. Basically all have:
- curved blades to fit around the head (Fig. 13.20)
- handles to apply traction.

In addition:

1 Some also have a curve to allow for the curve of the pelvis (Fig. 13.21)

2 If they do not have a pelvic curve, they may be straight-handled to allow rotation manoeuvres

3 A sliding lock to allow for an asymmetrically aligned head.

There are therefore two basic types. All have curved blades and handles for traction. In addition:
- Traction forceps incorporate **1**.
- Rotation and traction forceps incorporate **2** and usually **3**.

Indications for use

1 Poor progress in the second stage. No exact time limits but most would consider the longer limits as 2 hours in a primigravida and half that in a multi-

gravida. If an epidural anaesthetic is being used, these time limits are usually extended.

2 Clinical fetal distress.
- Alterations of fetal heart rate and rhythm.
- Passage of meconium.

3 Biophysical or biochemical signs of fetal hypoxia.
- On the fetal heart rate trace:
  — tachycardia or bradycardia
  — loss of baseline variability
  — late decelerations.
- On fetal blood sampling, scalp capillary blood: base deficit > mmol/l; pH <7.15 in second stage.

4 Maternal distress:
- A tired woman after a long first stage
- One who is frightened or has not had proper analgesia.

5 To prevent fetal morbidity:
- Very immature babies
- Delivering the head of a breech presentation.

6 To prevent maternal morbidity:
- Women with cardiac or respiratory disease
- Following a dural tap at attempted epidural injection.

Method

These methods are best learned by watching and helping in the labour ward. Here essentials only are given:
- Each blade of the forceps is slipped in turn along the obstetrician's cupped hand, holding back the vaginal walls in turn so that they lie alongside the baby's head.

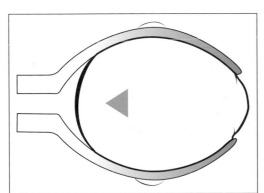

Figure 13.20 Cephalic curve of a pair of forceps to embrace a fetal head.

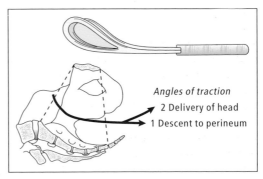

Figure 13.21 The pelvic curve of the forceps to fit the curved line of advance of a fetus through the pelvis.

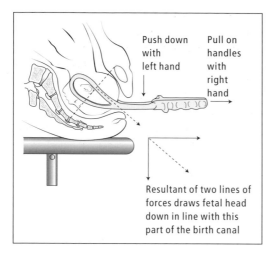

Push down with left hand

Pull on handles with right hand

Resultant of two lines of forces draws fetal head down in line with this part of the birth canal

Figure 13.22 Correct line of pull is achieved by use of two hands working in cooperation, thus performing the task more simply than a pair of axis traction forceps.

• The blades are locked together.
• Traction is applied in a downwards and backwards direction to follow the line of the curve of the birth canal (Fig. 13.22).
• For a rotation, forceps are applied on the sides of the baby's face and then rotated through 90° occipitoanterior and delivered by traction.

Complications

Maternal
• Most operative vaginal deliveries.
• Perineal tear: avoid by a properly sited episiotomy done at the right time; often an episiotomy will extend at a forceps delivery. Check for this at the apex of the episiotomy cut.
• Damage to vagina: occasional split of vagina where caught between descending head and ischial spines.
• Retention of urine: possibly caused by oedema at bladder neck. Responds to continuous drainage.
• Damage to anal sphincter and or rectal mucosa leading to occasional incontinence of flatus or faeces which can be very distressing.

Fetal
• Bruising to head: may go on to cephalohaematoma (rarer than Ventouse).

• Facial palsy: facial nerve in front of ear unprotected in fetus. May be compressed by forceps blade. Usually only temporary effect.
• Intracranial haemorrhage: if blades incorrectly applied or excessive traction used.

Failed forceps

An attempt to deliver with forceps, which is unsuccessful.

Reasons
1 Cervix not fully dilated
2 Misdiagnosis of position of head. Thought to be OA when it is OT or OP
3 Unsuspected disproportion.

Treatment
Get senior help in hospital. Then:
• If **1**, with mother and fetus well, await full dilatation.
• If **2**, rotate head and deliver.
• If **3**, caesarean section.

Caesarean section

Delivery of the fetus by surgical means through the abdominal wall.

Usage

Depends on availability of obstetricians and on the population served. In the UK 25% of all deliveries. The caesarean section rate has risen rapidly in the last 30 years. There are several reasons for this:
• The introduction of spinal and epidural anaesthesia has reduced the anaesthetic risks of the procedure. This has led to a lower threshold for doing a caesarean section in the second stage of labour rather than performing rotational/high cavity forceps deliveries, which lead to maternal and neonatal morbidity.
• The increased use of EFM has increased our awareness of fetal distress although most babies are born in good condition despite an abnormal CTG and/or low pH at fetal blood sampling.

• The reduction in the number of rotational forceps deliveries has led to a deskilling of obstetricians who do not feel confident to carry out these procedures.

• The evidence that breech presentation babies have a reduced morbidity and mortality if delivered by elective caesarean section.

• An increased number of women who have had a previous caesarean section.

• An increasing demand from women for elective caesarean sections with no medical reason.

The last group is difficult to deal with, because a first elective caesarean section does have a lower maternal morbidity than an emergency caesarean section but it is still higher than a normal vaginal delivery. In first pregnancies we do not have a reliable indicator for the outcome of labour and so we cannot guarantee that a woman will not end up with a caesarean section. Seventy per cent of women who go into spontaneous labour at term can expect to have a normal vaginal delivery. Many of the women who request caesarean section have a genuine fear of labour and/or motherhood, which may be based on past experiences of sexual abuse, poor mothering or other psychological problems. It is wise to refer them to a psychologist or midwife trained in these areas before agreeing to perform a caesarean section. All subsequent caesarean sections carry an increased morbidity.

Indications

Few are absolute and most are relative to the individual patient, the obstetrician and the obstetric environment. Generally, when the risks of vaginal delivery to the mother or baby are greater than those of abdominal delivery in any given circumstance, a caesarean section should be done:

• CPD

• Fetal distress in first stage of labour or a prolapsed cord

• Failure of labour to progress despite adequate stimulation

• To avoid fetal hypoxia of labour: pre-eclampsia; intrauterine growth restriction

• Antepartum bleeding: placenta praevia; abruptio placentae

• Poor past obstetric history

• Malpresentations: brow

• Malpositions: transverse lie, breech

• Death of mother in late pregnancy, a live fetus removed *peri mortem*.

The only absolute ones are gross disproportion, and the higher grades of placenta praevia.

In a British population, a hospital in this decade would have the following indications in differing proportions for operations:

• Fetal distress

• Pre-eclampsia

• Poor fetal growth

• Disorderly uterine action

• Breech, face and brow presentation

• Previous caesarean section.

Types of approach

• Lower segment operation: transverse approach through lower segment. In the UK, over 99% of operations are lower segment because:

— wound is extraperitoneal so less risk of intraperitoneal infection

— fewer postoperative complications.

— healing of scar is better because lower segment is relatively at rest in puerperium

— risk of rupture less in subsequent pregnancies.

• Classic operation: vertical approach through upper segment, performed:

— if lower segment unapproachable, eg fibroids

— if transverse lie

— if very small baby expected (24–28 weeks), lower vertical incision (De Lee's incision).

Anaesthesia

The operation requires an anaesthetic. The alternatives are:

• spinal block

• epidural block

• general anaesthetic

• infiltration of local anaesthetic agents.

Surgical technique

These surgical operations are best learned by watching and helping in theatre.

Perioperative complications

- Haemorrhage:
  — Worst if angles of transverse uterine incision extend into uterine vessels.
  — Always have blood grouped and saved with rapid access to 2 units of cross-matched blood. All labour/delivery wards must have 2 units of O-negative blood available at all times.
- Infection:
  — Watch asepsis and antisepsis
  — Give prophylactic antibiotics to all women.
- Abdominal distension:
  — Common for a day or so
  — Await events.
- Ileus:
  — Mild regional ileus may last 24 hours
  — Await events and avoid overloading the gut (keep on intravenous fluid for 24 hours)
  — Longer ileus may follow if there was a lot of handling and packing of the gut. Treat with stomach aspiration and intravenous fluids.
- Thromboembolism
  — Much higher risk after caesarean section than after vaginal delivery
  — Avoid thrombosis by:
    — TED (thromboembolic deterrent) stockings intraoperatively until woman fully mobilized
    — intraoperative compression stockings
    — postoperative subcutaneous low-molecular-weight (LMW) heparin continued daily until woman fully mobilized
    — early mobilization and leg exercises
    — keeping woman well hydrated postoperatively.
  — Avoid embolism by taking leg and pelvic signs seriously and anticoagulating early
  — Prevent thrombosis with prophylactic anticoagulation (subcutaneous heparin) in all women and particularly those women at higher risk:
    — aged >35
    — obese
    — past history of thrombosis, particularly if oestrogen associated (eg oral contraception)
    — anaemia.

Prognosis

Maternal

- *Mortality*: 1 : 3000 caesarean sections with causes mostly in the above complications group.
- *Morbidity:* subsequent pregnancies after a caesarean section may be affected:
  — if non-recurrent indication (eg fetal distress), two-thirds deliver vaginally
  — if recurrent indication (eg disproportion), only one-eighth deliver vaginally.

Hence patients who have had a caesarean section must have all subsequent pregnancies properly conducted in a hospital. Watch for dehiscence of uterine scar in late pregnancy next time. Take extra care if giving oxytocic stimulation.

Fetal

- *Mortality*: depends on indication; caesarean section reduces risk, but, if done for progressive fetal condition, it may be indicated only in the women with worst degrees of that condition and so fetal prognosis is worse, not from the surgical delivery but from the condition that indicated it.
- *Morbidity*: higher risk of retained lung fluid if delivered by caesarean section, especially before 32 weeks' gestation.

Obstetric emergencies

Presentation and prolapse of the cord

Presentation of the cord

During labour, loops of cord may be felt ahead of the presenting part; if the membranes are intact this is not dangerous. The cord will probably slip to one side when the presenting part comes down. However, if, in a live fetus, cord presentation is felt at a time of proposed artificial rupture of the membranes, that procedure is better postponed for an hour or so.

Prolapse of the cord

If the membranes rupture and the presenting part does not fit the pelvis well, the umbilical cord can be carried through the cervix by the flow of amniotic fluid.

Associated factors

Badly fitting presenting part:
- OP position
- Breech
- Face-and-brow presentations
- Transverse lie
- High head:
  — preterm delivery
  — small baby
  — multiparity.

Incidence

In 1 : 3000 of all deliveries.

Findings

Loops of cord may:
- pass through cervix and stay in vagina
- pass out of vulva.

Dangers

Fetus is put at risk of cutting off blood supply.
- Spasm of umbilical arteries from:
  — cooling
  — drying
  — altered pH
  — handling
- Mechanical compression between presenting part and maternal bony pelvis.

Diagnosis

- The fetal heart may show a sudden alteration in rate or rhythm soon after membrane rupture.
- Loops of cord appear at the vulva or are felt in the vagina at examination. Do *not* handle cord too much, just determine if the vessels are pulsating.

Management

If fetus mature and alive
- Deliver immediately:
  — if cervix <9 cm dilated, caesarean section.
  — if cervix >9 cm and favourable cephalic presentation in a multiparous patient, Ventouse delivery

  — if cervix fully dilated, Ventouse or forceps delivery.
- If immediate delivery impossible (eg prolapsed cord occurs outside a properly equipped obstetrical unit):
  — keep cord moist, warm and do not handle; if outside vulva, return cord to vagina
  — prevent compression of cord between the presenting part and the bony pelvis: put mother in lateral position or on all fours with pelvis raised on pillows; press up presenting part with the fingers in the vagina.

Keep these precautions until delivery about to occur, ie if the mother must travel in an ambulance, the doctor or midwife goes with her still doing a vaginal examination to continue to hold up presenting part.

Do not waste time trying to put the cord back into the uterus above the presenting part. Each attempt may allow more loops to come down and the additional handling increases spasm.

If fetus dead

There is no urgency because there is no increased risk to the mother. Allow events to proceed; the cord will not obstruct labour.

Prognosis

Maternal

Increased morbidity risks of surgical delivery.

Fetal

Depends where the woman is when the prolapse occurs and at what stage of labour. If the mother is in hospital and the prolapse is in the second stage, the fetal loss is <3%. Should she be at home with a first stage prolapse, figures as high as 70% loss occur.

Shoulder dystocia

Shoulder dystocia is an obstetric emergency. It occurs when the shoulders do not spontaneously deliver after the head. The anterior shoulder becomes trapped behind or above the symphysis pubis whereas the posterior shoulder may be in the hollow of the sacrum or above the sacral promontory.

Predisposing factors

- Previous shoulder dystocia
- Previous baby >4.5 kg
- Big baby clinically or on ultrasound scan (abdominal circumference >95th centile)
- Diabetic woman
- Obese woman (body mass index or BMI >30 kg/m²)
- Secondary arrest in labour augmented by Syntocinon
- Prolonged second stage.

Signs

- Fetal chin pulls back against the perineum
- No external signs of restitution
- Anterior shoulder fails to deliver with contraction.

Management

- Call for help.
- Change the maternal position:
  — McRobert's manoeuvre: flatten the bed, retract the woman's knees on to her chest as far as possible. This straightens the sacrum and maximizes the pelvic diameter. Apply gentle traction. If not delivered after 30 seconds try the following sequence with 30 seconds to try to deliver the baby with each one.
  — Place woman on all fours (shoulders move to oblique diameter).
  — Return to supine. External pressure—place hands, held as for cardiopulmonary resuscitation, on the mother's abdomen just above the symphysis pubis and apply pressure.
- Perform an episiotomy if not already done.
- Internal rotation: place hand behind the anterior shoulder and bring it forward; rotate the shoulders using the posterior shoulder.
- Deliver the posterior arm.
- Symphysiotomy: division of the symphysis pubis, supporting the hips so that they do not separate too quickly.

Risks

Maternal
- Vaginal trauma
- Bladder/urethral damage particularly if a symphysiotomy is performed
- Psychological trauma.

Neonatal
- Erb's palsy from brachial plexus injury
- Cerebral palsy from hypoxia
- Fractured humerus/clavicle
- Neonatal death.

All parents require sensitive and careful debriefing after shoulder dystocia. It is a frightening experience when a lot of doctors and midwives arrive suddenly, being asked to change positions with minimal explanation yet knowing there is something seriously wrong. They may also have to cope with a baby with a physical or learning disability.

Postpartum haemorrhage

Bleeding from the genital tract after delivery of the fetus.

Primary PPH

Definition

A blood loss in excess of 500 ml from the vagina within 24 hours of birth.

Incidence

Varies with use of oxytocic drugs. From 1% to 8% of all deliveries.

Causes

- Uterus does not contract and so prevent bleeding from placental site.
- Partly separated placenta: uterus cannot contract properly and so placental bed bleeds.
- Retention of separated placenta: lower areas of the uterus contract so that the placenta is trapped and cannot be expelled.

- Tears of the uterus, cervix, vagina or perineum.
- A clotting defect of blood.

Predisposing factors

- Overstretch of uterus: twins, polyhydramnios
- Long labour
- Deep anaesthesia or use of halothane
- Previous scar on uterus
- Morbid penetration of placenta
- Cervical contraction after oxytocic drugs
- Vaginal surgical delivery
- Hypofibrinogenaemia after abruptio placentae
- Disseminated intravascular coagulopathy.

Diagnosis

Since the definition of a PPH is a loss over 500 ml, an attempt should be made to measure blood loss at delivery. This is rarely accurate because of the following:

- Not all blood lost is collected:
  — some on sheets and floor
  — some still inside uterus (but lost from intravascular space).
- Other fluids often included accidentally:
  — urine
  — amniotic fluid
  — cleaning-up solutions.

Estimates are made and these are usually smaller in volume than the actual loss, sometimes as much as 50%. Therefore, give treatment on lower estimates of blood loss than would be done at a surgical operation.

Treatment

Prevention

Give oxytocic drug with delivery of baby, eg Syntometrine (ergometrine 0.5 mg and oxytocin 5 IU) i.m. This is the best way to prevent PPH. There may be an increased risk of retained placenta but that does not kill; PPH does (0.3/100 000).

Curative

- Give another dose of oxytocic (usually ergometrine 0.5 mg i.v.).

- Have blood taken for cross-matching and put up intravenous drip of Hartmann's solution.
- Give blood if loss over 1000 ml or woman was anaemic in pregnancy.
- Determine cause:
  — if placenta out: examine for completeness
  — if placenta not delivered: make arrangements for removal.

Uterine atony

- Massage uterus to stimulate contraction
- Syntocinon i.v. by continuous drip (40 IU/500 ml fluid)
- Bimanually compress uterus (Fig. 13.23)
- Injection of prostaglandin $PGE_{2\alpha}$ or carboprost directly into uterus or rectally
- Uterine artery embolization
- Hysterectomy.

As a result of the wider use of oxytocics in both prevention and treatment, the last two methods are rarely used. The last are exceedingly unusual.

Partly separated retained placenta

- Uterus is often well contracted.
- Try controlled cord traction again, being careful not to snap cord.
- Put up intravenous drip with Hartmann's solution while awaiting blood. Give blood if >1000 ml loss or patient was anaemic in pregnancy.

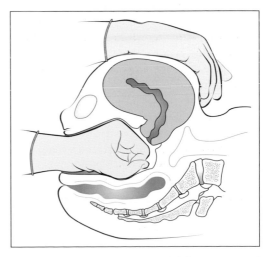

Figure 13.23 Bimanual compression of the uterus, wrapping it onto the clenched fist in the vagina.

- Empty bladder.
- If placenta still undelivered 30 min after birth of the baby, prepare for manual removal. Try one gentle, sterile, vaginal examination; placenta may be trapped by the closing cervix and an edge can sometimes be hooked down and the placenta gently eased out:
  — if an epidural is already acting, use this, otherwise a general anaesthetic is needed
  — try once more to remove placenta by controlled cord traction just before the anaesthetist induces sleep; sometimes separation has occurred in the meantime.
- Give a Syntocinon infusion and prophylactic antibiotics afterwards.
- Very rarely, the placenta may be abnormally adherent:
  — placenta accreta: villi just penetrate into myometrium
  — placenta increta: villi penetrate deeply into myometrium
  — placenta percreta: villi penetrate through myometrium to peritoneum.

Usually this is not possible to diagnose prospectively. If no plane of separation exists (and often there is little bleeding at the time) placenta accreta, increta or percreta must be thought of. Should the patient wish for no more children, the safest treatment is hysterectomy. If this is not possible, piecemeal removal is very dangerous and it is better to leave the placenta to atrophy with antibiotic control of infection.

Note: this is a very rare diagnosis made less often as the observer becomes more experienced.

Tears of genital tract

Heavy bleeding may occur from a tear of the cervix despite a well-contracted uterus and a completely expelled placenta.
- It is difficult to diagnose certainly and requires:
  — adequate general anaesthesia, unless epidural already acting
  — the woman in lithotomy position on a firm bed
  — good lights and good assistance

  — several sponge forceps and retractors (the vagina and cervix are soft just after delivery and tissues flop into the line of sight).
- Search cervix systematically using three pairs of ring forceps. If there is a tear:
  — check that it does not run up into uterus, especially if at 3 or 9 o'clock
  — suture with polyglycol absorbable material.
- Check lower uterine segment with fingers through the cervix. If a tear is found, either repair through abdominal incision or perform a hysterectomy.
- Check top end of episiotomy or tear which may go into posterior or lateral fornix: repair systematically.
- Check that no actively bleeding vessels in episiotomy or tear: tie them off separately.

Blood clotting defect

- Check that blood taken from an arm vein clots and stays clotted.
- Check:
  — platelets
  — coagulation studies.
- Treat appropriately by fresh frozen plasma (FFP): fibrinogen.
- Remember that such a state can allow secondary atony of the myometrium, so watch for that too as a cause of bleeding.

Effects of primary PPH

Rapid loss leads to hypovolaemic shock. If not corrected, this can cause the following:
- Death: about 8% of direct maternal deaths follow PPH; half of these are avoidable.
- Renal shutdown and consequent anuria.
- Damage to pituitary portal circulation causing necrosis and subsequent Sheehan's syndrome.
- Postpartum anaemia and chronic ill health.

Secondary PPH

This is abnormal vaginal bleeding that occurs after 24 hours following delivery. There is no volumetric definition; women usually present:

- with the passage of clots
- at 7–10 days with a resumption of fresh vaginal bleeding.

Causes

- Retained pieces of placenta
- Retained pieces of membrane
- Retained blood clot
- Infection of the residual decidua (endometritis).

Clinical findings

- Fresh red vaginal bleeding and clots
- A large uterus
- A tender uterus
- An open cervical internal os.

Risks

- Substantial bleeding.
- Infection:
  — septicaemia
  — blocked fallopian tubes.

Treatment

- Admit to hospital.
- Give intravenous broad-spectrum antibiotic cover, 24 hours preoperatively and continuing for a minimum of 3 days. This combats the bacteraemia that may occur and also reduces the risk of subsequent tubal damage.
- Carry out an evacuation of retained products of conception after 24 hours. This should be performed gently by a senior obstetrician because of the risk of perforation of the very soft uterus.

Massive blood loss

Rarely, a haemorrhage of 2–3 litres occurs suddenly at delivery. The woman's life will depend on a well-drilled team having a laid-down policy that should include a crash obstetric haemorrhage alert to the transfusion laboratory and the full obstetric and anaesthetic team.

Management

Massive loss from the woman's circulating blood volume of 2–3 litres in a few minutes. For practical purposes consider that it has happened if the woman has required more than 2 units of blood quickly.

In anticipation of blood loss all women are routinely grouped and screened for antibodies in the antenatal clinics. Furthermore all at high risk of haemorrhage during labour should be grouped and saved prospectively.

Action

- Put in two large-bore (at least 16 gauge) intravenous cannulae.
- Instigate the crash obstetric haemorrhage routine. Contact the duty obstetric registrar, if not already present, and the duty anaesthetic registrar. Call the obstetric consultant.
- Use one or more of the following fluids:
  — up to 2 litres of Hartmann's solution
  — up to 1.5 litres of Gelofusine
  — uncross-matched blood of the woman's group
  — cross-matched blood as soon as available
  — give O Rh-negative blood only as a last resort
  — in an emergency situation the use of blood filters and blood warming devices is not recommended; pressurized infusion bags should be used
  — give weight adjustment amount of FFP for every 6 units blood; the haematologist will advise on platelet replacement.
- Stop the bleeding. If the bleeding is from the uterus:
  — give 0.5 mg ergometrine (or Syntometrine) i.v. and set up 40 units Syntocinon in 50 ml Hartmann's solution to run at 4 ml/min
  — start bimanual compression of the uterus (see Fig. 13.23); if trauma, repair uterus/cervix/vagina
  — intrauterine injection of PGE_2 through abdominal wall up to five times every 5 min.
- Contact the blood bank. Send at least 20 ml blood for further cross-matching. Ask for at least 6 units of cross-matched blood.

- Inform the duty haematologist of the clinical situation, the rate of blood loss and the clotting problems.
- Insert a central venous line to monitor fluid replacement.
- One person should be assigned to record keeping and should record the following:
  — pulse
  — blood pressure
  — maternal heart rate, preferably from an ECG
  — central venous pressure
  — urine output
  — amount and type of fluids that the woman is given
  — drugs that the woman has received.
- Contact the interventional radiologist to perform uterine artery embolisation (see Fibroids).
- Prepare for theatre if appropriate.
- Before proceeding to hysterectomy, the following should be considered:
  — direct intramuscular injection of 0.5 mg PGE_2 into the exposed uterus
  — uterine artery embolization
  — Open the broad ligament and ligate the uterine artery on each side
  — Ligate internal iliac arteries.

The flying squad

Every major hospital doing obstetrics in the UK used to have available obstetricians and midwives who could be taken urgently to any patient who presented with an obstetric emergency outside the hospital environment. In some teams, which covered a larger area, an anaesthetist was included. The squad used to represent the patching up of a domiciliary and GP unit service.

Much of the real service has become a resuscitation one, the woman being brought to a state suitable for transfer back to the hospital where definitive treatment takes place. Problems at delivery have almost disappeared and the squad was being called inappropriately. A quarter of patients are given intravenous therapy but <1% had uncross-matched blood. Many of the calls related to normal women who had just delivered. The ambulance service transports such women but no flying squad is needed, but rather a community midwife or a paramedic.

The flying squad was introduced because private transport was rare, telephones were unusual and it was hard to get to the hospital. All that has changed and now, every time obstetricians, midwives and anaesthetists have to leave the centre to look after an individual, it leaves the larger number of women at that hospital with a diminished service.

Now paramedics in the ambulance services are trained in advanced resuscitation. They go to the home or GP unit and bring the woman safely into hospital.

A few flying squads persist in rural areas, but by 2004 virtually all had been closed down for the reasons discussed above.

Multiple pregnancies and deliveries

The human species is designed to have one baby at a time. Other multiples are rare (Table 13.4) and vary with racial characteristics inside the species (eg there is a higher incidence in West Africa than in Europe).

The differences between actual and theoretical figures are probably a result of the reducing birth rate, more births to older women and fewer to

Table 13.4 Rates of multiple pregnancies per 1000 deliveries in England and Wales in 1995 compared with the biologically expected rate

	Actual	Theoretical
Twins	13.6	12.5 (1 : 80)
Triplets	0.44	0.16 (1 : 80²)
Quadruplets and higher orders	0.014	0.02 (1 : 80³)

those of higher parity (both having increased multiple pregnancy rates). Higher rates in the UK are now caused by ovarian stimulation and assisted conception with a trebling of triplets with in vitro fertilization (IVF).

Twins

Types (Fig. 13.24)

Monovular twins (monochorionic/di- or monoamniotic)

Monovular twins are produced from one ovum fertilized by one sperm. After the two-cell division, instead of going into the four-cell stage, the blastomere divides into two separate cell bodies that go on to two individuals. Thus, there is common chromatin material; sex and physical characteristics will be the same, producing identical twins.

Binovular twins (dichorionic/di- or monoamniotic)

Binovular twins are from two separate ova fertilized by two different sperm. These ova are shed in one menstrual cycle and most likely to be fertilized after one intercourse, although they can be at separate times with different fathers. The two blastomeres develop separately and have different chromatin material. They can, therefore, be of different sexes, having no more in common than any other members of the same family. They are non-identical twins. Early ultrasound can help differentiation.

Incidence

Monovular twins have an incidence of 3 or 4 : 1000 worldwide and there is only a slight familial tendency. Binovular twins may have a family history on the maternal side. It is these that account for racial and maternal age variations. Binovular twins are more common than monovular ones (4 : 1). Binovular twins are more common if:

- maternal family history of non-identical twins
- >35 years
- After replacement of two, three or more fertilized ova at IVF.

Differentiation of twins

- Sex: if of different sexes, obviously binovular. If of one sex, may be either.
- *Placenta/chorion*: if two separated placentae, will be binovular; if one placenta, may be monovular or binovular (Fig. 13.25). Check septum between sacs

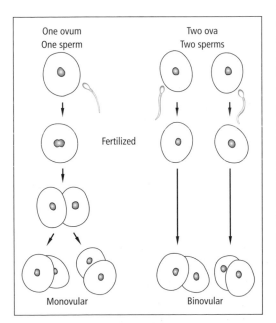

Figure 13.24 Biological differences in monovular and binovular twins.

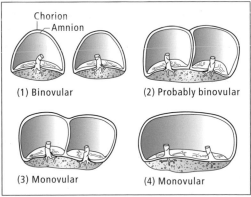

Figure 13.25 Placental types in twinning. Often the intervening membranes can be seen in early pregnancy on ultrasound and the two types of twins differentiated.

Table 13.5 Differentiation of twins by checking placentae

Septum	Placenta type	Twin type
(4) None	Monoamniotic Monochorionic	Monovular
(3) Amnion only	Diamniotic Monochorionic	Monovular
(2) Amnion and chorion	Diamniotic Dichorionic	Binovular or monovular
(1) No common septum	Diamniotic Dichorionic	Binovular

by peeling amnions from each other (Table 13.5). This can be detected on the ultrasound scan and is called the lambda sign.

- *Blood groups*: if doubt in dichorionic types, check the ABO, Rh, Duffy, Kell and MNS antibodies.
- Fingerprints: if different, binovular.
- *DNA fingerprinting* with probes identifying about 60 dispersed sequences of variable size.

Diagnosis of twins

History
- Suspicion on family history especially maternal non-identical twins.
- Suspicion on past obstetric history of twins.
- Suspicion from excessive vomiting in early pregnancy.

Examination
Examination from 20 weeks onwards shows a uterus that is bigger than expected. At first a lot of limbs are felt and later, about 30–32 weeks, more than two separate poles determined (eg two heads and one breech).

Investigation
Ultrasound at 6–7 weeks may show two or more sacs. The embryos can be seen in these at 7–8 weeks. The differentiation of mono- from binovular can often be made by expert examination of the dividing membranes.

Commonly one of a pair of twins diagnosed early does not develop and is absorbed: the vanishing twin syndrome.

Without ultrasound, twins may not be diagnosed until delivery on rare occasions. Although embarrassing to the attendants, this usually does not affect the second twin unless Syntometrine was given inadvertently at the birth of the first baby. This could jeopardize the O_2 supply to the second twin and so his or her delivery should be expedited.

Management of twins

Complications in pregnancy
- Miscarriage more frequent
- Preterm labour more common (50% before 37 weeks)
- Pre-eclampsia more common (×3)
- Risk of anaemia increased
- Iron deficiency
- Folic acid deficiency: polyhydramnios more common (×10 with monovular twins)
- Risk of APH increased:
  — abruptio placentae
  — placenta praevia.

Management in pregnancy

- Diagnose early by bearing it in mind (one diagnoses only what one thinks about); often ultrasound will give the result before the clinical suspicion.
- Give extra iron and folic acid supplements and see that the woman takes them: check blood more often for haemoglobin levels.

Complications in labour

- Delay in delivery of the second twin is associated with a higher mortality.
- PPH is more common.
- Prolapse of umbilical cord is more common.
- Mechanical collision of leading parts (or locking of a breech–cephalic) as they both enter the pelvis. This is very rare.

Management in labour

- Always plan for hospital delivery.
- Ensure that the first twin is longitudinal. Most common combinations of presentations show that both twins lie longitudinally 90% of the time and the first twin is a cephalic presentation in 80% (Fig. 13.26). Non-cephalic presentations are common if early preterm labour. If the first twin is transverse, do a caesarean section.
- Check for cord prolapse when membranes rupture (often early in labour).

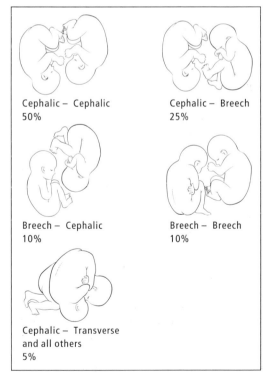

Cephalic – Cephalic
50%

Cephalic – Breech
25%

Breech – Cephalic
10%

Breech – Breech
10%

Cephalic – Transverse
and all others
5%

Figure 13.26 Presentation of twins at time of mature delivery (after 36 weeks).

- Progress is usually uneventful. Monitor both fetal hearts and have an intravenous drip running.
- An epidural anaesthetic is useful because it allows rapid anaesthesia for any manoeuvres that may be required for the second twin in the second stage.
- Deliver the first twin appropriately. Have an anaesthetist and a paediatrician in the labour ward. Make sure that nobody inadvertently gives Syntometrine to the mother at this point.
- Clamp cord of the first twin and divide. Hand baby to competent assistant or paediatrician in case resuscitation is required.
- Immediately check the lie of the second twin. If longitudinal, check presenting part. If oblique or transverse, convert to longitudinal:
  — external version: usually easy for uterus is lax, or
  — combined external and internal version: rupture membranes and bring a leg of the fetus down through the cervix. This produces an incomplete breech presentation but it is at least longitudinal.
- The second twin is best delivered within 60 min of the first. Usually uterus starts contracting again about 5 min after first delivery. If it does not do so spontaneously, use intravenous oxytocin augmentation. Very little is needed. Rupture membranes of second sac and deliver appropriately.
- Give Syntometrine with delivery of the second twin and continue oxytocin infusion for another hour.
- Deliver placentae as soon as uterus is contracted after delivery of the second twin, because retained placentae and PPH are common.

Outcome

Maternal
Higher risk:
- The complications of pregnancy, eg pre-eclampsia
- The complications of delivery, eg anaesthesia and PPH.

Fetal
- Risks to the first twin are twice, and to the second twin, about three times those of single births. Causes of death:

— immaturity}
— hypoxia}
— risks of operative delivery } Especially the second twin (only last band)

• Neonatal risks are jaundice or anaemia after intrauterine shunting of blood inside the placenta, leading to twin-to-twin transfusion in monovular twins.

Triplets

Rarely results from triovulation:

• Usually binovular twins with one fertilized egg dividing into two individuals or assisted conception.

• Usually born at an even more immature stage than twins and have double the risks.

• The complications and management are as for twins. As a result of the immaturity of the fetuses, delivery is commonly by caesarean section.

See www.nice.org.uk/nicemedia/pdf/ IntrapartumCareSeptember2007mainguideline.pdf

Chapter 14

Puerperium

In the puerperium the mother is returning to her pre-pregnant state. The various organ systems take different times but most physical restoration has occurred by 6 weeks. During this time, one should aim at:
- restoring maternal health and preventing illness
- maintaining infant health and preventing illness
- establishing infant feeding
- educating the mother about her child's and her own future health.

Physiological changes in genital tract

Uterus

Uterine bulk reduces by involution after withdrawal of oestrogens so that the organ is back in the pelvis by 10–12 days. The following occurs:
- Thrombosis of blood vessels
- Autolysis of cellular cytoplasm of myometrium
- Regeneration of endometrium within 6 weeks

The uterus never quite returns to nulliparous size but close to it. The cervix is normally stretched at

Lecture Notes: Obstetrics and Gynaecology, 3rd edition. By Diana Hamilton-Fairley. Published 2009 by Blackwell Publishing. ISBN: 978-1-4051-7801-3.

delivery and the external os is split after a delivery.

Vulva

After stretching, tissues revert to non-pregnant state with the following differences:
- Less fatty tissue in the labia
- Episiotomy or tear area leaves a scar that might be tender.

Management of first week

Observations

- Temperature: watch for pyrexia.
- Pulse rate: watch for transient tachycardia associated with thrombosis.
- Blood pressure: check especially if pre-eclampsia occurred in pregnancy.
- Uterine size: check daily reduction by abdominal palpation.
- Lochia: loss from vagina in the first days is the shedding of the decidua. Starts red with fresh blood but pales over 2 weeks to yellow–white. This may last for weeks.
- Urine output: normal diuresis starts within 24 hours and lasts about 3 days. If no urine has been passed after 6 hours palpate abdomen for enlarged bladder indicative of urinary retention.

- Bowels: often constipation. Avoid too long a gap for a very hard stool is painful. Provide fibre and extra fluids to give bulk to stools.
- Haemoglobin: check level about day 2 even if blood loss at delivery is recorded as minimal. Give oral iron if below 11 g/dl. Re-advise on diet.

Pain relief

Uterine contractions

- After-pains (contractions) are variable, painful and need analgesia.
- Warn the woman that they are coming so that she is prepared.
- Often felt more in multigravidae; worse after successive deliveries.

Perineal

- After the local anaesthetic/epidural wears off, the episiotomy will hurt. Further, oedema and burning may make sitting uncomfortable. Give analgesics, local heat and, if oedematous, ice packs.
- Check that sutures are not cutting in.

After caesarean section

This is a major abdominal operation and requires strong regular analgesia once the spinal or epidural has worn off. Diclofenac (a non-steroidal anti-inflammatory drug or NSAID) is often inserted per rectum at the end of the operation so that there are therapeutic levels of analgesia present when the regional block wears off. This can be supplemented with regular paracetamol and morphine derivatives as needed.

Bed rest

A balance must be struck between resting in bed to recover from the work of labour and resting so much that stagnation of blood leads to deep vein thrombosis.

Exercises

In association with bed rest, graduated exercises restore muscle tone to stretched areas and maintain venous flow in limbs and pelvis. They are aimed at:

- breathing exercises
- legs to prevent stagnation of blood in veins
- abdominal wall to restore tone of rectus muscles
- pelvic floor to restore levator ani.

Exercises are best taught by a physiotherapist in a clinical setting either antenatally or on the postnatal ward. Fifteen minutes twice a day should be set aside for these for some weeks or months. Pelvic floor exercises should be continued for life to prevent prolapse and urinary incontinence problems.

Psychological support

Having a baby is a major life event that changes a woman's way of life, and her role and responsibility within the family and society, and may affect her relationship with her partner. In the first few days circulating levels of oestrogen, progesterone and other steroidal hormones reduce rapidly and can have a profound effect on a woman's mood. In addition she is learning to breastfeed (see Chapter 15) and meet the needs of her newborn child. Women with different emotional backgrounds respond variously. Most women find a balance between the excitement and pleasure of the event, on the one hand, and the worry and responsibility of looking after the baby, on the other. Watch for this and prevent excessive worry by:

- adequate explanation of any baby problems
- ensuring good sleep
- pain relief
- support in the care of the baby.

Discharge home

The length of postnatal stay in hospital is determined by social and financial factors as well as by medical ones. The length of stay is reducing and the community services are supposed to take up their share of looking after those whom the hospital discharges. Recent national guidelines in the UK have recommended that all women should be visited regularly for the first 28 days and followed as needed for the first 3 months.

Many maternity units now offer a woman a named midwife/group of midwives who will provide full antenatal care, come into hospital, provide intrapartum and postnatal care both in the hospital and at home. Increasingly women looked after in this way are going home a few hours after delivery if mother and baby are well. Units are providing birth centres that are run by midwives, which may be co-located to an obstetric unit or some distance away. Guidelines must be in place for safe and rapid transfer of the woman if the labour, delivery or immediate postpartum phases do not proceed normally. The care offered by these systems has shown an increase in normal delivery rates with no increase in perinatal or maternal mortality for women with no risk factors. Most importantly the feedback from women looked after in this way shows much greater satisfaction than the older, more fragmented, medically led models. Women with risk factors should receive the same model and level of care but share their antenatal care with obstetricians and deliver in an obstetric unit with 24-hour obstetric, anaesthetic and paediatric cover.

Fifty per cent of women now leave the hospital by day 2 under planned discharge schemes evolved between the hospital and the local community midwives and general practitioners. Those who had uncomplicated caesarean sections go home at 3–5 days.

Advantages of earlier discharge

• Satisfaction: by providing better postnatal support in the community from midwives and health visitors women feel more confident about going home and being able to access appropriate advice as needed. Unfortunately resources have not been adequate to provide this ideal level of service to all women and this is reflected in the large differences in satisfaction ratings between those who are supported and those who are not.
• Leaves more beds available for those with antenatal/postnatal complications, allowing intensive care for the fetus or mother.
• Reduces the risks of hospital cross-infection. This was a rapidly diminishing factor in the UK but outbreaks of gastroenteritis and haemolytic streptococcal infection do still occasionally happen. The increasing numbers of bacteria that are resistant to antibiotics has led to an increase in hospital-acquired infection in recent years. Fortunately it has not been significant in maternity units but there is no room for complacency.

Disadvantages of earlier discharge

• Lack of rest: household duties soon demand the woman's attention.
• Poor housing conditions: if the woman is unsupported or from the lower income groups, she may be better kept in hospital for a little longer. This is a diminishing problem in the UK but a small proportion of homes (5–10%) are still considered to be unsuitable for early discharge.
• Medical problems after delivery may be missed. This is unlikely if proper community cover is given so that women who go home are visited by midwives and GPs by arrangement. In fact less than 2% of early discharged women are re-admitted for medical problems.

Problems in the puerperium

Over half of maternal deaths associated with pregnancy and childbirth occur in the first few days of delivery. Although rare, it is a measure of the need for vigilance; postnatal women should be seen each day for the first 10 days by a qualified doctor or midwife. Ideally a postnatal visit should be at about 6 weeks; this should be by the family practitioner if the delivery was straightforward or at the hospital if there were complications.

Psychological problems

The baby blues

Many women feel weepy and depressed 3–5 days after delivery but this is usually short-lived. Factors that prolong the baby blues are:
• postpartum pyrexia
• anaemia of <8 g/dl

- inadequate sleep
- delayed healing of the episiotomy or caesarean section wound
- delay in establishing breastfeeding
- decline in sympathy, congratulations and attention of friends and family as the time from childbirth increases.

Depression

Baby blues merge with serious depression. There is not a specific form of depression that is related solely to pregnancy and childbirth. The factors that aggravate depression are:
- a background predisposition due to previous history or family history
- a conflict in the responsibilities of looking after a new baby
- hormone changes acting on predisposition to depression
- fantasies
- anxiety and guilt
- residual pain
- sleeplessness.

   The signs of depression in the early days are recurrent bouts of weeping for no reason, anxiety, withdrawal, not responding to the baby and its needs, sleeplessness (even when the baby sleeps).

Treatment
- Involve a psychiatrist
- If no psychotic delusions, can be managed as an outpatient
- Oral antidepressants.

Postpartum psychosis

This is a rare condition that affects less than 1 in 500 women. It is potentially life threatening to both the mother and the baby.

Symptoms
- Rejection of the baby
- Delusion
- Confusion
- Agitation.

Management
- Admit the mother and baby to a special ward in the psychiatric unit
- Ensure 24-hour supervision
- Give appropriate psychotherapy drugs. Some use electroconvulsive therapy.

Postpartum psychosis is recurrent (about 20%) but chances are decreased by a gap of 2 years or more between pregnancies.

Infections

The following are the common infections of the puerperium:
- Infections of the genital tract
- Urinary tract infection
- Breast infections
- Wound infection (caesarean section/episiotomy)
- Endometritis.

Genital tract infection

An ascending infection that largely involves the placental bed. Unlike pelvic inflammatory disease (PID) it spreads directly through the uterus to the parametrial tissues.

   The most common organisms are *Escherichia coli* and *Streptococcus faecalis*.

   Rarely women can develop overwhelming sepsis from group A haemolytic streptococci (puerperal fever). They are often well or have a low-grade pyrexia with flu-like symptoms before becoming acutely unwell and developing multiorgan failure within a few hours, often leading to death. Although rare in the UK there are always cases reported in each triennial review of maternal deaths.

Diagnosis
History
- Puerperal pyrexia—temperature >38°C twice
- Offensive discharge
- Low abdominal pain
- Passage of clots and a return of red lochia
- Systemic symptoms associated with the pyrexia.

Examination
- Raised temperature and pulse
- Bulky uterus
- Tender uterus
- Offensive lochia (often bleeding with clots)
- An open internal cervical os.

Investigations
- Hb: may be reduced
- White cell count: raised with a neutrophilia
- Raised C-reactive protein
- High vaginal or endocervical swab: may grow the organisms
- Blood cultures to exclude septicaemia.

Management
- Admit to hospital
- Evacuation of retained products of conception under antibiotic cover.

Broad-spectrum antibiotics should be used to cover the bacteraemia and subsequently for 5 days.

Complications
Acute
- Parametritis
- Salpingitis
- Broad ligament abscess
- Peritonitis
- Septic thromboembolism.

Longer term
- Infertility
- Menstrual irregularities and pelvic pain.

Urinary tract infections

These are common in the puerperium because of:
- bladder stasis/urinary retention
- oedema of the bladder base
- periurethral bruising from vaginal trauma
- diminished bladder sensation
- catheterization in labour.

The common organisms are *E. coli* and *Proteus* spp.

Diagnosis
History
- Dysuria

- Frequency of micturition
- Loin pain if pyelonephritis supersedes
- Systemic symptoms such as pyrexia and tachycardia
- May be asymptomatic and recognized on routine midstream urine (MSU) sample. This should be performed on all patients who have been catheterized in labour.

Examination
- Raised temperature
- Tender suprapubically or in the renal angle.

Investigations
- MSU
- White cell count
- C-reactive protein
- Nitrites and leukocytes on dipstick
- Blood cultures if temperature >38°C.

Management
- Bed rest
- High-fluid, light, solid diet
- Broad-spectrum antibiotics until the results of culture and sensitivity are known; then be specific.

Complications
- Pyelonephritis
- Exacerbation of the baby blues.

Breast infection

This usually enters through a break in the skin (cracked nipple). It is usually confined to one quadrant of the breast. Most commonly it is caused by *Staphylococcus aureus*.

Diagnosis
History
Painful area of one breast.

Examination
- Raised temperature
- Erythematous segment of the breast
- If an abscess, brawny swelling or even fluctuation.

Investigation
Bacteriology of expressed breast milk from the affected side.

Management
Without abscess
- Supportive brassière
- Continue breastfeeding on other breast and empty the affected breast with a breast pump
- Give broad-spectrum antibiotic such as flucloxacillin orally.

With abscess
- Incise under a general anaesthetic
- Circumareola incision
- Break down septa and leave a drain through dependent part
- Adequate supportive brassière
- Appropriate intravenous antibiotics.

Thromboembolism

The postpartum period is the most common time in pregnancy for a thromboembolism because of the following:
- Increased coagulation: the increase in clotting factors from pregnancy remains, although plasma volume reduces to normal within a few hours of delivery.
- Stasis: many women have been immobilized in pregnancy, during labour or during the immediate puerperium.
- Damage to venous endothelium:
  — uterine veins: after uterine sepsis
  — deep leg veins: weight of legs compresses veins if immobilized.

Diagnosis
History
- Calf pain
- Unilateral leg oedema.

Examination
- A low-grade postpartum pyrexia
- An unexplained maternal tachycardia
- Tenderness over the deep veins of the calf
- Positive Holman's sign (calf tenderness on dorsiflexion of the foot).

Investigations
- Doppler ultrasound:
  — simple continuous wave Doppler ultrasound will fail to show flow in the femoral vein
  — colour flow Doppler may demonstrate the clot in the veins.
- Venography: this is the definitive test using image intensifiers and low-viscosity contrast medium.

Management
Prevention
- Early mobilization: all women are encouraged to be up as soon as they wish. Non-weight-bearing exercises used for postoperative mothers.
- Prophylaxis is usually given to women who have had a previous history of thromboembolism or are at moderate to high risk:
  — compression (TED [thromboembolic deterrent] stockings worn during labour or caesarean section)
  — subcutaneous low-molecular-weight heparin (LMWH).

Treatment
- Anticoagulate immediately with full-dose, subcutaneous LMWH to prevent further extension of the thrombosis with the risk of pulmonary embolism and allow earlier recanalization of the clotted veins.
- Long-term anticoagulation with warfarin for 12 weeks.

Pulmonary embolism

The most dangerous destination of a clot embolus from the leg or pelvic veins is in the pulmonary circulation:
- Mild cases follow microemboli. Dyspnoea and slight, poorly defined pleural pain. The condition resolves in a few days with no specific treatment and may not even be diagnosed.
- Severe cases arise from clot from the:
  — soleal veins: clot extends to popliteal vein and breaks off (30%)
  — uterine and ovarian veins: a thrombophlebitis with a friable clot after mid-pelvic sepsis (20%).

In 50%, no clinical signs of the origin exist before the pulmonary embolism.

Diagnosis

History

Pre-existing deep vein thrombosis (in half the cases only).

EARLY

- Acute tachypnoea
- Faintness
- Tachycardia
- Sudden-onset pleuritic chest pain.

LATER

- Chest pain
- Haemoptysis.

Examination

EARLY

No physical signs beyond dyspnoea.

LATER

- May be cyanosis
- Local signs of pulmonary underperfusion
- Right heart failure.

LATER STILL

- Pleural signs.
- Collapse of a pulmonary lobe.

Investigations

Often no positive tests early. Next day:

- X-ray:
  — raised diaphragm on affected side.
  — consolidation and infiltration of lung(s).
- ECG: rhythm disturbance.
  — lead I: S-wave inversion
  — lead III: T-wave inversion and deep Q wave
  — leads V1, -2, -3, -4: T-wave inversion
  — excludes cardiac infarction.

Arterial blood gases

- Lung ventilation–perfusion studies with radioactive albumin to show ischaemic areas.
- CT of chest

- Left and right heart catheterization to show reversal of pressures.

The last is only used in specialist thoracic units.

Management

Two-thirds of those dying do so within 2 hours, so act quickly on suspicion, not awaiting the sophisticated tests even if they are available.

Immediate treatment

- External cardiac massage if required
- Positive pressure O_2 by intubation if necessary
- Heparin (see below)
- Emergency embolectomy is only performed in hospitals with their own thoracic units with bypass facilities and rarely used.

Definitive treatment

If resuscitation is successful, give the following:

- Anticoagulants (more intravenous heparin):
  — 25 000 units immediately
  — 25 000 units 6-hourly for 24 hours.
  This is to prevent further emboli.
  At the same time start warfarin oral therapy controlled by prothrombin time.
- Thrombolytics (streptokinase). Actively accelerate lysis of existing clot:
  — 500 000 units immediately
  — 100 000 units hourly for 72 hours.
- Embolectomy (mortality rate 25%). Useful if:
  — thoracic unit in the same hospital
  — no response to streptokinase
  — too ill for streptokinase
  — contraindication to streptokinase, eg recent surgery, peptic ulcer or hypertension.

Both high-dose heparin and streptokinase have high risks of starting bleeding. Not indicated unless embolus is thought to be life threatening. If started, reduce to conservative dosage in 2–3 days and continue for 4–6 weeks.

Secondary postpartum haemorrhage

Any considerable fresh bleeding occurring in the puerperium after 24 hours. This is dealt with in Chapter 13.

Previous diseases continuing into the puerperium

Pre-eclampsia and eclampsia

When these conditions occur before delivery, their ultimate treatment is delivery of the baby. Usually the woman gets better rapidly after the placenta has been delivered and the normal diuresis starts to remove the water/salt overload. A few women stay as bad or worsen in the first few days of the puerperium. Management is the same as in pregnancy (see pp. 135–6). Postpartum eclampsia has a high mortality rate.

Diabetes

Delivery may have been operative and for a day immediately after the woman may be on intravenous therapy. Remember that insulin requirements drop very sharply in the puerperium so that many women with diabetes are at their pre-pregnant levels of insulin by 2 days into the puerperium. Infection of any wounds is more likely and breastfeeding may be an irregular drain of carbohydrates, making insulin balance more difficult.

Heart disease

The first 24 hours of the puerperium are dangerous, because the post-delivery shunting of blood from the uterine vessels may lead to pulmonary oedema and subsequent right-sided cardiac failure. After that the risk is reduced.

Puerperal infection could release bacteria that might colonize on any damaged endothelium in the heart (acute bacterial endocarditis). This is more likely to follow a congenital heart disease than rheumatic conditions, but antibiotic cover is often provided for either into the puerperium.

Ovarian tumours

These are more likely to undergo torsion in the puerperium because of the lax abdominal wall and the diminishing uterus. Surgery is recommended for any ovarian masses >10 cm diameter.

Chapter 15

The newborn

Evaluation at birth

The most usual assessment of the newborn recorded is the Apgar score (Table 15.1), which mixes two precise observations (heart rate and respiration) with three more subjective ones.

It is not a guide to prognosis but a description of the baby's condition at birth and response to resuscitation.

If there are any problems of respiration, a sample of cord blood is taken for pH and base deficit estimation.

Immediate management

Temperature

Newborn babies cool rapidly and need to be kept warm:
- Dry and wrap in a warmed, sterile, cotton blanket.
- Room temperature after birth should be 23–25°C.

Infection

All babies are at a higher risk of infection:
- Wipe baby clean of vernix, blood and meconium after birth.

Lecture Notes: Obstetrics and Gynaecology, 3rd edition. By Diana Hamilton-Fairley. Published 2009 by Blackwell Publishing. ISBN: 978-1-4051-7801-3.

- Wash eyes, face, skin, flexures and genitals at each nappy change.
- Regular cleaning of umbilical cord stump until separation.

Examination

All newborn babies should be examined soon after delivery and a detailed examination repeated within the first 24 hours of life. The first examination is often done by the doctor or midwife in charge of the delivery, the second by a paediatrician (Box 15.1).

Cord care

- Reclamp cord with plastic clip.
- Keep dry after washing.
- No dressings, because the stump dries quicker if exposed to air.
- It should separate on about days 8–10.

Blood glucose

Small-for-dates, preterm and infants of mothers with diabetes are at risk of hypoglycaemia. BMStix should be checked regularly in these babies and any others at risk. If 2 mmol/l or less, a paediatrician should be informed.

Screening tests

- Two blood spots on day 6:
  — Guthrie test, to detect raised level of phenylalanine indicating phenylketonuria;

Table 15.1 Apgar score performed at 1, 5 and 10 minutes after birth

Sign	Score 0	Score 1	Score 2
Heart rate	Absent	<100	>100
Respiratory effort	Absent	Irregular	Good, crying
Muscle tone	Flaccid	Some limb tone	Active
Reflex irritability	None	Cry or grimace	Vigorous cry
Colour	White	Blue	Pink

Box 15.1 Suggested items to be checked at first examination

General observations
- Breathing pattern and rate
- Neurological behaviour, cry and movements
- Skin pallor and cyanosis

Head
- Anterior fontanelle: tension
- Eyes: check epicanthic folds and for subconjunctival haemorrhages
- Lip and palate: check for cleft

Upper limbs
- Count digits and note interdigital webbing
- Palmar creases

Chest
- Auscultate for:
(a) Respiratory sounds
(b) Heart sounds: a faint heart murmur heard during the initial examination is usually innocent. Check daily if murmur heard

Abdomen
- Umbilicus: check two arteries and one vein
- Umbilical hernia
- Palpate abdomen for masses
- Groins:
  (a) Femoral pulses
  (b) Hernias
- Anus: check patency

Genitalia
- Female: clitoris size
- Male: hypospadias, undescended testes and hydrocele

Back
- Myelomeningocele
- Midline hairy patch, suggesting spina bifida occulta
- Straight spine: any kyphosis or scoliosis

Lower limbs
- Examine hips for congenital dislocation
- Number of digits
- Talipes deformities of ankles and feet

Measurements of body size
- Weight
- Occipitofrontal head circumference
- Crown–heel length

— thyroid-stimulating hormone (TSH) assay. Raised level indicates hypothyroidism.

If either test is positive, paediatric evaluation is needed:

- Babies of Rh-negative mothers should have blood group, haemoglobin, Coombs' test and bilirubin on umbilical cord blood at delivery.

• Babies at high risk for inherited disorders from a positive family history should be seen by paediatricians early and necessary treatment undertaken, eg cystic fibrosis, clotting disorders, inborn errors of metabolism.

The newborn after delivery

If a preterm or at-risk infant is to be delivered, an experienced paediatrician should be on hand.

As soon as the infant is born, assess its condition. A shorthand analysis is in the Apgar score. The three essential states may be:

1 *Healthy*: pink; effective regular respiration.

2 *Inadequate breathing*: irregular, shallow or gasping respiration.

3 *Terminal apnoea*: white; floppy; no attempt to breathe.

Care of the second and third stages is in the hands of the paediatrician (see Newell S, Darling J (2007) *Lecture Notes: Paediatrics*, 8th edn. Blackwell Publishing, Oxford).

Healthy

• If upper airway contains meconium, blood or mucus, then laryngoscope and aspirate trachea and larynx under direct vision.

• Wrap in a blanket and hand to mother.

Inadequate breathing

• If not already present, call paediatrician urgently. Carry out the following:
  — facemask O_2
  — gentle peripheral stimulation
  — oropharyngeal suction
  — dry and cover the body with warm towels.

• If the infant does not respond to this by 1–1.5 min (ie respiration not established and heart rate falling below 60 beats/min) start inflation breaths; extend neck, hold jaw forward and apply facemask closely to face to obtain a tight seal and give five 500 ml intermittent positive-pressure ventilation (IPPV) breaths through the mask before commencing cardiac massage while continuing mask ventilation at about 30 breaths/min, 100% O_2.

• If the infant still remains blue with inadequate respiration and a falling heart rate at 2–2.5 min, laryngoscope, aspirate any mucus or meconium under direct vision, and intubate. Give IPPV at pressures of 20 cmH_2O (a little more if lungs are stiff) and a rate of 30/min.

• As soon as the infant improves with any of the above (ie heart rate 140 beats/min, spontaneous respiration and pink in colour) remove endotracheal tube; watch for respiration to be established.

• Analgesics such as pethidine or morphine given to the mother late in labour depress respiration in the infant. Naloxone can be given (10 µg/kg estimated weight i.v. or i.m.). Do not give naloxone to the baby of a drug-dependent mother because this may cause withdrawal, fits or death.

• There is no indication for analeptic drugs in the management of birth asphyxia.

• Preterm babies need intubation earlier than term babies.

• Do not perform IPPV with a mask on very small babies.

Terminal apnoea

• Do not delay resuscitation if, at this stage, the infant is still pale, limp and apnoeic with a heart rate of less than 100.

• If not there, call paediatrician urgently.

• Laryngoscope, aspirate under direct vision and intubate. Give IPPV: rate 30/min, 20–30 cmH_2O with 100% O_2:
  — may require naloxone if mother given pethidine.

• If still apnoeic, assume birth asphyxia likely and give sodium bicarbonate i.v. and adrenaline via endotracheal tube under supervision of paediatrician.

• Cord blood at birth to estimate pH and base deficit.

• Admit to neonatal unit if:
  — poor response to resuscitation
  — base deficit >15 mmol/l.

- Let mother hold baby before transfer to neonatal unit, if possible.

Feeding

Babies are best breastfed; in the UK 68% of mothers do at first and 30% are still breastfeeding at 16 weeks. Mothers should be given advice in the antenatal period when breastfeeding should be encouraged.

Women with HIV are advised not to breastfeed because it increases the rate of vertical transmission between mother and baby. In areas where the water is not clean and the woman does not have access to boiled and disinfected water, the risk of gastroenteritis may outweigh that of acquiring HIV and so she may still be advised to breastfeed.

Breast

Mothers who wish to breastfeed put the baby to the breast for a few minutes at each side in the labour ward or certainly within 4 hours of birth.

- The infant will initially obtain only a small amount of colostrum when he sucks but this contains anti-infective substances. By sucking, the infant stimulates the production of more colostrum and then milk.
- Most of the feed is obtained within the first 3–5 minutes. The time that the baby is on the breast is not proportional to the amount of milk received.
- Baby takes the nipple towards the back of the mouth, not just between the gums.
- The most satisfactory method of breastfeeding is on demand. A rigid regimen of feeding is not to be encouraged. Infants who are initially fed on demand usually settle down within a few weeks to a regular pattern of feeding every 3–4 hours. In general, hungry babies cry and it is difficult to overfeed a breastfed baby.
- If lactation is insufficient in the first few days, breastfeeding should not be abandoned. Help and guidance should be given to the mother by one midwife, as often breastfeeding is not established until mother and baby are at home and in the second week.

Factors that help breastfeeding

- Motivation: encouragement at antenatal classes
- Good midwife or health visitor with plenty of time to advise
- Adequate fluid in mother's diet
- Baby awake and mother comfortable
- Change nappy before feeding to have a contented baby
- Proper brassière to hold breasts correctly.

Factors that hinder breastfeeding

- Mother does not really wish to feed
- Inverted, retracted nipples
- Poor fixation on the nipple
- Child with deformity of palate, tongue or lips.

Advantages of breastfeeding

- Breast milk protein, fat and solute content designed for human babies
- Promotes infant–mother bonding
- Contains anti-infective agents: active white cells, macrophages, IgA, IgG and lactoferrin
- Eliminates risk of infection from dirty bottles
- Cheap and always available on demand.

Problems in first week

- Engorged breasts: days 5–10 when breastfeeding is uncomfortable
- Cracked nipples
- Excessive air swallowing during first morning feed: too rapid flow of milk.

Formula or bottle milk

All cows' milk preparations in the UK are low solute milks. They have sodium and protein concentrations similar to those in human milk and most have added vitamins. Only these preparations should be used in newborn infants.

- A normal full-term infant receives about 60 ml/kg on the first day of bottlefeeding. This should then be increased to 150 ml/kg/day by the end of the first week. This is usually divided into 6 feeds/24 hours, eg 75 ml in each feed for a 3-kg baby.
- Make up feeds according to instructions. If feeds are made up for 24 hours, keep in refrigerator.

- Wash bottles and teats, then sterilize with dilute hypochlorite solution.
- When feed is due, place bottle in pan of hot water or microwave and warm milk to temperature acceptable to back of hand. However, feeding at room temperature does not cause any problems.
- Solids should start around 4 months or earlier if the baby can take them and weighs more than 6.5 kg.

Problems

- Protein, fat and solute load not exactly the same as human breast milk
- Lacks anti-infective properties of breast milk
- Teat hole is too large (too much milk) or too small (too little milk)
- Dirty bottles may lead to infections
- Cost of formula milks.

Neonatal jaundice

Nearly all babies become mildly jaundiced after 3–5 days. This is due to the breakdown of red blood cells with haemoglobin F while they are replaced with red blood calls with haemoglobin A. For most babies this is a self-limiting condition that requires no treatment. If the jaundice persists or the baby becomes deeply jaundiced, sleepy and refuses to feed, the bilirubin level should be checked. Using a neonatal bilirubin chart the value is plotted and the baby may require phototherapy for a few days.

Rhesus negative babies or babies born with an ABO/other red blood cell (RBC) antibody incompatibility with their mother may become severely jaundiced within 24–48 hours of birth. If the bilirubin levels become very high, they may require an exchange transfusion to prevent bilirubin being deposited in the supraventricular nuclei of the brain, causing kernicterus. Kernicterus is associated with deafness, delay in development and sometimes fitting.

Statutory duties of the health professionals after birth

As well as the moral obligations of doctors, midwives and health visitors, statutory duties are laid down for each in relation to a woman who is pregnant, in labour or recently delivered. The woman may book for her delivery at a variety of sites; basically in an institution, a midwifery-led unit or at home. The woman has a legal right to choose where she wants to deliver and the midwifery services have to back this up. It is the duty of the services to provide these options safely. Deliveries away from home are safe if the woman is properly assessed for risks and the woman appropriately advised. The supervisor of midwives in the health district has a duty to provide a midwife wheresoever a woman wishes to deliver and however inadvisable this might be on medical or midwifery grounds. It is wise not to refuse a woman a home/out-of-hospital delivery when she first raises the issue because it is vital that she receives the best antenatal care, and conflict about the site of delivery early in pregnancy could adversely affect this care. Discussions should continue through pregnancy and most women with complex needs who would be safest in hospital will agree with this over time.

GPs rarely provide intrapartum care in this country, although a few continue in remote communities here and across the world. They may not wish to cover the obstetric adventures of the woman who does not take advice and they have no obligation to do so. If a midwife looking after a pregnant or labouring woman runs into difficulty, she usually calls upon the emergency duty GP or local hospital maternity unit. If the woman refuses transfer, the GP has an obligation to attend and help. Perhaps that help will be passed on swiftly to the nearest hospital, but the doctor on duty must advise if called, although he or she may disapprove of the proceedings.

After the delivery there is an obligation for the woman to be under the care of a midwife for 10 days, although visiting may not be daily. At this point there is a handover to the health visitor who takes on the care of the mother and the child. Health visitors are first-rate community workers but they have to look after the whole spectrum of life and, with an increasing load of older people, it is difficult for some health visitors to fit in all that they would wish to do for the recently delivered woman and her baby. Recent recommendations advise that the midwife should continue to visit for up to 3 months for women at increased need and 28 days for less serious complications. The midwifery service is currently understaffed, particularly for postnatal care so that many women are not visited every day for the first 10 days with little chance of extending beyond the 10 days.

Part 4

The Mature Woman

Chapter 16

Abnormal vaginal blood loss

There are many Latin words to describe abnormal vaginal bleeding. It is better to use Anglo-Saxon and describe the symptoms as *heavy periods* or *prolonged periods* but the classic terms are still in use and need definition:

- *Menorrhagia* is an excessive loss of blood (>80 ml) with regular menstruation.
- *Metrorrhagia* is prolonged bleeding from the uterus.
- *Metro-menorrhagia* is heavy and prolonged periods.
- *Polymenorrhoea* is frequent menstruation.

  These may be associated with the following:
- Complications of early and undiagnosed pregnancy.
  — miscarriage
  — ectopic pregnancy
  — hydatidiform mole.

  A pregnancy test should be performed if there is any doubt.
- Foreign bodies in the uterus: intrauterine contraceptives.
- Psychosomatic causes, eg a severe emotional shock, may induce irregular bleeding.
- An abnormal bleeding tendency may be present such as leukaemia or Hodgkin's disease.

Lecture Notes: Obstetrics and Gynaecology, 3rd edition. By Diana Hamilton-Fairley. Published 2009 by Blackwell Publishing. ISBN: 978-1-4051-7801-3.

- Hyper- or hypothyroidism may be associated with menorrhagia or irregular bleeding.

Intermittent/intermenstrual bleeding

The causes of non-cyclical abnormal vaginal bleeding not associated with menstruation include:
- *lesions of the cervix*: polyps, carcinoma, ectropion (see Plates 13)
- *lesions of the body of the uterus*: endometritis, fibroids, polyps, adenomyosis, carcinoma, sarcoma (see Plates 7, 8).

  Treatment is with hormones, especially in menopausal and postmenopausal women. Breakthrough bleeding may occur with synthetic progestogens given for oral contraception or for treatment of pelvic disorders.

Menorrhagia

The range of normal menstrual loss is 10–80 ml per cycle. If >80 ml, this is considered excessive. More commonly, diagnosis is made on the woman's history:
- Increase in the number and thickness of pads or tampons used to more than 10 per day (5 ml/regular sized tampon)
- Starting to pass clots in the menstrual flow
- Use of a pictorial blood loss assessment chart which gives a semiquantitative measure of loss.

Up to 30% of women in the later part of menstrual life complain of heavy periods. Only a half of these actually lose more than 80 ml blood per period. The diagnosis, however, rests on the woman's history rather than scientific measurement.

The level of haemoglobin is generally lower in women aged between 15 and 50 than in men; this difference is accounted for by blood loss and the consequent iron deficiency associated with menstruation and child bearing. Menorrhagia or metrorrhagia can lead to anaemia, but many women with true heavy loss are able to respond to the chronic repeated demand on their bone marrow, although they may require iron therapy.

Aetiology

Menorrhagia commonly is a presenting symptom in:
- fibroids if increase uterine mucosal area (submucous, polyp)
- adenomyosis (endometrium within the uterine muscle wall (see Chapter 17))
- endometritis
- incorrectly controlled hormone therapy (including oral contraception).

Less commonly, it is associated with:
- endometrial polyps
- an intrauterine device (IUD)
- recent tubal ligation (usually secondary to stopping the contraceptive pill which has kept periods artificially light)
- functional ovarian tumours
- disorders of clotting (e.g. von Willebrand's disease).

Menorrhagia is not caused by idiopathic thrombocytopenic purpura.

After full examination and investigation (ultrasound scan, full blood count [FBC], endometrial biopsy in women over 40) in about 50% of women with true menorrhagia, no obvious pathology is found. This is *dysfunctional uterine bleeding* (DUB), implicating a malfunction of the endocrine controlling systems. A better name would be *menorrhagia of unknown origin*.

Clinical course

Although menorrhagia is most commonly found in those aged over 35 years, it can occur at any stage in female life up to the menopause. The causes and management may be classified according to age group.

Birth to 18 years of age

See Chapter 4.

Women aged 18–40 years

In this group true dysfunctional bleeding is uncommon and the most likely cause of abnormal bleeding is some complication of pregnancy or polycystic ovary syndrome (PCOS; see Chapter 4). Occasionally heavier periods follow tubal ligation for sterilization. Endometrial biopsy is rarely needed in this group because the possibility of malignant disease is unusual.

Women aged >40

All the organic causes of bleeding, including malignant disease, may occur and it is essential to exclude them.

Investigation

FBC: a haemoglobin of <11.5 g/dl is indicative of heavy menstrual loss.

Transvaginal ultrasound shows:
- Endometrial thickness should be <12 mm in perimenopausal women.
- Endometrial thickness should be <5 mm in postmenopausal women.
- Endometrial polyps: these can be better visualized by putting 10–20 ml 0.9% saline into the cavity (see Plate 7).
- Fibroids.
- Ovarian pathology in women with PCOS.

Endometrial biopsy should be done in:
- women aged >40
- women with abnormal endometrial thickness
- women with endometrial polyps.

This may be done in the outpatient department by using a thin tube that can suck the endometrium into itself by creating a vacuum, or by the use of a biopsy forceps. With appropriate skills, passing these causes little discomfort, about the same as fitting an IUD. This avoids admission and the general anaesthetic for dilatation and curettage (D&C). However, a fuller curettage is indicated if:

• it is impossible to pass the curette because of a tight cervix
• the woman is anxious and cannot relax
• there is a high risk of malignancy of the endometrium.

Hysteroscopy may accompany the curettage in the outpatient department if the gynaecologist is skilled and properly equipped. It is excellent at showing endometrial polyps and submucous fibroids (Plate 8), which could be missed by blind curettage. In many cases an organic diagnosis will be made and appropriate treatment be given.

Cervical smear to exclude carcinoma *in situ* or cervical intraepithelial neoplasia (CIN) (see Chapter 19).

Among women without organic disease, three main patterns of the endometrium are seen on histological examination:

1 *Atrophic* (postmenopausal).

2 A *mixed pattern* with proliferative and secretory endometrium with possible endometrial polyps. This is associated with irregular shedding of the endometrium because the normal mechanism of ovulation is disordered so that the endometrium is irregularly or excessively shed.

3 *Hyperplasia* of the endometrium may involve the glands or the stroma or both. *Cystic hyperplasia* is common in perimenopausal women. There is usually amenorrhoea followed by prolonged bleeding from the hyper-oestrogenized endometrium. A similar pattern is seen with an oestrogen-secreting tumour of the ovary. There is no great risk of cystic hyperplasia going on to carcinoma of the endometrium. Atypical hyperplasia is, however, more likely to be associated with endometrial carcinoma, the risk depending on the degree of atypia.

Management of dysfunctional uterine bleeding

Treatment should never be given without accurate diagnosis except perhaps in girls under 18 with puberty bleeding. All the above investigations should yield a normal result before commencing treatment. Blind hormone treatment is particularly dangerous as malignant disease may be masked.

Drug therapy

This is the first line of treatment because it:
• retains the uterus, a major factor for most women
• avoids surgery with general anaesthesia
• is more convenient, being administered in the outpatient department or GP surgery
• is much cheaper:
— to the health service
— to the woman.

Drug treatment may be non-hormonal (first line) or hormonal (second line) (Boxes 16.1 and 16.2).

Surgical therapy

Based on removal of the endometrium or the uterus with its endometrium.

Curettage
• Removes outer layers of endometrium but leaves the basal layers from which new tissue arises in a month or so.

> **Box 16.1 Non-hormonal treatment**
>
> Taken during menses hence no problem if accidental pregnancy is present
> *Prostaglandin synthetase inhibitors*
> Reduce uterine prostaglandins
> *Fenamates*
> Mefenamic acid 500 mg 6-hourly during menstruation
> Avoid if peptic ulceration
> *Antifibrinolytic agents*
> Reduce abnormal fibrinolysis
> Avoid if history of thrombosis
> Tranexamic acid 1 g 6-hourly during menstruation
> Ethamsylate 500 mg 4-hourly during menstruation

Box 16.2 Hormonal treatment

This aims at imitating or restoring the normal endocrine cycle

Norethisterone	5 mg three times a day for 6–9 months
Medroxyprogesterone acetate	Best for those with anovular cycles
	Cheap and good for emergency treatment: 10 mg three times a day for very heavy bleeding
Danazol	200 mg daily continuously for 3–6 months
	Derivative of testosterone so anti-oestrogenic at hypothalamus and at endometrium
	Expensive. May cause weight gain and androgenization
Oral contraceptive	Dose according to brand but probably best to use cyclical combined oestrogen (30 μg) and progestogen (0.25 mg)
	Practical, cheap and easily available
Mirena IUS (intrauterine system)	Progestogen IUS 75 μg/day to uterine lining only

---

- Ineffective as a treatment: one or two menses may be less heavy but are soon back to previous levels or heavier.

Local ablation

- Balloons, heated with 80°C water (thermal ablation)
- Microwave local destruction (microwave ablation)
- Free flowing heated water to 98°C (hydroablation).

Transcervical ablation

- Under vision through a hysteroscope, endometrium is destroyed:
  — with electrocoagulating loops
  — with a laser.
- At present, uses general anaesthesia but needs only 1 day or less in hospital:
  — uterus retained although lining (mostly) gone
  — after a year, 30% have amenorrhoea and another 60% report lighter blood loss
  — if it fails (10–20%), can proceed to either repeat ablation or to hysterectomy.
- It is not a minor operation:
  — requires manipulative skills
  — requires expensive equipment
  — risks of perforating uterus (1%)
  — risks of artery damage and bleeding (<1%)
  — risks of damaging bowel (<1%).
- However, saves time and hospital stay:
  — early return to normal activity
  — keeping uterus makes it popular

— contraception is still required unless there is complete amenorrhoea.

Hysterectomy

Removal of the uterus stops periods.

Abdominal hysterectomy

- Major procedure with general anaesthesia
- Abdominal scar to heal
- Hospital stay 4–6 days
- Risks of damage to ureters <1%
- Risks of damage to the bladder <1%
- Risks of damage to the bowel <1%.

Vaginal hysterectomy

- Needs to be a mobile, adhesion-free uterus
- Uterus not greatly enlarged
- Helps if there is some prolapse.

Laparoscopy-assisted hysterectomy

- Smaller abdominal incision
- Needs skilled laparoscopic surgeon
- Does the difficult part of a vaginal hysterectomy from above ligating tubes, ovarian suspensory ligament and round ligament via laparoscopy; then an easy vaginal removal
- Has all the complications of laparoscopic surgery.

Hysterectomy does not have to be accompanied by removal of ovaries. Increasingly the uterine arteries are also ligated laparoscopically and the uterus removed, leaving the cervix. The uterus is morcellated so that it can be extracted from the abdominal cavity through a 1-cm incision.

Indications for oophorectomy

- If ovaries abnormal
- If family history of ovarian cancer
- Consider if >45 years old and/or perimenopausal. Full informed consent is essential.

Retain:

- if menses cycling regularly
- if ovaries healthy at surgery
- if patient wishes.

Atrophic vaginitis

Secondary to a lack of oestrogens postmenopausally, the epithelium becomes thin, smooth and shiny with subepithelial haemorrhages. Low-grade infection from pathogens, which can more easily penetrate the surface, may occur.

Symptoms

- Vulval soreness
- Superficial dyspareunia
- Pink discharge
- Introital shrinking.

Physical signs

Red shiny epithelium with skin cracking and subcuticular haemorrhages. Occasionally causes postmenopausal bleeding. It is important to exclude other causes such as carcinoma.

Treatment

If there is secondary infection, antibiotics to which the organism is sensitive may be given. Topical oestrogen creams or pessaries can be used, eg dienoestrol or Premarin once or twice a week. This is enough to thicken the epithelium and reduce the pH, but insufficient to produce excessive endometrial stimulation.

Endometrial polyps

If the endometrium hypertrophies under oestrogen stimulation, areas of it may protrude above the surface, producing a sessile or eventually a pedunculated polyp. This may not be shed at the time of menstruation, but forms a site for persistent symptoms and signs.

Symptoms

There may be intermenstrual spotting or postmenstrual spotting.

Signs

There would be no signs, but an ultrasound and hysteroscopy would show the polyp.

Management

Endometrial polyps should be removed. Those inside the uterus will mostly require an anaesthetic and have to be twisted off with a polyps forceps or diathermy loop, although small ones can be removed in outpatients. Should the endometrial polyp stalk be long and the polyp present at the cervix, it is probably wise not to remove it in outpatients, because this could lead to heavy bleeding. A curettage with hysteroscopy should be performed at the same time to allow removal of any other polyps that are higher up and exclude any associated atypia/malignancy.

Pre- and postoperative care

Gynaecological operations are best learnt in the operating theatre, preferably acting as a scrubbed assistant, but the pre- and postoperative care must be understood by a wider range of medical personnel than just the surgeon.

Preoperative care

History

A complete history is taken with special attention to any recent illness. The date of the last period should be noted, to ensure that the patient is not pregnant. Confirm that a smear test has been done within the last year and is normal. Drugs and medicines recently taken should be noted—these may include hormones, especially oral contraceptives, antibiotics and tranquillizers.

Examination

A general examination is made. The heart and lungs are examined and blood pressure measured. Examination of the abdomen and pelvis follows. The legs are inspected for varicosities.

Investigations

Investigations include an examination of haemoglobin. Except in an emergency, it is unwise to carry out major surgery with a haemoglobin level <10.5 g/dl, or minor surgery <8.5 g/dl. In women of black or Asian origin, a test for haemoglobinopathies is essential.

The blood group and rhesus factor are determined and serum saved in the laboratory. If there is a probability that transfusion will be needed during the operation, blood is cross-matched in readiness.

The urine is tested for human chorionic gonadotrophin (hCG), albumin, nitrites and sugar. If there is a suspicion of a urinary infection, a midstream sample is sent for bacteriological examination. Renal function tests are advisable if there is a suspicion of abnormal kidney function.

An X-ray of the chest may be taken if indicated. Urography and magnetic resonance imaging (MRI) are done before operations when the ureters may be involved, as in Wertheim's hysterectomy. An ECG is advisable in patients with any suggestion of heart disease. Other investigations may be suggested by the examination or the nature of the case.

A pregnancy test should be performed before surgery.

Preparation

The patient should be weighed on admission or in the outpatient clinic. Shaving of the vulva has now generally been abandoned for minor cases, although most surgeons prefer it for major vulval and vaginal surgery. Postmenopausal women with prolapse may be helped by preoperative treatment with oestrogen, given before admission in the form of oestrogen by mouth or vaginal cream. Antibiotics, eg metronidazole or co-amoxiclav, are usually given before major elective surgery.

Thromboprophylaxis: TED (thromboembolic deterrent) stockings should be worn intraoperatively and until the woman is fully mobilized. During major surgery Flowtron boots that inflate and deflate regularly should be used during the operation. Daily prophylactic doses of low-molecular-weight heparin should be considered for all women at moderate-to-high risk undergoing major surgery, during and after surgery.

The patient should be nil by mouth for at least 6 hours before the operation. If the operation may involve the intestines or rectum, the bowel is emptied and prepared by the use of sodium picosulfate 10 mg/sachet or other suitable preparation.

A physiotherapist should visit every patient, ideally before the operation, and certainly everyone for major surgery. He or she can teach breathing and leg movements for the postoperative period.

Valid consent must be given in writing for the operation by the patient herself. This must be clearly and legibly countersigned by a doctor, who should have explained the operation and its possible sequelae. Girls aged 16 or over sign consent for the operation on their own behalf; for those under that age, the consent of a parent or legal guardian is usually necessary except in an emergency. There may be difficulty in the case of a girl under 16 requesting a termination of pregnancy and insisting that her parents are not to be informed. In such a case, the doctor will have to exercise discretion and act in what he or she considers to be the girl's best interest utilising the rest of Gillick Competency (see Chapter 5).

At the time of obtaining consent for the operation, an explanation should be given of the procedure that is contemplated, and its nature and effects, including possible complications. These should be written on the consent form. In the case of a married woman, her husband's consent is not legally necessary in the UK for operations that lead to sterility such as hysterectomy or sterilization, but it is important that counselling of the couple takes place. It should be made clear in the case of operations for sterilization or vasectomy that the operation should be considered irreversible; on the other hand, it must be emphasized that a few failures occur with sterilizations (1:300). This advice should be recorded in the case notes as well as on the consent form.

Counselling in general is important because many women do not understand the anatomy of their pelvic organs and have unnecessary fears about the effects of operations, in particular their effects on sexual function. Explanation, if necessary illustrated by a model or diagram, will help to dispel these fears.

Postoperative care

A period of recovery is required after any surgery. After *minor operations,* such as hysteroscopy, the patient can go home on the same day. She should not drive or operate machinery for 2 days after general anaesthetic. She must be warned to expect some bleeding for up to 14 days after the operation. More profuse bleeding can follow deep cauterization or conization of the cervix; this may on some occasions be enough to require readmission and possible suture of the cervix. These women should be advised to refrain from intercourse for 6 weeks.

After *major surgery* such as uncomplicated hysterectomy or prolapse repair, patients are encouraged to get up from bed and move about on the day after the operation. Breathing exercises and leg movements are started from the day after the operation. The length of stay in hospital varies but many can leave after 3–6 days. Before departure a clear explanation of the operation and the prognosis must be given by a doctor. An adequate period of convalescence at home is necessary before returning to work and normal activity.

The patient may be examined 6 weeks after the operation. She must be encouraged to return to normal life. Intercourse may be resumed as soon as the vagina is healed. If the ovaries have been removed premenopausally, the woman should be offered oestrogens by tablet, patch or implant. Patients treated for carcinoma must be followed up carefully by gynaecological oncologists.

Postoperative complications

During the first 12 hours after an operation, the patient must be carefully observed for the following:
- Respiratory failure or obstruction to the airways
- Shock
- Haemorrhage
- Cardiac failure.

She should be nursed in a recovery unit until she has recovered consciousness and only then returned to a general ward. The pulse rate and blood pressure should be taken and charted every quarter of an hour for the first 2 hours; thereafter every few hours for the first 12 hours, but longer if there is any anxiety.

Pain must be relieved by adequate doses of analgesics such as morphine or pethidine. Patient-controlled analgesia, with the woman controlling the flow of weak solutions of analgesia intravenously, is very useful for recovery from elective gynaecological surgery. Addition of promazine or chlorpromazine increases the effect of analgesics and helps to prevent postoperative vomiting.

Haemorrhage

1 *Primary,* occurring during the operation and requiring immediate transfusion.

2 *Delayed,* occurring during the immediate postoperative period: generally a result of a slipped ligature or a bleeding vessel in the vagina or cervix. Blood transfusion is given and the patient returned to the operating theatre to deal with the haemorrhage.

3 *Secondary,* occurring up to 14 days after operations and generally from the vagina or cervix, but occasionally from the abdominal wound. Infection is commonly associated, but suture of the bleeding area and blood transfusion may still be needed in all but the slightest cases. After cauterization of the cervix there is generally some bleeding about days 10 and 12 and patients should be warned to expect this.

4 Anaemia is common after gynaecological operations and should be prevented with a correct diet and iron therapy.

Respiratory tract

Complications of a general anaesthetic include sore throat, tracheitis, bronchitis, bronchopneumonia and massive collapse of the lungs. Breathing exercises should be given after general anaesthetics. Pulmonary infection should be treated with antibiotics. Chest symptoms after the first week sometimes indicate pulmonary embolism.

Urinary tract

Retention of urine is common after gynaecological operations and it may be complete or partial. A bladder scan should be performed to calculate the urinary residual post-micturition. Complete retention of urine often occurs after hysterectomy or repair of prolapse. Rarely unexplained retention occurs after a minor operation such as hysteroscopy.

If there is more than 150 ml urine in the bladder, immediate single episode catheterization should be performed. If it must be repeated, an indwelling catheter has to be put in for a few days. Some surgeons prefer suprapubic catheterization.

Partial retention of urine is common after surgery for prolapse and a scan should be performed for residual urine 5 days after surgery. Catheter drainage should continue until the residual urine is <200 ml.

Cystitis and pyelonephritis are very common after gynaecological operations. A catheter specimen or a midstream specimen should be examined for evidence of infection after all major operations and suitable treatment given.

Poor or absent urine output may result from obstruction to the ureters, which may be accidentally injured, ligated or obstructed by a haematoma; it may also be reflex blockage. Warning is often from a unilateral loin ache and a slight temperature. It is a very serious complication and must be dealt with urgently, if necessary with relieving surgery by a urologist.

Incontinence of urine through the urethra sometimes occurs after catheterization and in elderly women; it is usually transient. Persistent incontinence suggests a fistula. Urinary fistulae may be vesicovaginal or ureterovaginal. These may be caused by trauma at surgery, haematoma formation or difficult obstetric delivery. They also result from malignant disease.

An ureterovaginal fistula may follow operations, especially Wertheim's hysterectomy, if the ureters are extensively dissected so that their blood supply is imperilled and they become devascularized.

Venous thrombosis

Two types can occur after surgery.

Phlebothrombosis

This is primary venous thrombosis and generally begins in the deep veins of the calf; predisposing causes are:

- trauma
- anaemia
- stasis commonly due to immobility
- high oestrogen levels.

Thrombophlebitis

This is caused by infection, generally in the pelvic veins initially and spreading to involve the iliac veins. *Pulmonary embolism* can follow thrombosis and if massive is rapidly fatal. Small emboli cause pulmonary infarction.

Prevention of thrombosis and embolism consists of:
- the use of pneumatic boots and leggings during the surgery
- elasticated stockings worn before, during and after surgery
- early mobilization
- avoidance of anaemia
- prompt treatment of infection
- prophylactic low-dose heparin before and just after surgery.

The contraceptive pill should ideally be stopped 4–6 weeks before major elective surgery.

In established thrombosis, low-dose heparin at 1.5 mg/kg should be given as a single or divided dose. Warfarin is started with a loading dose of 10 mg for 2 days followed by a daily dose that is determined by the clotting time. In proven deep venous thrombosis (DVT) this should be continued for 3 months and, if there was a pulmonary embolism, for 6 months (see Chapter 14 for investigation).

Chapter 17

Pelvic pain

Many diseases causing lower abdominal symptoms are gynaecological in origin. The general surgeon and gynaecologist must both be trained to recognize and deal with them. When available, consultation will take place, but delay and mortality are linked and acute abdominal conditions do not leave time for leisurely consultations. If the condition is obviously gynaecological in origin, it is best dealt with by gynaecologists because they are more used to conservation of genital tract tissue, particularly the ovaries.

Acute intra-abdominal emergencies present with pain, shock, vomiting or abdominal distension. The first of these is the most common in gynaecological conditions.

Pain

Pain in pelvic organs may arise from:
• inside the organ with irritation of its lining or stretch of its walls
• stretch of the visceral peritoneum over the organ
• involvement of the parietal peritoneum in proximity.
For example, an ectopic pregnancy can cause pain from:

Lecture Notes: Obstetrics and Gynaecology, 3rd edition. By Diana Hamilton-Fairley. Published 2009 by Blackwell Publishing. ISBN: 978-1-4051-7801-3.

• damage to the muscle of the tube by trophoblast invasion and bleeding
• stretch of the peritoneum from the broad ligament over the fallopian tube at the site of the pregnancy
• blood spilt on to the peritoneum by the rupture of the tube or ovarian cyst (acute) or trickling from the outer end of the tube (chronic). The pain may be referred down the anterior part of the leg (via L1–2) or the shoulder tip if the blood irritates the diaphragm (via the phrenic nerve).

The first two origins of stimuli are mediated by the autonomic nervous system with poor localization; hence non-specific pain in the pelvis results.

The parietal peritoneum is innervated by the somatic nervous system and localization may be more specific. The peritoneum of the pouch of Douglas, however, has a poor nerve supply and is often undemonstrative. As this is the area in which the tubes and ovaries spend much of their time, it makes pain localization in the abdominal wall difficult in pelvic conditions in the earlier stages, but signs are easier to detect on pelvic and rectal examination.

Shock

A sudden deterioration in a woman's vital state may be characterized by:

- a rise in pulse rate
- a fall in arterial and then diastolic blood pressure
- pallor
- faintness and later unconsciousness.

This may result from either:

- true hypovolaemia, eg a ruptured ectopic pregnancy with 2 litres blood in the peritoneal cavity
- relative hypovolaemia, eg excess of autonomic stimulation after peritoneal irritation with a sudden release of pus or blood.

Pallor, sweating, agitation and restlessness are traditional indications of shock, of which pallor is the most important for prognosis in the gynaecological field. Fainting and unconsciousness come later in shock and may be considered as signs of more extensive involvement. Gynaecology tends to deal with younger people who can withstand hypovolaemia for longer. The tachycardia and low blood pressure may be sudden in onset and are often a sign of significant intraperitoneal loss. Alternatively they may faint and then recover and appear stable as they compensate for the acute loss.

Nausea and vomiting

These happen rarely in non-pregnant gynaecological conditions but have a number of causes:

- Stimulation of a large number of nerve endings of the peritoneum overlying an affected pelvic organ, eg torted ovarian cyst.
- The direct action of toxins on the central nervous system from infective organisms. Pelvic inflammation often becomes localized early and toxins are released intermittently into the general bloodstream.
- Vomiting is a common accompaniment of early pregnancy. Many gynaecological conditions happen in early gestation so vomiting might be nothing to do with the acute condition in the pelvis but more to do with the human chorionic gonadotrophin (hCG) produced by the pregnancy trophoblast.

Abdominal distension

Distension is unusual in gynaecological conditions but common in alimentary tract ones, particularly those of the large bowel. In consequence, if distension is present, it is probably a result of an associated bowel problem rather than a gynaecological one. It is important to auscultate the abdomen when distension, guarding and /or rebound is present to exclude intestinal obstruction or an ileus.

Diagnosis

The triad of history, examination and investigations applies here as anywhere else in medicine. This section should be read in conjunction with the account of making a gynaecological diagnosis in Chapter 2.

History

Women in severe acute abdominal pain do not like having long histories taken. Hence, the questions must be tailored to the situation.

Pain

- Characteristics of the pain site, time and nature.
- Relationship of pain to various body functions, eg vaginal bleeding or micturition.
- Past gynaecological or obstetric events.
- Menstrual history, ie details of last menstrual period.
- Symptoms of a possible pregnancy, eg nausea, vomiting, breast changes

Examination

A general examination must cover a number of points:

- Paleness (conjunctival assessment)
- Pulse rate
- Arterial blood pressure
- Temperature.

Abdominal examination helps to localize pelvic causes.

- *Observation* will show old scars and the degree of distension; the site of the pain can be elicited from the woman at this point.
- *Gentle palpation* of the abdomen leading to the lower pelvic zones may help localization further.

- *Firmer examination*: if tenderness allows; this will reveal guarding or any rebound tenderness.
- Many pelvic abdominal conditions do not have specific localizing signs in the abdomen and so any opinion should await the performance of a bimanual vaginal examination.
- A *speculum examination* should be performed. This may be painful so it should be done gently and slowly. Any vaginal discharge or bleeding through the cervical os should be noted and swabs taken from the posterior fornix and cervical canal for bacterial culture and identification of *Chlamydia*.
- At *bimanual vaginal assessment* tenderness from a pelvic organ will obviously limit the thoroughness of the examination because the woman will guard if there is pain on moving the cervix. This is called cervical excitation (Fig. 17.1); moving the cervix to the side of an ovarian or tubal mass will cause intense pain by a further stretch of the overlying peritoneum. Moving the cervix towards the opposite side will decrease the pain by releasing the tension of the peritoneum. Masses of over 5cm should be palpable and the following should be recorded:
  — size
  — site (ovarian, uterine, anterior/posterior/right/left)
  — consistency (cystic/solid)
  — regularity
  — mobile or fixed.
- *Rectal examination* may be needed but usually one can assess acute problems in the pouch of Douglas at a vaginal assessment. If structural changes are sought in the back of the pelvic cavity, the rectal examination is useful, eg endometriotic lesions on the uterosacral ligaments, or to differentiate from appendicitis.

Investigations

There are a few investigations that help:
- Haemoglobin to check on chronic bleeding.
- Differential white cell count to assess inflammation.
- Urine cells and organisms to diagnose urinary infection.
- Urinary hCG levels to check for pregnancy.
- High vaginal swab and cervical swab to test for genital tract infection.
- Ultrasound: extremely useful to check the pelvic organs, particularly using a vaginal probe. Then the transmitter and receiver are within a centimetre or two of the affected organs.
- MRI/CT may help to identify the site and nature of a pelvic mass.

The vaginal ultrasound examination gives far more precise images of pelvic organs and tissues.
- Changes in ovarian morphology and size:
  — cysts (nearly always spherical)
  — polycystic ovary syndrome (not a cause of pelvic pain as such)
  — irregular masses.
- Fallopian tube:
  — occasionally a swollen tube from a pyo- or hydrosalpinx is identified as a sausage-shaped mass that may have fine septa (see Plate 9)
  — ectopic pregnancies may be diagnosed (see Chapter 8).
- Uterine size can be detected:
  — the thickness of the endometrium is shown
  — the presence of a pregnancy sac can be detected as early as 5 weeks, and embryonic parts and fetal heart beats by 6 weeks from the last menstrual period.
- Fibroids of the uterus.
- Pouch of Douglas fluid can often be detected in as low a volume as 7 ml. This might indicate blood loss from an ectopic pregnancy.

Often a combination of ultrasound with other tests is helpful, eg in the UK now, many unrup-

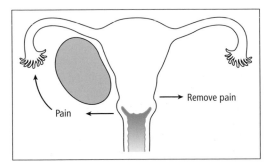

Figure 17.1 Cervical excitation: moving the cervix pushes the uterus, so altering the tension on the overlying peritoneum and causing pain.

tured ectopic pregnancies are diagnosed at ultrasound in symptomatic women who have an empty uterus but a thickened endometrium and fluid in the pouch of Douglas in the presence of raised urinary hCG levels.

Conditions to be considered

We diagnose what we are thinking of and it is helpful to have a checklist (Table 17.1).

Pelvic organs (Table 17.2)

Vagina

Vaginal trauma

Intercourse occurring forcibly or after a long interval of abstinence can cause damage to the vaginal tube:
- Lower end: usually obvious but may be labial or fourchette.
- Upper end: vaginal guarding to prevent the easy passage of the speculum—hence hard to see.
- Haematoma: paravaginal or paracervical haematoma.

The obvious point needed in the history may not be volunteered readily. Treatment is by vaginal repair under anaesthesia.

Uterus

Uterine fibroids (Plate 10)

Alternatively named myomas or leiomyomas, uterine fibroids are the most common of all pelvic tumours. They are benign fibromuscular swellings, arising in the muscle wall of the uterus. Fibroids are oestrogen sensitive.
- *Submucous*: lying immediately beside the endometrium and enlarging the surface of the uterine, cavity often leading to menorrhagia. Fibroids may become pedunculated forming polyps that can extrude through the cervix (Plate 8). The pain is commonly associated with menses and menorrhagia. It is usually crampy as the uterus contracts to try to expel the mass occupying its cavity.
- *Intramural*: the most common site for fibroids, surrounded by smooth muscle, enlarging the uterine wall and distorting venous drainage. The pain is usually constant and severe, and caused by degeneration. It may last for some weeks while the process of degeneration takes place. Once it is complete the fibroid initially looks cystic on a scan and then calcifies, shrinking in size as it does so.
- *Subserous*: fibroids just beneath the peritoneum on the outer uterine surface (Fig. 17.2). May be on an elongated stalk (pedunculated) with a risk of torsion; may grow into the broad ligament. These swellings can also undergo degeneration.

Degeneration

Uterine fibroids frequently outgrow their blood supply and degenerate.
- *Hyaline*: an aseptic necrosis with loss of muscle cell structure. This may lead to calcification.
- *Cystic*: a sequel to hyaline change with subsequent breakdown and cyst formation giving a honeycomb appearance.
- *Fatty*: in which partial necrosis results in the development of fatty substances, which may subsequently undergo calcification (visible on X-rays and ultrasound).
- *Red*: necrobiosis, particularly encountered in the mid-trimester of pregnancy or the early puerperium. This breakdown of blood supply by thrombosis leads to necrosis and suffusion with red blood cells.
- *Sarcomatous*: rare malignant change reported in 0.2–0.4% of fibroids examined in asymptomatic older women *post mortem*.

Symptoms
- *None*: a pelvic swelling is found incidentally on examination.
- Occasional *tightness* of waistband of clothes.
- *Pressure*: bladder compression causing daytime frequency and occasionally impaired urinary stream. In the supporting ligaments it causes backache and overall sensation of pelvic heaviness. If posterior it may cause rectal pressure and constipation.
- *Pain*: associated with red degeneration or torsion of subserous pedicles. Dysmenorrhoea may indicate the presence of a submucous fibroid.

Table 17.1 Differential diagnosis of acute abdominal/pelvic pain

Condition	History	Examination	Investigation	Ultrasound scan
Ectopic pregnancy	• Pain—sudden onset, constant, shoulder tip • Other—sudden collapse, period of amenorrhoea, minivaginal bleeding	Rebound, guarding BP↓, P↑, T < 37°C VE—unilateral Cx excitation, uterus small for dates, os closed	Hb = or ↓ WBC = hCG +ve	Empty uterus Free fluid in POD ?Adnexal mass
Acute salpingitis	• Pain—gradual onset, constant, generalized, bilateral • Other—vaginal discharge, irregular menses	Guarding? rebound T > 37.5°C, BP =, P↑ VE—bilateral Cx excitation	Hb = WBC↑ hCG −ve +ve HVS	NAD ?? Free fluid
Fibroid degeneration	• Pain—gradual onset, constant, generalized • Other—? menorrhagia	Tender over fibroid T 37–37.5°C, VE—no Cx excitation, enlarged uterus	Hb = WBC = or ↑ hCG −ve	Fibroid seen in uterine wall with cystic areas
Ovarian cyst accident:				
Torsion	• Pain—sudden onset, constant, may be getting less • Other—vomiting	Rebound, guarding T 37–37.5°C, BP =, P↑ VE—unilateral Cx excitation, adnexal mass	Hb = or WBC = or ↑ hCG −ve	Echogenic mass seen separate from uterus ?Free fluid
Rupture	• Pain—sudden onset, constant, getting less • Other—? irregular menses	Rebound, guarding T 37°C, P, BP =, VE—generalized tenderness only	Hb = WBC = hCG −ve	Free fluid in POD No cyst seen
Haemorrhage	• Pain—sudden onset, constant, becoming less	Rebound, guarding T 37°C, BP =, P↑ VE—unilateral Cx excitation, adnexal mass	Hb = or ↑ WBC = hCG −ve	Echogenic cyst Free fluid if ruptured
Appendicitis	• Pain—gradual onset, right-sided • Other—anorexia, no BO, nausea/vomiting	Rebound, guarding, right-sided tenderness T 37–37.5°C, BP =, P↑ VE—NAD PR—empty rectum, right-sided tenderness	Hb = WBC ↑ hCG −ve	NAD
Pyelonephritis	• Pain—loin pain, colicky • Other—nausea, vomiting, rigors, dysuria	Loin tenderness T > 37.5°C VE—NAD	Hb = WBC ↑ hCG −ve MSU +ve	Renal pelvicalyceal dilatation Pelvis—NAD
Obstruction	• Pain—intermittent, generalized, colicky • Other—nausea, vomiting, anorexia, bowels not open	Rebound, guarding, distension No BS. T 37°C, VE—NAD PR—empty rectum	Hb = WBC = or ↑ hCG −ve	Pelvis—NAD AXR—dilated loops with fluid levels

BP = blood pressure; T = temperature; P = pulse; VE = vaginal examination; PR = rectal examination; NAD = no abnormality detected; AXR = abdominal X-ray; Hb = haemoglobin; WBC = white blood count; hCG = pregnancy test; MSU = mid-stream urine; HVS = high vaginal swab; POD = pouch of Douglas; Cx = cervical; BS = bowel sounds.

	Organ	Condition
Non-pregnant	Vagina	Trauma
	Uterus	Fibroid:
		Torsion
		Degeneration
		Adenomyosis
		Endometritis
		Pyometra
	Fallopian tubes	Salpingitis
		Pyosalpinx
		Torsion
	Ovaries	Tumours
		Simple cyst
		Torsion
		Bleeding
		Rupture
	Peritoneum	Endometriosis
Early pregnancy	Uterus	Abortion
		Impacted retroversion
		Red degeneration of fibroids
	Fallopian tubes	Ectopic pregnancy
		Torsion
	Ligaments	Round ligament
		Stretch
	Extra-pelvic	Vomiting in pregnancy
		Pyelonephritis
		Appendicitis
		Rectus haematoma

Table 17.2 Pelvic diseases that may present as acute abdominal emergencies

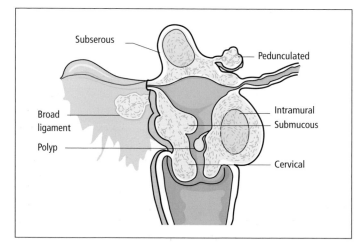

Figure 17.2 Uterus with fibroids.

- *Menstrual disturbances*:
  — menorrhagia: heavy bleeding
  — metrorrhagia: prolonged menses
  — irregular, intermittent bleeding: often associated with polyps and other surface lesions.
- Subfertility and *miscarriage*: intramural and submucosal fibroids can interfere with implantation and therefore reduce the chances of successful pregnancy with an increased risk of miscarriage and preterm delivery. Subfertility may arise if the fibroids block the isthmic portion of the tube.

Investigations

Ultrasound: to define the location, dimensions and consistency.

Diagnosis

Bimanual palpation reveals hard rounded non-tender often bosselated mass, moving when the cervix is displaced.
- Grow fast in pregnancy.
- Shrink:
  — at the menopause
  — with anti-gonadotrophic hormone therapy.

Pathology

Fibroids may be single or multiple (occasionally numbering >100) and vary in size from a seedling to a football. They form a pseudocapsule by compressing surrounding uterine muscle, a process helpful to the surgeon at myomectomy.

Aetiology

Cause is unknown:
- Rarely found under the age of 30 years
- More common in African–Caribbean populations
- More common in nulliparous women and those with low fertility
- Often a family history.

Differential diagnosis
- Pregnancy: particularly if fibroids have been softened by cystic degeneration.
- Ovarian tumour: often cystic, unilateral and does not move with cervical displacement.
- Adenomyosis: more commonly causes uniform diffuse and tender uterine enlargement.

Conservative management

The needs and condition of the woman must be paramount in discussing the options for treatment:
- If the fibroids are small and asymptomatic, no treatment is required except annual examination with or without ultrasound monitoring. This is used particularly in women >40 because fibroids do not grow after the menopause and may shrink.
- If she is keen to have children in the future medical treatment with a gonadotrophin-releasing hormone (GnRH) agonist for 6 months is advised as first-line therapy because the withdrawal of oestrogen will reduce the size of the fibroids, but its effects are not long lasting and the fibroids will grow back.
- Pain: requires analgesia.
- Uterine artery embolization under radiological control: a cannula is passed into the uterine arteries via the femoral artery. The uterine arteries are embolized by injecting tiny silicon particles, causing the fibroids to degenerate. Pain relief is essential for 48 hours. In women with large/multiple fibroids there is an increased risk of hysterectomy compared with surgical treatment. Pyrexia and abscess formation can occur. It is not recommended for women who wish to preserve their fertility, although live births have been reported after the procedure.
- Heavier and longer periods with anaemia are the most common indication for proceeding to surgery.

Surgery
- Transcervical resection of submucosal fibroids: using an operating hysteroscope the fibroid is resected with diathermy. To reduce the risk of bleeding/absorption of the distension fluid a GnRH agonist is given for 6–8 weeks before the procedure. Perforation of the uterus is a risk that may cause damage to other organs; fortunately this is rare.
- Myomectomy: in young women whose families are incomplete or when there is a personal desire to retain the uterus. The procedure is often vascular and may cause scarring, with adhesion formation impairing fertility. If the fibroids are numerous it may be impossible to remove them all, and growth

of the remainder may cause problems in the future. Women undergoing this procedure should be warned that the surgeon may have to proceed to a hysterectomy and consent to the possibility of this (1% risk). This risk is reduced through the use of a tourniquet intraoperatively around the uterine and ovarian arteries and/or the use of a vasoconstrictor such as pitressin.

• Abdominal hysterectomy: suitable when family is complete with women over the age of 40 or when the uterus is grossly enlarged and distorted by multiple fibroids.

• Vaginal hysterectomy: when fibroids are small and few in number and there is an associated prolapse of the uterus.

Effects on child-bearing

• Implantation over a fibroid may lead to spontaneous miscarriage.

• Pain may develop from red degeneration.

• Preterm labour may develop if the fibroids are large, multiple and/or undergo red degeneration.

• Dysfunctional uterine contractions may follow the interruption of smooth waves of electrical stimulation by masses of inert, non-myometrial tissue.

• The pelvis may be obstructed causing malpresentation or even obstructed labour. This is unusual because most fibroids usually move up as the uterus grows in pregnancy.

• Postpartum haemorrhage and retained placenta are more common.

• Management in pregnancy is conservative.

The aim should be to secure a vaginal delivery. If a caesarean section becomes necessary, the incision in the uterus should be made around the fibroids. They should not be removed or incised as severe haemorrhage may develop, leading to the need for a hysterectomy.

Uterine adenomyosis

Adenomyosis is a condition where endometrial glands of stroma are found within the uterine musculature. If localized to one site, it is called an adenomyoma. It is like diffuse endometriosis in the muscle of the uterus (Fig. 17.3).

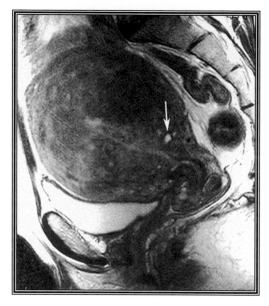

Figure 17.3 MRI of adenomyosis. Diffuse enlargement of the uterus with multiple areas of fibrosis (arrow).

Pathology

The uterus is enlarged and thick walled with no pseudocapsule formation, unlike fibroids. The endometrial glands sometimes do not all menstruate, as they derive from the basal layer of the endometrium.

Symptoms

This condition is most frequent in women aged 35–40, with reduced fertility. The symptoms usually are:

• dysmenorrhoea
• menorrhagia
• dyspareunia
• subfertility
• miscarriage.

Signs

A uniformly enlarged uterus that is rarely larger than 12 cm. It is tender on palpation, particularly premenstrually. It often coexists with intra-abdominal endometriosis and fibroids. Commonly there are multiple small fibroid like masses (<2 cm in diameter) spread throughout the uterus. These are fibrotic reactions to the bleeding from the endometrial glands and form the adenomas.

Differential diagnosis

- Uterine fibroids
- Early pregnancy
- Uterine infection.

Treatment

- Conservative use of progestogen therapy, eg nor-ethisterone 10–20 mg daily
- Danazol 200–400 mg daily (very rarely used now)
- Gonadotrophin analogues: buserelin or goserelin
- Intrauterine system (IUS) releasing levonorgestrol.

All hormone regimes aim to suppress menstruation, but each carries side effects and sometimes cannot be used for more than some months at a time. This condition is associated with an increased incidence of breakthrough bleeding while on any of these treatments.

Surgery

Abdominal hysterectomy is the treatment of choice, although occasionally resection of the affected area can be considered. This is often not acceptable to women who still wish to have children.

Endometritis

The condition is usually acute and associated with ascending infection. The disease may result from:

- post-abortal infection
- criminal (illegal 'back street') abortion
- post-curettage/evacuation of products of conception
- intrauterine device infection
- post partum, particularly after caesarean section. It rarely results from blood-borne tuberculosis.

Findings

ACUTE INFECTION

- Irregular bleeding
- Offensive vaginal discharge
- Uterine tenderness.

CHRONIC INFECTION

Occasionally secondary amenorrhoea and secondary infertility, caused by the development of intra-uterine adhesions leading to partial or complete occlusion of the uterine cavity (Asherman's syndrome).

Pyometra

- Infection leading to pus formation may be associated with blocking of the fallopian tubes and the cervix.
- Pyometra are more common in older women.
- A bag of pus builds up pressure and distends the uterus causing:
  — pain from the stretch of the muscle wall
  — occasional acute bursts of toxaemia as a bolus of pus is forced into a vein and so to the vascular network
  — chronic infection with low-grade temperature and malaise
  — occasionally pus is forced through the cervix to produce a purulent or blood-stained discharge.
- Many pyometra are associated with cancer of the endometrium (see Chapter 20).

Any woman with such symptoms should have a hysteroscopy and a dilatation and curettage (D&C) under appropriate antibiotic cover to exclude endometrial malignancy.

Fallopian tubes

Torsion of the fallopian tube

This rare cause of lower abdominal pain is usually associated with ovarian torsion on a long pedicle. Treatment is by laparotomy or laparoscopy and depends upon the degree of devascularization of the tube and ovary:

- If on unwinding the tissues are healthy, they are best conserved with a securing suture to the side wall of the pelvis to prevent retorsion.
- If the tissues are devitalized, the ovary and tube must be removed.

Salpingitis (see Plate 9)

An ascending infection from the vagina through the cervix is the usual cause of salpingitis. It is often associated with:

- intercourse
- transcervical surgery (D&C or evacuation)
- intrauterine foreign bodies such as an intrauterine device (IUD)
- retained products of conception
- very rarely, blood-borne infection.

Acute salpingitis

The fallopian tubes become red, swollen and distorted, often obstructed at the abdominal end so a pyosalpinx forms, later becoming a hydrosalpinx (see Plate 9). Peritoneal inflammation with adhesions to the serosal surface occurs, leading to pelvic abscess and, if severe, to septicaemia. The condition is usually bilateral. The destruction of the cilia later leads to infertility. Chronic hydrosalpinges may become reinfected.

Clinical features
- Pyrexia, often with a temperature >39°C
- Tachycardia
- Dehydration.

Abdominal examination
- Lower abdominal pain with guarding
- If parietal peritoneum is involved, rebound tenderness
- Distension.

Vaginal examination
- Cervical excitation pain (bilateral)
- Tender, normal-sized uterus
- Fullness in the fornices and tenderness over the tubes
- Vaginal discharge.

Investigations
- Organisms may be isolated from cervical discharge.
- Gonorrhoea (see Chapter 6).
- *Escherichia coli*, haemolytic streptococci and staphylococci are often found in the puerperium and post-abortion.
- *Clostridium perfringens* may thrive on dead tissue, eg placental products.
- *Chlamydia* is a common secondary organism.
- Leukocytosis (in excess of $20 \times 10^9/l$).

- Laparoscopy is the only certain way of making a true diagnosis. Remember to take serosal swabs.

Differential diagnosis
- *Appendicitis*: pain is usually central then radiating to the right iliac fossa; the fever is lower.
- *Ruptured ectopic pregnancy*: if there is intraperitoneal bleeding, symptoms such as faintness and shoulder tip pain. Tenderness tends to be unilateral and a pregnancy test is usually positive. There is no pyrexia.
- *Ovarian tumour torsion*: the pain is localized and unilateral. Pregnancy test is negative and there is no pyrexia. Ultrasound will confirm.
- *Pyelonephritis*: the pain is usually associated with loin tenderness and there are pus cells in the urine.
- *Intestinal obstruction*: usually associated with colicky pain and abdominal distension. X-rays show fluid levels.

Treatment
CONSERVATIVE
- Sit the patient upright in bed.
- Set up intravenous infusion.
- Administer broad-spectrum antibiotics until the high vaginal swab (HVS) microbiology and sensitivity reports have been returned.
- Drugs such as clindamycin, co-amoxiclav, cephradoxyl and metronidazole are suitable. Continue the antibiotics after the acute phase for 2–3 weeks with doxycycline.
- Provide analgesia and fluids.
- Refer to genitourinary clinic with partner for treatment and contact tracing (see Chapter 6).

RADICAL
- Exploratory surgery should be contemplated if diagnosis is in doubt.
- Use only minimal interference, eg drainage under antibiotic cover.

Chronic salpingitis

Chronic salpingitis is usually a sequel to acute or subacute infections, but is often associated with a lower-grade purulent organism, eg *Chlamydia*.

Pathology
- Thickened fallopian tubes
- Fibrosis
- Hydrosalpinges
- Pelvic floor peritoneal adhesions.

Symptoms
- Persistent recurrent episodes of low abdominal pain
- Deep dyspareunia
- Congestive dysmenorrhoea
- Heavy periods
- Subfertility.

Investigations
- Ultrasound scan of pelvis
- Laparoscopy: if there is no recent acute episode, dye installation with antibiotic cover.

Long-term sequelae
- Subfertility
- Ectopic pregnancy.

Ovaries

Ovarian masses/cysts
History
Enlargement of the ovary often occurs without any symptoms, because the ovaries are tucked away in the pelvis and can expand without causing very much pressure on surrounding organs until they get quite large. Pain is not a usual association nor is vaginal bleeding, except with the few hormone-producing ovarian cysts, which are rare.

Symptoms
When ovarian cysts do produce symptoms they are varied:
- *Abdominal distension*: this is usually noticed by the woman herself with an increase of waist size or when washing in the bath. Usually the cyst has to be >14 cm in diameter before she notices it and often, in the mildly plump, it could be missed until 20 cm.
- *Pressure* on the rectum, bladder or lymphatic system producing appropriate pressure or back symptoms.

- *Pain*: this is usually associated with complications of cysts:
  — torsion
  — rupture
  — haemorrhage.
There is peritoneal irritation leading to a degree of shock and a tendency to abdominal muscle guarding. Torsion is usually accompanied by vomiting.
After resuscitation, a laparoscopy is usually required. In skilled hands, minimal access surgery through a laparoscope can deal with an obviously simple ovarian cyst, which has either undergone torsion or bled. If there is doubt about whether the cyst is malignant, most surgeons prefer to open the abdomen at laparotomy and perform a formal removal.
- *Hormone secretion*: this happens only with a few rare cysts. They may synthesize either:
  — oestrogens—leading to menstrual upset (eg granulosa cell tumours)
  — androgens—leading to masculinization, including amenorrhoea (eg arrhenoblastoma).

Examination
The woman may look cachectic and show signs of weight loss if presenting with malignant tumours of the ovary. Otherwise, there are few general signs:
- The *abdomen* may appear enlarged. If there is gross stretch of the abdominal wall, there may be shiny skin with possible oedema and peau d'orange.
- *Palpation* may allow a firm ovarian cyst to be felt. If there is ascites or the cyst is lax, it might be difficult to delineate it.
- *Percussion* may demonstrate central dullness with resonance of the flanks. However, if ascites is present, this sign is lost and shifting dullness may replace it.
- *Auscultation* is usually not helpful.
- *Pelvic examination* may reveal a tumour or pain.
  If benign, the mass can be felt separate from the uterine body and may be freely mobile. If it is fixed, infection, endometriosis or malignancy should be suspected.

Investigations

Ultrasound of the abdomen can detect masses and ascites; with smaller masses, a vaginal probe approach is even better at delineation. X-rays are not very helpful unless calcification is present (eg dermoids).

Tumour markers should be measured in the following circumstances:

• *Premenopausal women*: cyst >5 cm in diameter that persists for more than 6 weeks and/or has both solid and cystic elements; hCG, LDH (lactate dehydrogenase) and AFP (α-fetoprotein) should be measured in addition to those for postmenopausal women.

• *Postmenopausal women*: any cyst >5 cm or one <5 cm that persists for >6 weeks, measure Ca-125, Ca-19.9 and carcinoembryonic antigen or CEA (see Chapter 20).

Features of common tumours

It is difficult to classify ovarian masses precisely, because the ovary has several histological tissues in it and each can contribute to ovarian tumours. Many are simple variations of normal physiology.

Functional cysts

These are commonly an incidental finding on ultrasound scans performed for other reasons. They are spherical, echo-free areas within the ovary. They can be safely ignored in premenopausal women unless they are >5 cm in diameter and persist for >6 weeks.

Follicular cysts (Fig. 17.4 and Plate 11)

These consist of unruptured and enlarged graafian follicles and a normal ovary commonly contains one or more small cysts (<5 cm in diameter). They are not neoplastic and tend to disappear by resorption of fluid. These cysts rarely exceed 15 cm in diameter and are lined with one or more layers of granulosa cells, which degenerate in long-standing cysts. There may be difficulty clinically in distinguishing a follicular cyst from a small serous cystadenoma.

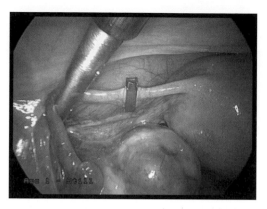

Figure 17.4 Left follicular cyst at laparoscopy.

Corpus luteum cysts

These are lined with luteal cells derived from the granulosa layer. The corpus luteum of pregnancy may reach 3 cm or more in diameter. Sometimes, apart from pregnancy, the corpus luteum persists, becoming cystic and causing amenorrhoea, followed by bleeding. Haemorrhage into a corpus luteum can cause pain and the symptoms and signs may resemble those of ectopic pregnancy.

Haemorrhagic cysts

A haemorrhagic cyst may result from bleeding into a graafian follicle or corpus luteum. Sometimes acute symptoms result, leading to laparotomy. Removal of the ovary may be performed unnecessarily in young women. All that is required is haemostasis of the affected area after shelling out the haematoma.

Theca luteal cysts

Theca luteal cysts are found in association with raised hCG levels:

• hydatidiform mole
• choriocarcinoma
• gonadotrophin therapy.

Both ovaries are enlarged (10 cm or more) with multiple cysts lined by luteal cells. The ovaries return to normal when hCG levels reduce.

Benign ovarian cysts

Serous cystadenoma

This benign tumour contains fluid that is rich in protein, resembling blood serum. It often contains papillary growths, each with a connective tissue core and a covering of cubical cells, similar to those that line the cyst. In larger cysts, papillae are always present and in some cases grow rapidly, almost filling the cyst and giving the appearance of a solid tumour.

Bilateral tumours are often seen and malignant change is frequent. The histological diagnosis of malignancy is occasionally not easy and may have to be made on the clinical features.

Mucinous cystadenoma

The most common of the benign new growths, this contains viscous mucin, the secretion of the lining of the tumour. The cyst grows slowly and may reach a very large size, filling the abdominal cavity. Tumours >100 kg have been reported (ie heavier than the woman from whom they are taken).

It is multilocular, each loculus being lined with tall columnar epithelium, which may be ciliated and can proliferate to form papillary folds. Goblet cells are found among the epithelial cells.

Malignant change occurs in about 5%.

Pseudomyxoma peritonei

This is a rare condition whereas mucinous tumours are common; it may occur if the contents of a cyst leak or are spilled into the peritoneal cavity. Epithelial cells lining the cyst proliferate and produce a mucinous ascites, the whole peritoneal cavity becoming filled with viscid mucinous material. The condition arises also from a mucocele of the appendix and thus may be found in males as well as females.

Fibroadenoma

A benign tumour that occurs in about 3% of women with an ovarian tumour. It arises from connective tissue as a solid non-encapsulated tumour, which may be bilateral and can grow to 20 cm. The normal ovary is compressed but not invaded. The histological appearance is that of a benign tumour composed of whorls of fibrous connective tissue, resembling the ovarian stroma. These tumours are associated with:

- ascites
- hydrothorax—only occasionally
- hydropericardium.

This association is Meigs' syndrome and is also found with a Brenner, granulosa cell or theca cell tumours. The effusions into the serous cavities disappear when the tumour is removed.

Brenner tumour

A rare tumour found mostly in postmenopausal women, often discovered accidentally *post mortem* because it remains small and symptomless. It is a mostly solid tumour with nests of epithelial cells resembling transitional epithelium enclosed in dense fibrous tissue. Cavities arising in the epithelial nests contain mucin-like mucinous cystadenoma. A Brenner tumour is sometimes found in a mucinous cystadenoma. Meigs' syndrome may occur.

Germ cell tumours

This is a group of primitive germ cell tumours. The best known is the *dysgerminoma*. This rare tumour arises from primitive undifferentiated sex cells; histologically identical tumours are found in the ovary (dysgerminoma) and in the testicle (seminoma). They consist of epithelial cells arranged in alveoli separated by septa of fibrous tissue infiltrated with round cells, resembling lymphocytes. The epithelial cells are large and round or polygonal, similar to spermatocytes. It may happen in young patients and is liable to malignant change in both sexes. Dysgerminoma is more common in individuals with infantile genitalia and in males with undescended testicles, but it also occurs in normal individuals. The tumour secretes gonadotrophin so that a positive pregnancy test may be obtained.

Endodermal sinus tumour or *embryonal carcinoma* may occur with dysgerminoma.

Dermoid or benign teratoma

This common tumour of the ovary makes up 15% of all ovarian tumours. It occurs mainly between 15 and 30 years of age and is the most common tumour in this age group because it develops from an unfertilized ovum by parthenogenesis and thus occurs mostly in the reproductive period. These tumours are often multiple and bilateral (10%).

A dermoid is a thick-walled cyst with solid parts, rarely exceeding 20 cm in diameter. It does not adhere to surrounding structures so torsion is common. The cyst is lined by squamous epithelium and contains:

- a fatty sebaceous secretion resembling sebum
- hairs
- sebaceous glands
- hair follicles
- teeth
- cartilage
- gastrointestinal epithelium
- nervous tissue
- thyroid tissue.

Malignant change sometimes occurs in the form of squamous epithelioma or embryonal carcinoma in one of the elements of the tumour.

Hyperthyroidism can follow in a benign teratoma consisting mainly of thyroid tissue.

Solid teratoma

This is a very rare tumour. It has a variety of primitive tissues with ectoderm, mesoderm and endoderm all represented so that the tumour consists of masses of embryonic cells of all varieties in a bizarre histological pattern. It is highly malignant.

Gonadoblastoma

This tumour occurs in abnormal gonads and in individuals who are sex chromatin negative. It consists of large germ cells similar to those of a dysgerminoma and small cells similar to granulosa cells. It may show hormonal activity and may become malignant.

Granulosa cell tumour

The cells resemble granulosa cells, being polygonal with deeply staining nuclei. They tend to be arranged in rosettes; clear space may be seen between them and strands of connective tissue run between the granulosa cells. Malignant change may occur and they secrete oestrogens.

Granulosa cell tumours may occur at any age. In infants and young children they are a rare cause of precocious puberty with uterine bleeding. In adult women, granulosa cell tumours cause profuse and irregular uterine bleeding from a hyper-oestrogenized endometrium, often of metropathic type. An ovarian tumour must not be overlooked when considering these symptoms. In postmenopausal women irregular uterine bleeding is caused, with oestrogenization of the uterus, vulva and vagina. A hyper-oestrogenized endometrium is found and there may be malignancy with associated carcinoma of the uterus.

Thecoma

This is a solid tumour that is usually 5 cm in diameter but may grow to 15 cm, although this is rare. It resembles a fibroma and Meigs' syndrome can occur. Yellowish fatty areas that show up in sections stained for fat are scattered among the fibrous tissue cells. These are theca lutein cells. A mixed granulosa cell tumour and thecoma also occurs.

Thecoma occurs mainly in women >30. It may present with a pelvic mass or uterine haemorrhage or both; ascites and pleural effusions may be seen. There is a high incidence of carcinoma of the endometrium in association with thecoma.

Sertoli–Leydig cell tumour

Often called androblastoma or arrhenoblastoma, this tumour causes virilism from its testosterone metabolism, but it is rare. The tumour may be cystic or solid and is potentially malignant. The cells consist of undifferentiated mesenchyme, and may be arranged in tubules as in the testicle.

Ovarian infections

Pure oophoritis is rare. However, the ovary is often involved in general pelvic infection. The condition of salpingoparametro-oophoritis is probably a better description of what is usually called a pelvic abscess. Certain viral conditions such as mumps can affect the ovary, and can cause ovarian swelling and some upset in ovulation, although this is very rare. Unlike such infections in the male, this is usually temporary.

Dysmenorrhoea

Dysmenorrhoea or pain associated with menstruation occurs in two main forms:

1 Primary spasmodic
2 Secondary, congestive or acquired.

Spasmodic dysmenorrhoea

This is very common; most normal women have some discomfort at the onset of menstruation. In dysmenorrhoea, pain is severe during the first hours or days of the period. It may be:

- continuous or spasmodic like colic
- accompanied by vomiting and fainting
- felt in the pelvis and lower back
- radiating into the legs
- diarrhoea.

Cause

The pain is probably caused by excessive prostaglandin production producing contractions of the uterine muscle in the first days of menstruation. There is rarely any pathological cause found.

It is associated with adenomyosis (p. 248).

Management

- Simple analgesics: non-steroidal anti-inflammatory drugs (NSAID), paracetamol and codeine or a combination of these may be used. Mefenamic acid 500 mg three times a day gives good pain relief in many cases.
- Hormone treatment includes oral contraception to inhibit ovulation and thus cause painless bleeding. One of the low-dose oral contraceptives may be preferred, although women sometimes object to contraceptives being given. The best effect follows hormones that inhibit ovulation. Given for a few months at a time they cause no ill effects and improvement may continue when treatment is stopped.

Secondary, congestive or acquired dysmenorrhoea

This is rare before age 25 years and uncommon before 30.

Symptoms

Pain begins before menstruation and may be relieved when bleeding starts. It is felt in the pelvis and back and made worse with exertion. Other symptoms such as menorrhagia and dyspareunia may be present.

This type of dysmenorrhoea usually occurs with a physical cause:

- Chronic pelvic infection
- Endometriosis
- Acquired fixed retroversion of the uterus
- Fibroids.

Endometriosis

Endometriosis is the presence of endometrium outside the uterus. This tissue responds to the hormone variations in the cycle, as does normally sited endometrium.

Endometriosis is most commonly a disease of women in the second half of their reproductive life, between 30 and 45 years, and tends to regress at the menopause or even before. The greatest incidence is in women who are childless or have few children; full-term pregnancy leads to regression of the condition, though miscarriage or early termination does not. Endometriosis is most common in women of European origin.

Pathology

Deposits of endometriosis consist of endometrial glands and stroma. The tissue bleeds in response to hormone cyclical changes, but there is no escape for the blood, which becomes encysted; infiltration of surrounding structures such as bowel occurs with subsequent fibrosis. These endometriotic areas vary in size from a pinhead to a large cyst with tarry material—the chocolate cyst. Perforation and leakage from chocolate cysts in the ovaries are very irritant and lead to dense adhesions.

The cause of endometriosis is unknown, but the following are hypotheses:

- Retrograde spread of collections of endometrial cells shed from the uterus at menstruation passing along the fallopian tube to the peritoneal cavity. This would account for by far the highest incidence of endometriosis occurring in the pelvis.
- Blood or lymph borne embolization.
- Metaplasia of islands of totipotential coelomic epithelium.

255

• Altered immunological recognition of endometrial tissue allowing acceptance of emboli of endometrium in these.

Probably a combination of the first and last theories is the most likely.

Sites

Endometriosis is most common in the pelvis. It is very occasionally found in bizarre sites such as the pleura, umbilicus, caesarean section scars, diaphragm, arm, leg or kidney, but these cases are rare.

Ovaries

The ovaries are a very common site for the disease, which may take the form of:
• numerous endometrial cysts containing blood
• a large chocolate or tarry cyst, densely adherent to the surrounding tissues
• bilateral cysts and adhesion formation, which may lead to the ovaries becoming stuck together-kissing ovarles (Plate 12).

Histological examination does not always reveal typical endometrial glands because these may have been destroyed in large cysts.

Pelvic peritoneum

The pelvic peritoneum is very often affected over the back of the uterus, fallopian tubes, uterosacral ligaments and pouch of Douglas. Peritoneal deposits often present as widespread blue-black nodules with scarring and puckering of the peritoneal surface. Adhesions may form between these and the back of the uterus, causing fixed retroversion.

Uterine ligaments

The uterosacral ligaments and the rectovaginal septum are commonly involved. Endometriosis in the round ligament may be found inside the abdominal cavity or may present as a tumour in the groin if the inguinal end of the ligament is involved.

Bowel

The intestines and rectum may all become infiltrated with endometriosis. The most common result is that fibrosis in the wall of the bowel leads to stricture formation and thus to obstruction. Bleeding into the bowel lumen is uncommon.

Urinary tract

Endometriosis may occur in the bladder, leading to haematuria and painful micturition. Fibrosis around the ureters can follow long-standing endometriosis, leading to obstruction of renal flow.

Abdominal wall

Endometriosis may occur as an isolated lesion at the umbilicus probably by travelling up a patent urachus; this presents as cyclical bleeding. It occurs in scars after operations on the uterus, particularly where the cavity of the uterus is opened, such as myomectomy or caesarean section.

Perineum and vagina

Deposits of endometriosis may be seen in perineal scars and in the vaginal wall, although these are surprisingly uncommon.

Classification

Endometriosis is classified into stages to allow comparison between clusters and grade response to treatment (Table 17.3).

Clinical features

Symptoms

The symptoms of pelvic endometriosis depend on the site and the activity of the disease:
• *Pain*: three main types of pain are found:
— *congestive dysmenorrhoea* begins with menstruation; it is felt in the pelvis and lower back
— *ovulation* pain is sometimes severe in midcycle

Table 17.3 Classification of endometriosis from the American Fertility Society

Size of deposits	<1 cm	1–3 cm	>3 cm
Peritoneum			
Superficial	1	2	4
Deep	2	4	6
Ovary			
Right superficial	1	2	4
Deep	4	16	20
Left superficial	1	2	4
Deep	4	16	20
Adhesions			
Ovary			
Right film	1	2	4
Dense	4	8	16
Left film	1	2	4
Dense	4	8	16
Tube			
Right film	1	2	4
Dense	4	8	16
Left film	1	2	4
Dense	4	8	16
Pouch of Douglas			
Partly obliterated	4→		
Completely obliterated	40→		
Score			
1–5	Minimal		
6–15	Mild		
16–40	Moderate		
>40	Severe		

— *dyspareunia* is felt deep in the pelvis due to pressing on the uterosacral ligaments and recto-vaginal septum during coitus.

• *Infertility* may be the main complaint, caused by:
   — ovulation occurring into closed-off areas of fibrosis
   — damage to tubal fimbria
   — kinking of tubes by adhesions
   — blockage of tube by deposits of endometriosis in the wall.

• *Disturbances of menstruation*: menorrhagia may occur if deposits are in the myometrium. Shorter cycles and episodes of prolonged bleeding may occur (adenomyosis).

Other symptoms from endometriosis may be:
• haematuria
• dysuria
• intestinal obstruction
• pain on defecation
• occasionally a chocolate cyst may rupture, causing symptoms and signs of an acute abdomen.

Physical signs

The most typical clinical picture is that of fixed retroversion of the uterus with enlarged, tender ovaries adherent behind it. Deposits in the utero-sacral ligaments may be palpable as tender nodules. Laparoscopy is essential to establish the diagnosis.

Differential diagnosis

• *Chronic pelvic infection* most closely resembles pelvic endometriosis, with dysmenorrhoea, menorrhagia, sterility and dyspareunia being identical, but the history and laparoscopy findings are different and pelvic inflammatory disease (PID) pain is rarely cyclical.
• *Fibroids* of the uterus are often associated with endometriosis, and the differential diagnosis may be difficult.

Treatment

Treatment of pelvic endometriosis is essentially conservative because the condition:
• tends to occur during the reproductive period
• does not become malignant
• tends to regress at the menopause.

Hormone therapy

This is successful in many cases. The diagnosis must first be made at laparoscopy and if there are large chocolate cysts these should be drained/removed; local areas of endometriosis can be coagulated with laser/diathermy through the laparoscope.

Danazol inhibits pituitary gonadotrophin secretion and in adequate doses will suppress menstruation. The initial dose is 200 mg daily in divided doses, increasing up to 600 mg daily as required. Treatment should be given initially for 6 months. There may be androgenic effects:

- acne
- hirsutes
- weight gain due to fluid retention.

It is important to be sure that the woman is not pregnant and it must be stressed that danazol is not a contraceptive.

Progesterone used to be the major therapy, using norethisterone starting on the fifth day of menstruation with 10 mg daily and increasing up to 40 mg daily. Nausea, vomiting, weight gain and fluid retention occur, although a cure is unusual.

An alternative progestogen, medroxyprogesterone acetate 10–30 mg daily by mouth, can suppress menstruation for 6 months. If breakthrough bleeding is troublesome, the dose should be increased.

Side effects are common with hormone treatments, but, in patients who persist, regression of the endometriotic lesions occurs and pregnancy may become possible, though ovulation may be delayed for several months after treatment.

Synthetic substitutes of GnRH and their agonists are inhibitors of ovarian function. Two weeks' treatment (subcutaneously or nasal spray) reduces follicle-stimulating hormone (FSH) and luteinizing hormone (LH) concentrations and leads to lower oestrogen levels. Treatment for 3–6 months gives relief. Side effects may be:

- headaches
- hot flushes
- depression
- loss of bone density if treatment is >6 months.

Surgery

Lesions may be treated at laparoscopy by diathermy or laser. Increasingly laparoscopic surgery is being used to remove areas of peritoneum that are affected by endometriosis, as well as larger masses that may be found in the rectovaginal space or on the uterosacral ligaments. Laparotomy may be indicated in:

- pelvic masses >5 cm
- acute rupture of a cyst
- intestinal obstruction.

Conservative surgery is always performed if possible, aiming to leave the uterus and normal ovarian tissue.

In intractable cases, and especially among women who do not want children, wider surgery may be needed. Hysterectomy with bilateral salpingo-oophorectomy may be performed for intractable menorrhagia and dysmenorrhoea or when there are fibroids or adenomyosis. Some ovarian tissue may be left if not actually involved in the destructive process.

Premenstrual tension

Premenstrual tension occurs most usually in the second half of the menstrual cycle. It consists of a cluster of behavioural symptoms and physical signs that come in the second half of the cycle with abolition immediately after menstruation.

Symptoms and signs

- Irritability
- Depression
- Lassitude
- Insomnia
- Lack of concentration
- Oedema with fluid retention
- Abdominal swelling
- Swollen fingers and ankles
- Weight gain.

Migraine can occur during this phase or at the onset of menstruation. The symptoms tend to come on 7–10 days premenstrually, after the luteal phase has been established. Women may become more accident prone and there is an increased prevalence of suicide. Some women who suffer from premenstrual tension have endogenous depression exacerbated at this time.

Aetiology

Hormonal

- Timing in cycle in luteal phase
- Improved in absence of cyclical ovarian activity

- Renin–angiotensin system
- Reduction of endogenous opioids
- Changes in monoamine neurotransmitters.

Probably a combination of the second and third factors.

Treatment

- Explanation and reassurance.
- Progestogens: may be deficient in second half of cycle so replace them.
- Oestrogens: to suppress ovulation.
- Oral contraceptive: combined preparation of both of the above; works for some.
- Danazol: stops ovulation; beware unwanted androgenic side effects.
- Evening primrose oil: may effect essential fatty acid metabolism.
- Pyridoxine (vitamin B_6): may affect dopamine and serotonin metabolism. Benefit weak: beware overdosage and neuropathy with long-term treatment.
- Antidepressants: during the premenstrual phase may help. More severe cases need psychiatric treatment. Fluoxetine has been shown to be the most effective.

The variety of medication emphasizes how little the cause of this syndrome is understood. Treatments may be a matter of trial and error.

Abdominal organs

Pyelonephritis

The woman presents with ill-defined abdominal pain, pyrexia and shivering. The diagnosis differs from an acute abdominal problem because the pain is often around the side in the loin and tenderness is then high up in the costal angles.

Examination of the urine for pus cells and organisms reveals the diagnosis. Treatment is conservative with bedrest, fluids and appropriate antibiotics.

Very rarely a ureteric stone may present in pregnancy. If this sticks in the ureter, it causes pain by stretch of the ureter from dammed-back urine (renal colic). Pethidine is helpful both for its

analgesic properties and because it is an antispasmodic.

Appendicitis

This occurs equally commonly in early pregnancy as during any other 9 months of a young woman's life. It is a young person's disease.

Diagnosis can be difficult because the appendix rises up from its usual position in the right iliac fossa. The typical history of periumbilical pain moving to the right iliac fossa may not be given in pregnancy; the signs are confusing because the caecum with its attached appendix is pushed up the right paracolic gutter by the enlarging uterus. Remembering this, the examiner must seek the point of maximum tenderness higher in the abdomen.

Treatment should be by surgery and the surgeon in later pregnancy would do well to mark the site of maximum tenderness before the anaesthetic and incise there rather than over McBurney's point.

There used to be a higher mortality of appendicitis in pregnancy because of the reluctance of people to operate for fear of miscarriage. However, it must be realized that a progressing appendicitis carries a much higher risk to the fetus and mother than the problems of carrying out a surgical procedure under controlled anaesthesia.

Rectus haematoma

The deep epigastric arteries with their concomitant epigastric veins may be stretched by the growing uterus and occasionally, after a severe attack of coughing, one of these veins under tension may rupture. This leads to a haematoma that is very difficult to diagnose. If seen early, the pain is localized under one segment of one rectus muscle, but after a few hours this sign spreads. If seen very late, there may be anaemia due to loss of blood into the haematoma.

If diagnosed competently, surgical treatment is not needed. Occasionally, a laparotomy is performed and the diagnosis becomes obvious when the rectus muscles are separated before opening the peritoneum. Usually it is too late to ligate any of the veins. The operator need proceed no further.

Bowel problems

Should a gynaecologist open the abdomen and find a bowel or peritoneal problem, he or she would be wise to consult with a surgical colleague urgently. Although gynaecologists may have been trained once to do general surgery they do not practise such operations daily. Combined surgical and gynaecological operating would probably be better for the woman.

Chapter 18

Breast disease

In the UK, obstetricians and gynaecologists do not usually deal with breast problems. However, many women will mention that they have felt a lump when visiting the gynaecologist or in antenatal clinics. Breast disease is managed by specialist breast surgeons or general surgeons with an interest in breast surgery. This is partly a consequence of the work of Sir Hedley Atkins who set up the first specialist breast surgical unit in the world at Guy's Hospital.

Breast problems are extremely common, comprising one in six of all general surgery referrals. This is partly the result of a heightened awareness of breast cancer, which is the most common malignancy in the UK among women.

Breast history

The most frequent breast symptom is a lump. The particular features of a breast lump are usually ascertained during clinical examination but it is important to find out the following:
- *Time*: how long the lump has been there.
- *Pain*: whether it is painful. Breast pain is rarely associated with malignancy but may be severe and may interfere significantly with a patient's lifestyle.

Its site, distribution, severity, radiation, precipitating factors and relieving factors should all be asked about, but the effect that it has on a patient's lifestyle is the most relevant question.
- *Size*: whether it has changed in size. In particular, areas of benign breast thickening and nodularity may become more pronounced and more tender before each menstrual period.
- *Nipple discharge*: a common symptom that can be a sign of malignancy. It should be noted whether this is unilateral or bilateral, occurs spontaneously or only on expression from a single or multiple ducts, its colour and whether there is blood staining.
- *Nipple inversion*: can also be a sign of malignancy. The salient points are whether it is unilateral or bilateral and how long it has been present.
- *Nipple eczema*: should be distinguished from Paget's disease of the nipple. This often requires a skin biopsy.

Breast examination

Examination is carried out with the patient seated in good light and in a warm room. She should be stripped to the waist.

Inspection

Inspection involves comparing one breast with the other, particularly with regard to:

Lecture Notes: Obstetrics and Gynaecology, 3rd edition. By Diana Hamilton-Fairley. Published 2009 by Blackwell Publishing. ISBN: 978-1-4051-7801-3.

- symmetry
- preservation of the natural curved contour of the breast
- position and appearance of the nipples
- scars
- changes in the skin (erythema, peau d'orange, ulceration) and skin dimpling. It is quite common for one breast to be a little larger than the other but be sure to find out whether this is a recent change. Always look underneath the breast in the inframammary fold. Skin dimpling is a very significant sign because it is associated with malignancy in more than 95% of cases.

Palpation (Fig. 18.1)

Each breast should be palpated in turn, starting with the normal breast. Palpation is carried out with the palmar aspect of the index, middle and ring fingers. It is usually more sensitive to use the dominant hand. The impression of a breast lump is obtained by moving the examining fingers in a circular motion. The fingers should be pressed down gently but firmly and moved in a circular manner so that any underlying mass will be felt as something slipping under the fingers. The examining fingers and the patient's skin move more freely than a mass within the breast tissue, and the latter is therefore felt to slip under the fingers but over the stationary chest wall. A mass in the breast can be felt to move relative to the fixed structures of the underlying chest wall and ribs.

In the relatively uncommon instance where the breast mass is tethered to the underlying muscle there is significantly less mobility, and virtually no mobility when the underlying muscle is tensed (by pressing the hand onto the hip).

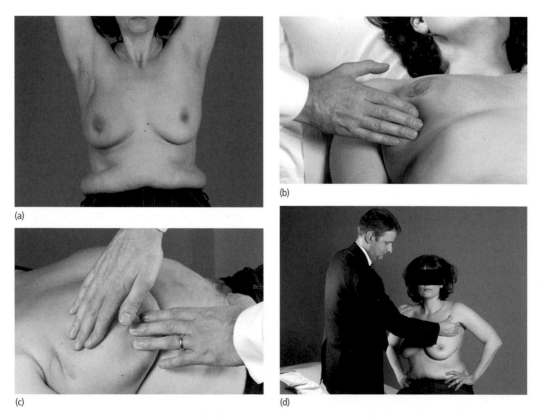

(a)

(b)

(c)

(d)

Figure 18.1 Breast examination. (a) Inspection. (b) Palpation using index, middle and ring fingers (e) Non-dominant hand stretching the skin. (d) Examination of the axilla.

A mass within the skin, such as a sebaceous cyst, does not slip under the fingers and is felt only by direct pressure that particularly identifies the edge of the lesion. Palpation of breast lumps is easier with the patient lying absolutely flat with the bed high enough so that the elbow of the examiner is at least flexed to 90°. It is important to examine the breast systematically so that none of the breast is missed. It is usually best to develop your own method for this. One way is to examine the breast a quadrant at a time and then specifically to feel the retroareolar area and the axillary tail. During examination the non-dominant hand can be used to stretch out the breast tissue, particularly the tissues in the lateral aspect of the breast.

Axillary nodes can be examined with either the patient sitting up (hands on hips) or lying supine (with the arm abducted to 45° and supported by the examiner). The boundaries of the axilla should be examined in turn:
- the medial boundary (lateral chest wall)
- the anterior boundary (the anterior axillary fold)
- the posterior boundary (latissimus dorsi)
- the lateral boundary (the upper aspect of the arm)
- the apex.

Lymph nodes draining the breast are usually situated in the medial, posterior or apical parts of the axilla. Sometimes a pathological axillary node lies particularly low in the axilla or in the axillary tail of the breast.

Lastly, the supra- and infraclavicular fossae should be palpated with the patient sitting up (preferably from behind). If metastatic disease is suspected the lower lung field should be percussed for the presence of pleural effusion and the liver palpated.

Benign breast disease

Breast cysts

Aetiology

All women will develop cysts in their breasts at one time or another. Usually they are too small to feel.

They develop under the influence of oestrogen and are therefore usually found only during the reproductive years or in women on hormone replacement therapy (HRT). They are not common between the ages of puberty and 25. Breast cysts develop by the dilatation of a breast duct.

Symptoms

Breast lump (sometimes of considerable size) that is frequently painful or tender.

Signs

Smooth, round, circular mass that may be visible. Breast cysts are usually tense and can feel remarkably hard.

Investigations

Breast cysts are best investigated with ultrasound, which can show any irregularity in the wall of the cyst. Mammography is generally not able to differentiate between a solid and a cystic mass (Fig. 18.2).

Natural history

Breast cysts often appear suddenly and equally may disappear relatively quickly. Some cysts, however, remain for a number of years. Breast cysts practically never become malignant. Rarely, they can develop *in situ* malignancy (intracystic papillary carcinoma).

Treatment

Breast cysts do not need any treatment unless they are uncomfortable, in which case they can be aspirated with a needle and syringe.

Fibrocystic change

Aetiology

Fibrocystic change, previously termed 'fibroadenosis', is a normal way that the breast develops with

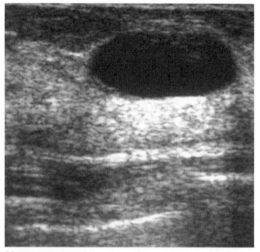

(a)

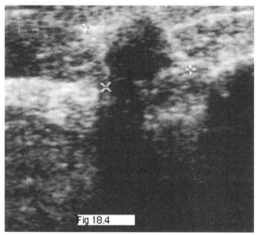

Fig 18.4

(b)

Figure 18.2 Ultrasound scan of (a) benign breast cyst and (b) breast carcinoma.

time and under the influence of the normal menstrual cycle. It involves an increase in the fibrous tissue of the breast stroma, together with the formation of multiple small and large cysts. It occurs to a greater or lesser extent in every woman and may be responsible for breast lumps.

Symptoms

Tender breast lump that varies with the menstrual cycle and becomes more prominent before each period.

Signs

A diffuse area of tender thickening or nodularity, only rarely amounting to a discrete mass with definable edges. The thickening may be approximately symmetrical with the same site in the opposite breast.

Investigations

Fibrocystic change shows as a diffuse increase in the density of the breast parenchyma on a mammogram. If the associated cysts are large enough these will appear as discrete, rounded masses. An ultrasound shows small and large cysts.

Natural history

Some women have more fibrocystic change than others, resulting in permanently lumpy breasts. This is more apparent in slim women. The changes generally resolve after the menopause.

Treatment

Reassurance only is required.

Breast pain (mastalgia)

Aetiology

The vast majority of breast pain is caused by either hormonal changes in the breast tissue or a chronic inflammatory condition of the major breast ducts close to the nipple—periductal mastitis. Breast pain is only very rarely associated with malignancy and then only when it is unilateral and localized to a specific site.

Symptoms

The pain is usually described as an aching, particularly in the lateral aspects of the breasts, radiating into the axilla and sometimes into the upper arm. The pain may be unilateral. It is often worse in the second half of each menstrual cycle, although mastalgia relating to hormonal changes can also frequently be non-cyclical. Hormonal breast pain does not respond significantly to standard analgesics. It is usually associated with marked tenderness and is helped by wearing a supportive brassière. The breast pain relating to periductal mastitis is non-cyclical, sharper and more transient, and frequently radiates through the nipple.

Signs

Breast tenderness. Patients with hormonal mastalgia often have denser and more nodular breast tissue.

Investigations

No investigations are necessary except in the case of unilateral and focal breast pain.

Treatment

Simple measures such as reducing the amount of dietary caffeine and taking regular starflower or evening primrose oil. Drugs that are helpful include tamoxifen (10 mg daily), danazol (100 mg daily) and bromocriptine (1 mg daily).

Nipple discharge

Aetiology

Nipple discharge may be caused by malignancy but is more frequently the result of either periductal mastitis (chronic inflammation involving a number of breast ducts) or a duct papilloma (usually involving a single duct). Periductal mastitis is much more common in smokers.

Symptoms

Periductal mastitis causes discharge of any colour (brown, green, clear, milky). It is often bilateral. A duct papilloma causes clear discharge that is usually unilateral. Breast cancer causes unilateral discharge. All three causes can be associated with blood staining.

Signs

• *Periductal mastitis*: multiduct, multicoloured discharge, usually bilateral.

• *Papilloma*: single duct, crystal clear discharge.
• *Carcinoma*: unilateral discharge, often with blood staining and associated underlying breast lump and/or nipple distortion.

Investigations

Mammography and ultrasound should be carried out to exclude malignancy. An ultrasound scan may demonstrate a large papilloma. Nipple discharge fluid can be sent for cytological examination.

Natural history

• *Periductal mastitis*: this is a chronic condition.
• *Duct papilloma*: a duct papilloma can cause profuse discharge, which is inconvenient for the patient.

Treatment

• *Periductal mastitis*: no treatment is available except for surgical total duct excision.
• *Duct papilloma*: breast duct microendoscopy and microdochectomy.

Fibroadenoma

Aetiology

A fibroadenoma is a solid mass arising in the breast of young women, particularly from the age of puberty to the mid-30s. It is also more common in postmenopausal women who take HRT. The aetiology is unknown, although there is undoubtedly a hormonal influence.

Symptoms

Painless lump. Some patients have multiple lesions.

Signs

Firm to hard, rounded or elliptical mass that is characterized by unusual mobility underneath the palpating fingers (colloquially known as a breast mouse).

Investigations

A well-defined mass with discrete clear margins on both mammography and ultrasound.

Natural history

Fibroadenomas do not become malignant. They may gradually increase in size and in this case they should be removed to definitely exclude a malignant mass that may have the same clinical features as a fibroadenoma.

Treatment

It is important to differentiate this solid mass from other solid masses in the breast such as a carcinoma. This should always involve at least needle aspiration cytology and, over the age of 30, preferably a core needle biopsy. If there is any doubt about the diagnosis the lesion should be removed surgically by excision biopsy. This latter operation can often be carried out under a local anaesthetic.

Breast abscess

Aetiology

A breast abscess can either be associated with lactation or periductal mastitis.

Symptoms

Painful, rapidly enlarging mass in the breast with associated pyrexia.

Signs

Lactational abscess may be very large and the borders may be quite indistinct so that the mass forms a prominent area of hardening of the breast tissue. Abscesses associated with periductal mastitis are found either in the retroareolar region or just around the areola. Breast abscesses are always associated with overlying breast erythema. There may be peau d'orange. This latter scenario mimics inflammatory breast cancer and this differential diagnosis should always be entertained.

Investigations

Breast abscesses are best shown by ultrasonography.

Treatment

Early in the development of a breast infection (whatever the aetiology) treatment with antibiotics may be successful in averting a frank abscess. Use either co-amoxiclav or flucloxacillin and metronidazole (anaerobes may be responsible). Once the breast abscess is >1 cm needle aspiration or incision drainage is usually required. Needle aspiration may need to be repeated.

Other benign breast lumps

- *Lipoma*: soft, rounded, quite difficult to feel, may have a distinct edge.
- *Hamartoma*: fairly soft, discrete, no malignant potential.
- *Phylloides tumour*: mimics a fibroadenoma and may be quite similar histologically. Phylloides tumours may grow to become very large. They may recur after excision if a small amount of the lesion is left behind and they should therefore be removed with a clear histological margin. There are malignant variants of phylloides tumours that develop into fibrosarcomas.

Breast malignancy

Epidemiology

Rates

The incidence of breast cancer in the UK is still increasing. In 1999 there were 40 000 cases diagnosed each year. The mortality from breast cancer has been falling since the late 1980s, which is thought to result from the therapeutic effect of tamoxifen and more recently the beneficial effects of the National Breast Screening Programme (Figs 18.3 and 18.4).

Risk factors

Genetic

Mutations in either of the two recognized breast cancer genes (*BRCA*-1 and *BRCA*-2) result in a very high chance of developing breast or ovarian cancer. Other genetic abnormalities associated with a higher than average breast cancer risk are Cowden's syndrome and ataxia telangiectasia.

Hormonal

The following are associated with a higher than average risk of breast cancer: early menarche, late menopause, no full-term pregnancies, full-term pregnancy occurring after the age of 40. Longer periods of breast-feeding and multiple full-term pregnancies are associated with a lower incidence of breast cancer. The oral contraceptive pill has practically no effect on breast cancer risk. HRT is associated with a small increase in the risk of breast cancer, which amounts to around 35% increase after 12 years of usage.

Environmental

Radiation (such as that associated with the fallout from the atomic bombs in Japan) is associated with all subtypes of breast cancer. Alcohol increases the risk of breast cancer in a dose-dependent manner. Diet has a large effect on breast cancer risk. Diets rich in fresh fruit and vegetables are associated

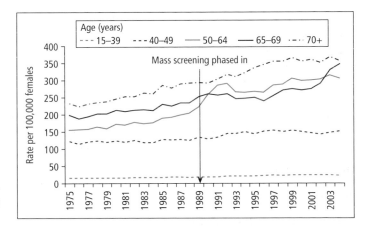

Figure 18.3 Age-standardized incidence of breast cancer in England and Wales (1975–2004).

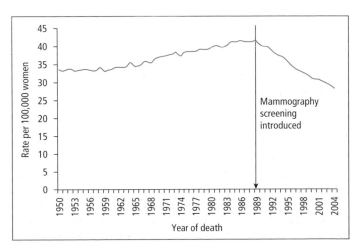

Figure 18.4 Age-standardized mortality rates from breast cancer in women aged 55–69 years in England and Wales.

with a much lower risk of breast cancer (50% reduction). This risk reduction is probably partly related to vitamin C intake. Smoking is not related to breast cancer. The lowest incidence of breast cancer occurs in Japan, the highest risk in western Europe and North America. Women migrating from one geographical region to another slowly develop the full breast cancer risk associated with their new environment.

Presentation

Breast malignancy most commonly presents with a painless lump. Skin tethering is highly suggestive of malignancy. The characteristics of a malignant lump compared with a benign lump are compared in Table 18.1. For breast cancers around the nipple, inversion or distortion of the nipple together with nipple discharge may be presenting symptoms. Infrequently, patients present with an enlarged axillary lymph node, with no obvious palpable mass in the breast. Other less common symptoms and signs of breast cancer are peau d'orange, distortion of the shape of the breast, generalized enlargement of the breast, focal breast pain and skin changes (erythema or ulceration). Paget's disease of the nipple is always associated with an underlying malignancy. This may be invasive or *in situ* disease. Paget's disease may look similar to nipple eczema, being dry and scaly or possibly beefy red and weeping.

Staging

- Stage 1: breast cancer confined to the breast.
- Stage 2: involvement of the breast and axillary lymph nodes.

- Stage 3: locally advanced disease involving the breast with muscle fixation or skin involvement.
- Stage 4: metastatic disease.

Breast cancer can be more accurately staged according to the TNM classification.

- **T** relates to the size of primary tumour:
  — T1 = 2–20 mm
  — T2 = 21–50 mm
  — T3 ≥51 mm
- **N** refers to the regional lymph node status:
  — N0 = node negative
  — N1 = mobile ipsilateral nodes
  — N2 = immobile, fixed or matted nodes
  — N3 = internal mammary node involvement
- The **M** classification whether there is metastatic disease that:
  — M0 = no detected metastases
  — M1 = metastatic disease.

Primary breast cancer is usually simply staged by performing the following:

- Chest X-ray to look for pleural or pulmonary disease
- Liver function test or a liver ultrasound to look for hepatic metastases
- Large tumours (>4 cm) or high-grade tumours (3) would in addition have staging involving a bone scan.

Investigation and diagnosis

Investigation of any breast lump is based on the principle of triple diagnosis.

- Clinical assessment
- Radiological imaging
- Cytological or histological verification.

Table 18.1 Clinical features of some common breast lumps

	Fibrocystic	Cyst	Fibroadenoma	Cancer
Tender	Yes	Yes	No	No
Discrete	No	Yes	Yes	Usually
Surface	No edge/surface	Smooth	Smooth	Irregular/smooth
Consistency	Normal to firm	Firm to hard	Firm	Firm to hard
Shape	Nodularity/ridge	Round	Round/ellipse/lobulated	Rounded
Overlying skin	Normal	Normal	Normal	Tethering
Multiple lesions	Yes	Yes	Yes	No

It is only if all these three types of assessment are entirely benign that a lump can be left without further investigation.

Invasive breast cancer shows up on a mammogram by producing either:
- a dense (white) mass or
- an area of distortion of the breast parenchyma or microcalcification.

On mammography, a malignant mass will appear spiculate with ill-defined edges. Breast distortion may occur without a mass, particularly in the case of a lobular carcinoma. Malignant microcalcification is focal, relatively fine and heterogeneous. The sensitivity of mammography for detecting a malignancy is around 85% (Fig. 18.5).

An *ultrasound scan* will show a malignant mass as an echo-poor focal area that interrupts the normal transverse breast architecture. The lesion is ill defined and usually taller rather than wider. There may be a dense acoustic shadow. The sensitivity of breast ultrasound for the diagnosis of malignancy is between 75% and 80%.

Needle cytology is carried out without local anaesthetic. The specimen, which usually amounts to just a drop or two of blood-stained tissue fluid, is spread onto glass microscope slides. These can be air dried. No immediate staining is required although this is carried out later in the laboratory. The breast cytopathologist requires five clusters of duct epithelial cells to be able to make a definitive

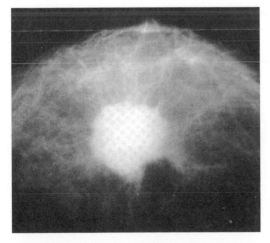

Figure 18.5 Mammogram revealing malignant mass.

diagnosis. An alternative to fine-needle aspiration cytology (FNAC) is core-needle biopsy. This is now being carried out much more frequently because it gives additional information about the architecture of the lesion. It is performed under local anaesthetic with a core-needle-biopsy gun and needle varying between 14 and 11 gauge. It is possible to perform cytological examination of the cells on the surface of the core by simply rolling the tissue core between two microscope slides. This gives an accurate answer in less than an hour (touch imprint cytology). A core biopsy will require at least 48 hours for histological examination.

Magnetic resonance imaging (MRI) may be used to diagnose breast malignancy. It is particularly sensitive (95–100%) but the specificity is much lower (65–70%). Examination needs to be carried out with contrast during the first half of the menstrual period. Benign breast lesions such as fibroadenomas may enhance, but the enhancement characteristics are generally different in benign compared with malignant lesions.

Treatment

General strategy

Breast cancer, when confined to the breast or the axillary lymph nodes, is curable. Metastatic breast cancer is not. More than 90% of patients present with primary breast cancer (stage 1 or 2) with no evidence of metastatic disease. However, at this stage micrometastases are probably present in some patients and these are often the patients who later relapse systemically. The treatment of primary breast cancer is therefore to eradicate the malignancy from the breast and axillary lymph nodes and to provide some type of systemic (adjuvant) treatment to try to eliminate any micrometastases. The presence or absence of micrometastases is not known in any one individual patient, although the likelihood of micrometastases can be estimated by taking into consideration the lymph node status and the size and grade of the tumour.

When considering the treatment of primary breast cancer, think of three anatomical boxes, each of which will receive its own treatment. The treatment strategy for each box has either no or only marginal impact on the other two anatomical areas and each should therefore be formulated independently. The treatment of primary breast cancer should therefore involve adequate treatment of:

- the breast itself (breast primary)
- the axillary lymph nodes
- the micro-metastases.

The treatment of a breast primary

Surgical treatment

The most effective modality utilized in the treatment of breast cancer is the surgical treatment of the primary. The aim of surgical treatment is to achieve complete removal of the primary lesion together with any satellite lesions and any associated ductal carcinoma *in situ* (DCIS). Mastectomy is one effective way of removing a primary lesion, although it is now well established that a lumpectomy, if carried out in conjunction with breast radiotherapy (breast conserving therapy), is as effective as mastectomy in terms of both local control and overall survival. Lumpectomy is not appropriate for large tumours (generally >4 cm), multifocal tumours (unless the lesions are small and closely applied to each other) or lesions associated with very extensive DCIS. For these cases and for patients who cannot, for one reason or another, undergo breast radiotherapy (serious heart or lung disease), mastectomy is the only safe option. In the case of large tumours primary chemotherapy (neo-adjuvant chemotherapy) can be employed at the outset to shrink the tumour to a size that is amenable to a lumpectomy and radiotherapy.

Opinion is still divided over the importance of clear surgical margins after breast lumpectomy. It is certain that widely involved margins are associated with a much higher rate of local recurrence. Focally involved margins or close margins (1 mm or less) are associated with a small increase in local recurrence rates compared with widely clear margins.

Mastectomy as performed by Halstead in the early part of the twentieth century involved removal of not only the breast but also the axillary nodes and pectoralis minor and pectoralis major. This was termed a radical mastectomy. It is now known that it is not necessary to remove either of the pectoral muscles because primary breast cancer only infrequently infiltrates the skeletal muscle. Removal of the breast and axillary lymph nodes is termed a modified radical mastectomy.

Breast radiotherapy

Radiotherapy to the breast after lumpectomy is a critical and irreplaceable part of breast-conserving therapy for primary breast cancer. If breast radiotherapy is not possible then mastectomy is the only safe alternative. The radiotherapy course takes 6 weeks and involves daily fractions (30 fractions). It is usually associated with a skin reaction that comprises erythema and sometimes peeling of the skin.

Breast radiotherapy can be given to the chest wall after a mastectomy. It is shown to be effective in reducing local recurrence rates in the patients with positive axillary nodes, high-grade tumours and large tumours. There is some evidence that irradiation of the supraclavicular fossa and internal mammary nodes, in addition to the chest wall, may produce a small improvement in overall survival.

Treatment of the axilla

All patients with primary breast cancer (stage 1 and 2) undergo surgery to the axilla. This achieves two main functions: first any lymph nodes involved with metastatic carcinoma are removed effectively avoiding the potentially serious problem of axillary recurrence. The incidence of axillary recurrence without any axillary treatment is around 30–35%, whereas after full axillary node clearance the risks of recurrence are around 1%. Axillary surgery is also very important in staging the axillae. The status of the axillary nodes is the best prognostic indicator that is currently available in patients with breast cancer, and the place of other aspects of treatment such as adjuvant systemic chemotherapy and chest wall radiotherapy are decided largely on the axillary node status. Not only is the presence or absence of axillary disease important, but also the number of axillary nodes that are involved provides more specific prognostic information that allows treatment to be customized to the individual patient.

Until recently standard axillary surgery comprised a full axillary node clearance to level 2 or 3. The levels are related to the medial extent of the dissection, level 2 being under pectoralis minor and level 3 the lymph nodes medial to this. Usually this operation removes between 10 and 50 lymph nodes. Axillary node clearance has proved itself to be a very effective cancer operation, but it is associated with significant morbidity. Currently around 60% of breast cancer patients are node negative, and for these women a full axillary clearance represents unnecessary over-treatment. For this reason, patients who are likely to turn out to be axillary node negative are increasingly being advised to undergo a new surgical alternative, termed 'sentinel node biopsy'. In this procedure only one or two lymph nodes are removed from the axilla greatly reducing the postoperative morbidity. All patients being considered for sentinel node biopsy should have a preoperative axillary node ultrasound with image-guided fine needle axillary clearance (FNAC) of any abnormal lymph nodes that are identified.

Sentinel node biopsy was first described in 1997 and is currently carried out in many centres throughout the UK, but is not yet universally available. In this technique blue dye and/or an isotope-labelled colloid tracer are injected close to the breast primary or directly into the retroareolar lymphatic plexus. The tracer is carried through the breast lymphatic system to the ipsilateral axilla where the first one or two lymph nodes in the axillary chain of lymph nodes become blue and radioactive. These 'hot' and blue nodes are termed the sentinel nodes. In theory if the sentinel nodes are clear of metastatic disease, all the other axillary nodes distal to them are also negative and a full axillary clearance is not required. Of course, if the sentinel node is affected by metastatic disease, a second operation is required to complete the axillary clearance. Sentinel node biopsy has the potential for avoiding axillary clearance surgery in more than 50% of patients with breast cancer, and as a consequence has become rapidly accepted

as a standard of care in institutions where it is available.

Patients who have proven axillary node metastasis or have a positive sentinel node biopsy should undergo a full axillary clearance. All the lymph nodes within the axillary fat up to the level of the axillary vein are removed. Axillary node clearance is associated with significant morbidity. The most serious problem associated with this type of the surgery is lymphoedema, which occurs to a variable degree but is serious enough to impact on a patient's lifestyle in around 15% of cases. Lymphoedema is more common in older woman and women who are overweight. Other problems following axillary node clearance include an alteration in the sensation of the skin of the upper arm due to interruption of the intercostobrachial nerve, pain in the arm and an increased susceptibility to serious infections in the affected upper limb. Less radical axillary node dissection may be undertaken (level 1), but it is not entirely clear whether this makes very much impact on the postoperative morbidity.

Adjuvant systemic treatment

Adjuvant systemic therapy aims to eliminate any micrometastatic disease that may be present but undetectable at the time of primary diagnosis. Adjuvant systemic treatment is given after primary breast surgery and involves hormonal treatment, chemotherapy or both.

Adjuvant chemotherapy

Adjuvant chemotherapy is usually given as soon after primary breast surgery as is safe (2–3 weeks). The combinations of chemotherapy drugs that are normally used are either FEC (5-fluorouracil, epirubicin, cyclophosphamide) or AC (Adriamycin/doxorubicin and cyclophosphamide). In younger node-positive patients the regimen may be switched to a taxane-containing combinations after the first three or four cycles. Usually six or eight cycles of this treatment are given with a 3-week gap between each cycle, meaning that chemotherapy continues for between 4 and 6 months. The common side effects include tiredness, nausea, hair loss, stomatitis and infection.

Adjuvant chemotherapy is much more effective in younger (premenopausal) woman and in women who are node positive. It is only occasionally used in woman over the age of 70 as there is little evidence of its efficacy in this age group. In younger women these drug combinations may cause infertility and this adverse affect needs to be very carefully discussed with the patient. A single cycle of IVF with embryo cryopreservation can be safely carried out prior to starting chemotherapy if this is a serious concern.

Adjuvant hormone therapy

Hormone therapy is effective in breast cancer because at least 75% of breast malignancies are composed of cells that depend primarily on oestrogen as a growth factor. These tumours are identifiable by immunohistochemical staining to reveal the oestrogen receptor. It is only breast cancers expressing the oestrogen receptor that are amenable to adjuvant hormonal treatment.

The most common hormonal agent used in the adjuvant setting is tamoxifen. Tamoxifen is a selective oestrogen receptor blocker that fortunately effectively blocks the oestrogen receptor in breast duct epithelial and breast cancer cells. Tamoxifen is used in the adjuvant setting for a period of 5 years after surgery. It has a generally benign side-effect profile and has only one significant drug interaction (with warfarin). Common side effects are menopausal symptoms such as hot flushes and night sweats. The two serious side effects associated with tamoxifen use are slightly increased incidence of endometrial carcinoma and a low incidence of deep venous thrombosis and pulmonary embolism. Adjuvant tamoxifen reduces the rate of breast cancer recurrence by around a third and also reduces the chance of developing a primary breast cancer in the opposite breast by 35–40%.

The aromatase inhibitor class drugs are now also widely used in the adjuvant setting. They have been shown to be slightly more effective than tamoxifen and are currently prescribed for women with node-positive disease. These drugs include anastrozole, letrozole and exemestane. They work by blocking the synthesis of estradiol from adrenal precursors in peripheral adipose tissue. Production of estradiol in the ovaries is not dependent on aromatase, so the aromatase inhibitor class of drugs is therefore effective only in postmenopausal woman. They have turned out to have a rather worse side-effect profile than tamoxifen, causing troublesome joint pains, but do not increase the incidence of endometrial carcinoma.

Measures that effectively reduce circulating estradiol in premenopausal women are also effective as adjuvant treatments. These include goserelin or bilateral oophorectomy. Goserelin is an LHRH (LH-releasing hormone) agonist that suppresses oestrogen secretion by the ovary. It is given by depot injection once a month. For premenopausal woman it can be given together with tamoxifen with enhanced effect. Goserelin or ovarectomy drastically reduces circulating estradiol in young women and both are associated with a significant reduction in bone density as well as other menopausal side effects.

Ductal carcinoma *in situ*

Pathology

It is now established that DCIS is the precursor lesion to invasive breast cancer. The individual cells are derived from the breast duct epithelium and are similar morphologically to those found in invasive breast cancer. The critical fact that differentiates DCIS from invasive breast cancer is the lack of invasion. The atypical cells that characterize DCIS remain within the breast ducts and as a consequence do not have the ability either to spread to the regional lymph nodes or to cause metastatic disease. As with invasive breast cancer DCIS is divided into three histological grades (low, intermediate and high grade). The higher grade of DCIS particularly can be associated with cell necrosis and subsequent secondary calcium deposition. This ductal microcalcification is detectable on mammography and is the most common way for DCIS to be diagnosed.

Natural history

The natural history of DCIS depends on the grade of the malignant change. High-grade DCIS is very likely to develop into invasive malignancy over a fairly short time. When it does so it develops into higher-grade invasive carcinoma (usually grade III). Low-grade DCIS (various types) may never turns into invasive carcinoma, the progression towards invasive disease is much slower and if invasive disease does occur it is usually of low grade (grade I).

Presentation and diagnosis

It is unusual for DCIS to form a palpable mass. Most patients who are diagnosed with DCIS have only a mammographic abnormality, usually consisting of microcalcification of the ductal type. This is typically focal, fine and heterogeneous, with branching forms. Suspicious microcalcification is further investigated with stereotactic core needle biopsy or mammotome biopsy.

Treatment

DCIS is confined to the breast. No treatment to the axillary lymph nodes is required. There is no chance of metastatic disease as long as there is no invasive breast malignancy. For this reason the treatment of DCIS does not involve adjuvant systemic treatment such as chemotherapy.

The principal treatment modality for DCIS is surgery and complete excision with clear margins is required. This may be achieved by local excision (for focal areas of DCIS measuring <4 cm) or by mastectomy (for extensive areas of DCIS). After local excision, breast radiotherapy further reduces the chance of recurrence. For patients with low-grade DCIS the chance of recurrence is anyway very low and radiotherapy is not usually given. It is, however, normally part of the treatment for high-grade DCIS. Patients with intermediate-grade DCIS may or may not have breast radiotherapy depending on the size of the lesion and the margins. Tamoxifen has been shown to further reduce the risk of recurrence for DCIS.

The recurrence rate for DCIS after mastectomy is 1%. The recurrence rate for high-grade DCIS after wide excision is between 25% and 30%. If radiotherapy is used in addition to local surgery the recurrence rate is approximately halved. Recurrence of DCIS is in the form of *in situ* disease in 50% of cases and of invasive breast cancer in the other 50%.

Breast cancer screening

Breast cancer screening using mammography is a good example of effective population screening. In the UK it has been offered to women between the ages of 50 and 70. Screening involves mammograms without clinical examination performed at 3-yearly intervals. Breast screening using mammography has proved to be effective between the ages of 40 and 50, but more frequent mammography (annual) is required. This is not currently part of the NHS screening programme.

Breast cancer screening using mammography can be made more sensitive in a number of ways. The mammograms can be double reported (reviewed independently by two radiologists) and the X-rays can be carried out in two perpendicular views on each screening visit rather than as a single view. These changes are expensive but are gradually being introduced into the National Breast Screening Programme. In the UK women over 70 can still elect to continue with mammographic screening but they have to request this by contacting the screening unit themselves.

Web links

More information on benign and malignant breast conditions can be obtained at www.breast-cancer-information.com.

Chapter 19

Screening for gynaecological cancer

Cervix

The best-known screening service is for carcinoma of the cervix; this should be a preventable disease because:

- there is usually a phase of premalignancy, dysplasia or intraepithelial neoplasia
- the cervix is a relatively accessible organ to examine
- cells can easily be obtained in the premalignant phase.

The biggest problem is getting women liable to develop a carcinoma of the cervix to take part in the screening.

Current position

In the UK screening is aimed at all women at risk from within 5 years of starting sexual activity (usually 15–20 years) to the age of 65 years. After this the development of premalignant lesions is rare.

The screening service for cervical cancer aims to recall women aged 25–50 years every 3 years and those aged 50–64 who have never had an abnormal smear every 5 years; in some high-risk areas the programme commences from age 20. It is possible that some carcinomas will grow very rapidly, but for the majority a cervical smear

performed every 3 years will pick up the pathological warning signs. Three-yearly smears detect 91% of the premalignant conditions. Increasing the smear frequency to yearly only improves the pick-up rate to 93%; trebling the workload thus improves results by only 2% (Box 19.1).

Smear tests are offered at most places where women attend for obstetric or gynaecological procedures. Thus they may be done at:

- GP surgeries
- antenatal clinics
- family planning clinics
- genitourinary medicine (GUM) clinics
- gynaecology outpatient clinics
- well woman clinics.

The average age group of women with premalignant conditions is gradually declining. Half of women diagnosed with cervical cancer are between the ages of 35 and 55. It rarely occurs in women younger than 20. Although cervical cancer does affect young women, many older women do not realize that the risk of developing cervical cancer is still present as they age. A well-organized computer-generated record system with an age–sex register (call–recall system from health authority) is essential; those who do not accept their invitation must be re-invited. There must also be some system of ensuring that the results are returned to the woman promptly. This is now achieved through computer technology so that each woman receives a letter saying either that her result is normal or that she should contact her doctor. All smear results are sent

Lecture Notes: Obstetrics and Gynaecology, 3rd edition. By Diana Hamilton-Fairley. Published 2009 by Blackwell Publishing. ISBN: 978-1-4051-7801-3.

to the woman's GP, irrespective of where the smear is taken. During 2006–7 3.4 million women of all ages were screened, most after a formal invitation. There has been a decrease in the percentage of eligible women who have been screened in the previous 5 years from 82% in 1997 to 79.2% in 2005–6. It is hard to explain this decline and it is not uniform across the country, with 71 of 152 primary care organizations screening 80% of their population.

This requires an enthusiastic primary care/GP service that is appropriately funded. In the UK, the National Health Service offers incentives to GPs to ensure that a high percentage (>85%) of those in the appropriate age groups have their smears at the correct intervals.

Box 19.1 The benefits and drawbacks to the individual woman of cervical screening

Advantages
1 Reassurance for most who have no premalignant changes
2 Reassurance to a few that any premalignant changes found are at a very early stage
3 Avoidance of radical treatments if the condition is picked up early
4 Produce an increased life expectancy

Disadvantages
1 Fear of finding cancer. This may sound illogical but it is true for most human beings
2 The anxiety generated while waiting for the results
3 The fear that comes from false-positive results

Taking a cervical smear

The smear can be taken by anyone competent to perform a vaginal examination; thus it can be done by a gynaecologist, a GP, a community clinic doctor, a trained midwife or a nurse. New technologies have been introduced recently that have altered the methodology. The Papanicolaou smear test, in which cells are spread out onto a glass slide at the bedside, sent to the laboratory, stained and read by a cytologist, is being replaced by liquid-based cytology (LBC) where the cells are suspended in a collection fluid, sent to the laboratory, separated so that cervical epithelial cells only are spread onto a slide and stained, before being read by a cytologist.

After discussion, the woman is positioned on the couch and a warmed speculum is passed to expose the cervix. If the sample is being prepared at the bedside a glass slide should be labelled before undertaking the examination. The slide is marked in pencil with the woman's name, date of birth, date of test and hospital number/NHS number if known. A spatula is then used to scrape the whole squamocolumnar junction (SCJ). If the external os is regular, the pointed end of a spatula can be passed into the canal and rotated by 360° (Fig. 19.1). If the cervical os is stenosed, the brush end of a cytobrush should be used (Fig. 19.2 and Plate 3). This is common after surgery to the cervix for cervical abnormality or in postmenopausal women.

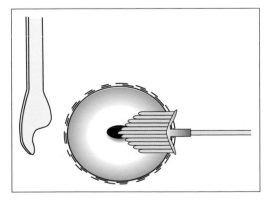

Figure 19.1 Smear taken from a nulliparous cervix with the broom (LBC) alongside the shaped end of an Aylesbury/extended tip spatula.

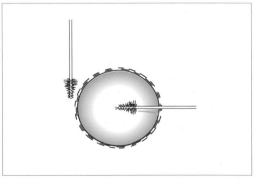

Figure 19.2 Smear taken from a stenosed cervix with the brush end of a cytobrush.

The most commonly used spatula is the Aylesbury spatula with its elongated beak to go up the cervical canal.

The material removed on the tip of the spatula should be smeared onto the glass slide and fixed immediately to prevent the cells drying in air. The slide can go straight into the fixative medium or be sprayed with the fixative aerosol, which dries rapidly, fixing the cells and nuclei. The slide can then go to the laboratory through the post or by messenger.

If LBC is being used a broom or an extended tip spatula or both should be used. The tip of the broom/spatula is placed into the cervical canal, rotating it *clockwise* through 360°. The broom/spatula is then put into the collection fluid and tapped on the bottom of the vial for 10 seconds to shake all the cells into the fluid. The vial is labelled as per the slide although a pre-printed label/black pen should be used rather than a pencil.

The cytopathologist will need certain basic information about the woman in order to interpret the findings carefully:
- The age of the woman
- Menstrual cycle and date of last menstrual period
- Any irregular vaginal bleeding
- Is she pregnant?
- Any current hormone therapy (including oral contraception)?
- Presence of intrauterine device
- Clinical state of the cervix.

Examination of the smear

Do not take a Papanicolaou smear during menstruation because red cells obscure the epithelial cells at microscopic examination. However, if the woman has irregular bleeding it is impossible to avoid this. A note should be made to the pathologist if this occurs. If LBC is used the red cells will be mostly removed during the preparation of the slide so the sample can be taken when menstrual loss is light.

At the laboratory the smear is stained and examined by cytotechnicians. If any abnormality is detected, the smear will be passed to a cytopathologist.

The introduction of LBC has had two major effects on the screening service:
1 An improved time to the result being available (2006–7 48% in 4 weeks, 74% in 6 weeks – compare 2005–6 32% and 56%, respectively)
2 The percentage of inadequate samples has fallen from >9% pre-2005 to 4.7% in 2007.

This has led to a reduction in the number of repeat samples requested, a reduction in the burden on the laboratory and a relief to women both psychologically and physically because it is not a test free of discomfort.

False-negative results

These occur when a woman has premalignant changes in her cells but these are not reported. Incidence is unknown but, from data on women who do develop carcinoma of the cervix, it is probably between 10 and 30%. Causes include:
- Error in taking the smear:
  — non-representative sample of cells
  — not from SCJ
- A misinterpretation in the laboratory itself
- Incorrect typing of the report from the laboratory.

False-positive results

This happens when the smear is reported as having a greater degree of malignant change than exists. This is caused by:
- misinterpretation by the cytologist
- infection
- pregnancy
- incorrect typing of results on the report
- incorrect interpretation of the report by the clinician.

In 2006–7 29.7% of women referred to colposcopy after more than one mild abnormality on their smear test had no significant pathology.

Grading the smears

Originally the grading of smears was according to the classification of Papanicolaou. This has changed so that cytological grading is different from histological grading. Cytologists grade the smear according to the appearances of the cells that they see. For a satisfactory smear they must receive a sample with cells from the SCJ – in other words cells that are undergoing metaplasia from columnar to squamous cells (Plate 13) because these are the cells most likely to undergo neoplastic change. The following features are assessed:

• Nuclear/cytoplasmic ratio (amount of cytoplasm should be twice that of the nucleus)
• Shape of the nucleus (poikilocytosis)
• Density of the nucleus (koilocytosis).
    Other features that may be present:
• Inflammation: the presence of leukocytes (removed in LBC)
• Infection: presence of *Trichomonas*, *Candida*, diplococci
• Evidence of mitosis.
    The cytologist will classify the smear accordingly:
• Insufficient for adequate assessment: no cells seen from the SCJ.
• Inflammatory: excessive numbers of leucocytes, *Candida* or *Trichomonas* seen.
• Borderline: some nuclear changes but indeterminate.
• Mild dyskaryosis: cells have irregular enlarged nuclei with a change in the chromatin pattern. The nuclear membranes may be slightly irregular.
• Human papillomavirus (HPV) only: DNA tests are now available to rapidly check cells for the presence of HPV-16 and -18. These can be done on LBC samples and identify a high-risk group of women who need more regular screening.
• Moderate dyskaryosis: as mild, but the nucleus is enlarged to <50% of the cell size.
• Severe dyskaryosis: the nucleus is enlarged to >50% of the cell size. The nuclei vary in size and shape and the nuclear membranes are irregular.
• Possible invasive carcinoma: mitotic figures seen.
The relationship of the degree of dyskaryosis to the histological findings at biopsy or removal of the affected area is not absolute.

All women with a smear showing mild/moderate/severe dyskaryosis/invasion should be referred to a colposcopy clinic where the cervix can be examined under magnification. Inflammatory smears should be treated with antibiotics or antifungal agents if appropriate and the smear repeated 3–6 months later. All women with a smear showing mild dyskaryosis or greater should be referred to colposcopy. Women with a borderline smear should have the smear repeated within 6 months. If the woman has two consecutive borderline or inadequate smears she should be referred to colposcopy. In addition, a woman who has had three abnormal smears in the preceding 5 years, which may not have been consecutive, should be referred for colposcopy if she has not already been seen in a clinic (Box 19.2). All women with moderate or severe dysplasia or evidence of invasive carcinoma should be seen in the colposcopy clinic within 6 weeks of diagnosis.

It is very important when telling women the result of their smear test to emphasize that they do not have cancer but that, if nothing was done, they could develop cancer in time. Treatment now will cure the problem in 98% of cases.

Colposcopy

A speculum is passed and the cervix visualized as for a smear. Acetic acid 4% is painted onto the surface of the cervix with a cotton-wool swab. Abnormal cells at the SCJ will stain white with this liquid because of their increased glycogen content (Acetowhite) (Plate 14). The speed and the density of the white colour are proportional to the degree of

---

Box 19.2 Indications for referral to colposcopy

Two consecutive borderline smears
Mild dyskaryosis
Moderate dyskaryosis
Severe dyskaryosis
Three abnormal smears in the preceding 5 years that may not have been consecutive if she had not already been seen in a clinic
Two consecutive smears inadequate for assessment (particularly in postmenopausal women)
(British Society for Cervical Cancer Prevention 2005)

abnormality. The abnormal areas are noted and drawn in diagrammatic form in the notes. Additional features that can be looked for that have been associated with microinvasive disease are:

- mosaicism (tile-like formation of the cells) (Plate 15)
- punctation (small dots on the surface of the cervix)
- new vessel formation (using a green light filter)
- the upper limit of the abnormality inside the cervical canal must be seen.

Iodine solution is then painted onto the cervix (Plate 16). Normal squamous epithelium will stain dark brown with this solution whereas abnormal cells and normal columnar epithelium will remain unstained. This delineates the area more accurately but does not give an idea of how severe the lesion may be so acetic acid should always be used first.

Once the lesion has been defined a biopsy is taken and the treatments, with a local anaesthetic cervical block, may be as follows:

- *Cryotherapy*: the abnormal area is frozen with a liquid nitrous oxide probe.
- *Laser*: suitable for small mild/moderate lesions where the limits are clearly visible on the surface of the cervix.
- *Large loop excision of the transformation zone (LLETZ)*: the abnormal area is removed using a red-hot loop (diathermy). This goes to a depth of 1 cm down the cervical canal, ensuring that the whole of the transformation zone is removed. An LLETZ is sometimes employed if the area is more extensive. Suitable for extensive, moderate or severe lesions with no evidence of invasion.
- *Formal cone biopsy*: this has to be undertaken under general anaesthetic. A specially shaped knife is used, bent inwards, so that a cone of the cervix is removed to a depth of 1.5–2 cm. This is useful in cases where microinvasion is suspected and is the most likely procedure to cause later problems in pregnancy: either cervical incompetence or cervical stenosis.

Cervical intraepithelial neoplasia

This is a purely histological diagnosis. Biopsies or samples from a LLETZ or cone biopsy are graded into:

- CIN-1: the outer third of the epidermis contains cells with a reduced cytoplasmic/nuclear ratio and increased nuclear density.
- CIN-2: the outer two-thirds of the epidermis contains abnormal cells.
- CIN-3: the entire depth of the epidermis contains abnormal cells but the basement membrane is intact.
- Microinvasion: the entire depth of the epidermis contains abnormal cells and there are small breaches in the basement membrane with abnormal cells invading to a depth of <3 mm.

After treatment, all women should have a repeat smear at 6 months and, if normal, check smears every year for 5 years.

Effectiveness of cervical screening

If cervical screening were totally effective, carcinoma of the cervix would be eliminated. Approximately 1300 women still die annually from this condition in the UK so the cervical screening programme has obviously not been completely effective. Countries with a more effective cervical screening programme than the UK's report a diminution in deaths from carcinoma of the cervix (Fig. 19.3).

In practice, no screening programme can, however, have perfect success in controlling disease because:

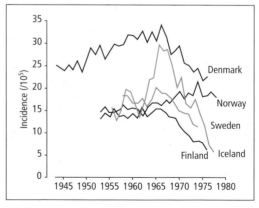

Figure 19.3 Incidence of cervical cancer in the Nordic countries. Norway was the only country with no cervical cancer screening programme.

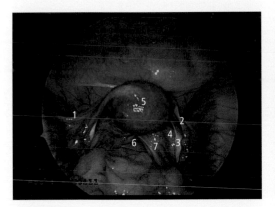

Plate 1 Normal anatomy: (1) round ligament, (2) fallopian tube, (3) ovary, (4) infundibular ligament, (5) uterus, (6) pouch of Douglas, and (7) uterosacral ligament.

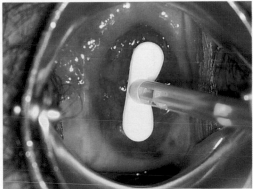

Plate 3 A cervical smear being taken with a cytobrush. The bright red area is an ectropion.

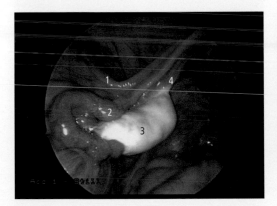

Plate 2 Normal tube and ovary: (1) round ligament, (2) fallopian tube, (3) ovary, and (4) infundibular ligament.

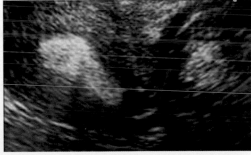

Plate 4 Hysterosalpingogram using ultrasound (HyCoSyR). The uterus is on the left with a bright endometrium, the white streak on the right is the tube.

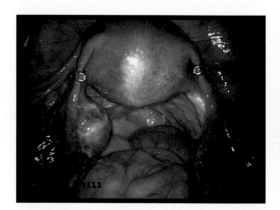

Plate 5 Sterilization. A Filshie clip is seen on each tube.

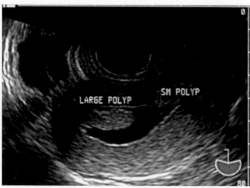

Plate 7 Ultrasound of a polyp with 0.9% saline in cavity.

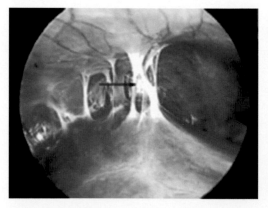

Plate 6 Fitz-Hugh–Curtis syndrome – adhesions from the liver capsule to the diaphragm – associated with chlamydial infection.

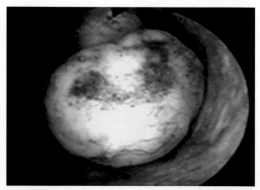

Plate 8 Fibroid polyp at hysteroscopy.

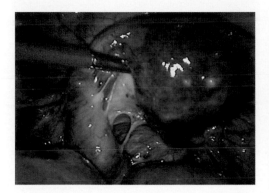

Plate 9 Pyosalpinx.

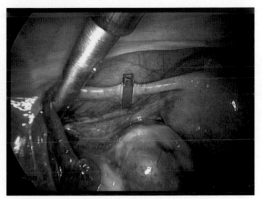

Plate 11 Filshie clip on left fallopian tube with follicular ovarian cyst at laparoscopy.

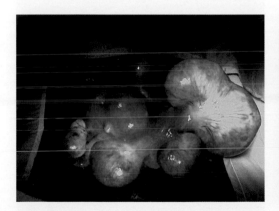

Plate 10 Fibroid uterus.

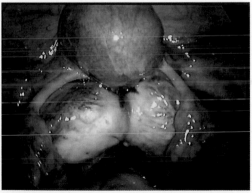

Plate 12 Kissing ovaries. Secondary to endometriosis. Note the dark areas of active endometriosis between the ovaries and the uterus.

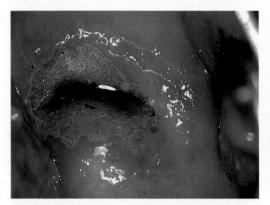

Plate 13 Cervical ectropion/squamocolumnar junction at colposcopy.

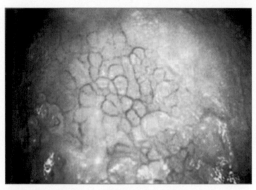

Plate 15 Mosaicism – outlining abnormal blood vessels.

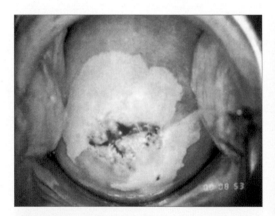

Plate 14 Dense acetowhite (CIN 3).

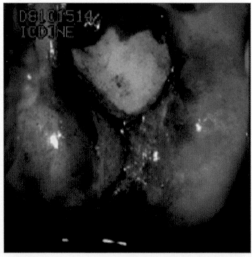

Plate 16 Iodine-negative area of abnormality.

- screening may not reach all the population at risk (20% of women have not been screened in the last 5 years)
- there will be false negatives
- the infrequency of screening may miss a rapidly progressive case
- treatment as a result of screening may be incorrectly given
- the treatment that follows screening may not be effective
- recurrences may occur after even apparently successful courses of treatment.

In reality, most women in the UK who now die from clinical carcinoma have never had a cervical smear.

Rapidly progressive cases are rare, but women with a carcinoma of the cervix can have had a normal smear performed within a year or so, although this is unusual. The more aggressive cases tend to occur in younger women and are often glandular in origin, giving rise to adenocarcinoma rather than the more common squamous carcinoma. Glandular abnormalities are more difficult to detect on routine screening.

Benefits of cervical screening

A screening programme should aim to benefit the individual first (see Box 19.1) and then society.

Society, however, can reap benefits or disadvantages from extending the cervical screening programme. If priority is given to cervical screening, monies have to be diverted from other resources and other services curtailed. In 2005 the screening age for the population was changed from 20 to 25. In 2007 20% of women between 20 and 25 continued to be screened, 0.6% had severe dyskaryosis and there were no cancers detected. Overall the change in prevalence of high-grade abnormalities was 0.1% between 2004 and 2007. The reduction in number of samples taken has therefore had no significant impact on the number of high-risk cases detected.

The cost/benefits of different aspects of cervical cancer screening can be assessed; an example is the frequency with which smears are taken. The financial benefits to society of a successful cervical screening programme would be the avoidance of expenditure in treating advanced cancer and the extra years of productivity of people who have survived.

A vaccine against HPV (Gardosil™) is being introduced for all girls aged 12–15 year from 2009 in the UK.

Conclusion

In the UK, the cervical screening programme has reduced the incidence of deaths from cervical cancer but it is by no means perfect. To achieve a 3-yearly smear for the 20 million women at risk (4 million per year over a 3- to 5-year recall programme), a more organized system of screening is now provided, but will take a few years to come into full effect.

Ovary

Cancer of the ovary is a significant cause of premature death in women (Fig. 19.4). It is often diagnosed late because of its lack of symptoms and it commonly spreads quickly and widely (see Chapter 20, p. 289–92). Hence, a screening test would be helpful. At present, two methods are possible:

1 Serum tumour marker CA-125:
  — 25% of those with ovarian carcinoma are positive 5 years before clinical diagnosis
  — 50% of those with ovarian carcinoma are positive 18 months before clinical diagnosis

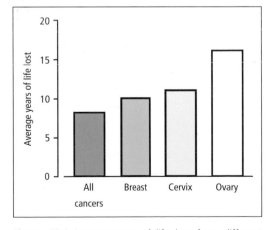

Figure 19.4 Average years of life lost from different cancers.

— additional serum markers for epithelial ovarian cancers include CA-19.9 and CEA. Tumours of embryonic origin produce high levels of α-fetoprotein (AFP), lactase dehydrogenase (LDH) and/or human chorionic gonadotrophin (hCG).

2 Ultrasound: high sensitivity for ovarian tumours, but:

— high false-positive rate leading to unnecessary surgery

— depends on experience and equipment that is not universally available

— needs expert ultrasonographers who are not widely available.

Hence, serum CA-125 is first screen and ultrasound the back-up. A modest increase in earlier diagnosis could reduce death rates. Combining the years since the menopause of the patient, the features of the ultrasound scan and the CA-125 gives a risk of malignancy index (RMI). If the CA-125 is >200 then there is a high risk of malignancy but it is not diagnostic.

Endometrium and vulva

Cancer of the endometrium and vulva tends to bleed early and/be visible and so is detected on clinical grounds. There are no useful screening programmes.

Breast

Screening for breast cancer—mammography—is considered in Chapter 18.

Part 5

The Older Woman

Chapter 20

Malignant gynaecological conditions

Cancer registries collect data about every new case of malignant disease diagnosed in that catchment population. In the UK, data come from:
- hospital inpatient statistics
- pathology registers
- radiotherapy registers
- oncological outpatient clinics
- colposcopy clinics.

Registries also get death certificates of all cancer deaths in their population, so giving a measure of the total incidence of gynaecological cancer. Mortality rates of malignant disease come from death certificates and are published by the Office of Population Censuses and Surveys (OPCS). Thus, there are two distinct sources of epidemiological data about malignant disease:

1 The living: prevalence and incidence rates
2 The dead: mortality rates.

In 2004, 3 gynaecological cancers featured among the 10 most frequent cancers among women. Some 6615 women were reported with new cases of carcinoma of the ovary, 2726 with invasive carcinoma of the cervix and 6438 with carcinoma of the body of the uterus. Thus, carcinoma of the ovary has overtaken that of the cervix in the last 20 years as the most common gynaecological cancer. In 1973 registrations for cervical and ovarian cancers were

Lecture Notes: Obstetrics and Gynaecology, 3rd edition. By Diana Hamilton-Fairley. Published 2009 by Blackwell Publishing. ISBN: 978-1-4051-7801-3.

4065 and 3819, respectively. Endometrial cancer is also on the increase largely as a result of the increase in the prevalence of obesity – a major risk factor for this cancer – over the last 20 years.

In 2005, the deaths (mortality rate per 100 000 women) reported of the same three cancers were 4447 (10.4), 1061 (2.6) and 1637 (3.5). No precise mathematical ratios can be derived because the data are from different populations in time; however, this provides an indication of the poor prognosis of cancer of the ovary compared with that of the cervix/uterus; over the years the prognosis for ovarian cancer has remained unchanged because it continues to present late and we have not developed an effective screening programme. The 5-year follow-up data are given in Table 20.1. These differences may represent:
- a real change in the prevalence of a condition
- a more complete reporting system
- better diagnostic facilities for making an early diagnosis.

There is a trend for increasing incidence of cervical cancer in younger women. There has been a 20-fold increase in the number of women aged <35 presenting with cervical carcinoma. Many of these will have adenocarcinoma rather than squamous cell carcinoma, which is harder to detect on routine screening and has a poorer prognosis. The numbers remain small and there is no evidence that the overall mortality for cervical cancer is increasing.

Table 20.1 Approximate 5-year survival rates for gynaecological cancer in Europe in 2004

Condition	5-year survival rates (%) by stage			
	I	II	III	IV
Carcinoma of the ovary	95	70	40	31
Carcinoma of the endometrium	96	65	50	26
Carcinoma of the cervix	92	70	51	16

The geographical incidence of carcinoma of the cervix was highest in central and southern America, decreasing as it crossed Europe and Africa to Asia and the Far East. This apparent trend no longer exists. There are many local variations, eg Portugal has a very high rate of carcinoma of the cervix whereas its close neighbour, Spain, has a very low one, yet their economic and social characteristics are very similar.

Gynaecological cancer mortality rates

The standardized registration rates of women dying in 2005 of three major gynaecological malignancies show an increase in ovarian cancer cases in a decade, and a reduction of endometrial cases, although cervical cancer cases stay the same. Such rates cannot be compared directly with incidence rates because the latter takes place many years before the former. Five-year survival rates after treatment may be a slightly more precise measure. As cervical carcinoma may recur up to 10 years, a time interval longer than 5 years may be required. The 15-year survival rate is currently about 40%. There are few recurrences of carcinoma of the endometrium after 5 years, so that index is a reasonable one; one can say that about two-thirds of women with endometrial cancer are cured.

The survival rate of carcinoma of the ovary is poor and probably reflects the fact that only about a fifth of diagnosed patients are cured. It may be in the future that, with more drastic surgery and chemotherapy, this might be improved, but it is still mostly a result of late diagnosis of the disease.

Subdividing these coarse 5-year survival rates into stages gives a better idea of the problem, eg in the UK most carcinoma of the cervix is either stage I or stage II when diagnosed compared with developing countries when it is stage III or even stage IV.

Cancer of the cervix

Cancer of the cervix arises most frequently from the squamous epithelium at its junction with the columnar epithelium; it is predominantly a squamous carcinoma. A columnar cell type arises from the cervical glands inside the cervical canal, an adenocarcinoma. Malignant change may also arise in a cervical mucus polyp.

Aetiology

- Mainly in the age group 45–55
- Rare in virgins
- Coitus increases the risk:
  — very early coitus
  — multiple sexual partners.
- Infection with the wart virus or human papillomavirus types 16 and 18 and certain herpes viruses
- Rare in nuns, and women of Jewish and Muslim origin (because their husbands have been circumcised)
- More frequent in the lower social class groups; possibly hygienic factors may play a part
- Cigarette smoking shows an associated higher risk
- Immunosuppression: post-transplantation, autoimmune disease, HIV.

Pathology

Of the growths 95% are squamous cell carcinomas from the squamocolumnar junction. About 5% are adenocarcinomas from the columnar cells inside the cervical canal.

Invasive cancers present as an ulceration of the cervix. In advanced cases, the cervix is replaced by an ulcerated, fungated mass of growth, which is fixed to the surrounding structures. Spread may be via:

- the vaginal fornices
- the bladder
- the body of the uterus
- the broad ligaments, which may cause obstruction of the lower ends of the ureters; a large blood vessel may be eroded causing severe haemorrhage
- lymphatic spread to the iliac, obturator, sacral, inguinal and para-aortic nodes
- the bloodstream, occurring comparatively late but possibly leading to metastases in the lungs, bones or elsewhere.

Symptoms

The symptoms of cervical cancer begin only when the surface of the growth becomes ulcerated. Hence, they present later with endocervical growths. The chief symptom is a watery *discharge* (often offensive) and blood-stained discharge or bleeding, particularly after coitus (postcoital bleeding). Later frank, sometimes severe and continuous *bleeding* occurs, with the patient rapidly becoming anaemic.

Physical signs

Early, the cervix feels hard and bleeds on touch. Later the cervix is ulcerated and friable. In advanced cases the vaginal vault is filled with an ulcerated mass and pieces of growth are detached by the examining finger; examination may provoke severe bleeding. In endocervical growths the cervix feels barrel shaped.

The cervical smear may contain frankly malignant cells, but not always because the surface cells are often dead and atypical.

Diagnosis

This depends on biopsy of the cervix. If the site and size of the lesion allow, a cone biopsy should be

taken to include all the squamocolumnar junction and most of the cervical canal.

Staging investigations

Staging for cervical carcinoma includes the following:

- Examination under anaesthetic, including rectovaginal examination to assess the size of the tumour, parametrial spread, extension into the rectovagina; septum
- Cystoscopy and sigmoidoscopy to assess bladder and bowel involvement
- Biopsy of the suspicious area
- Chest X-ray
- Intravenous urography (IVU).

Computed tomography (CT) or magnetic resonance imaging (MRI) may be offered if available to give further information on tumour size and nodal involvement, but does not alter the FIGO (International Federation of Gynecology and Obstetrics) staging which is determined by the above investigations.

Differential diagnosis

Mainly from:

- cervical ectropion
- cervical polyp/fibroid
- tuberculosis may present in a proliferative form
- other chronic granulomatous infections.

Staging

Box 20.1 shows the clinical staging of cancer of the cervix. This is a clinical classification; in fact 20% of stage 1 cases are found at subsequent surgery to have metastases in the lymph glands (ie would be stage 3).

Treatment of invasive carcinoma

The choice of treatment depends on many factors:

- The age and general condition of the patient
- The extent and type of the lesion

Box 20.1 Staging of cancer of the cervix

Stage 0   Intraepithelial carcinoma (carcinoma *in situ*). The growth remains within the epithelial layer of the cervix

Stage 1   Cancer clinically confined to the cervix

Stage 2   Growth has spread to the upper two-thirds of the vagina or into the parametrium but not as far as the pelvic wall

Stage 3   The growth has spread to the lower third of the vagina or into the parametrium as far as the lateral pelvic wall

Stage 4   Metastases have formed beyond the pelvis or growth has involved the bladder or the rectum

---

• Ideally, all patients with cancer of the cervix should be seen by a gynaecological oncologist and a radiotherapist for consideration of all the factors of the individual case.

Renal function should be assessed by blood urea and IVU. Urinary infection is often present and should be treated. Anaemia may also need treatment.

Ultrasonography and CT may help identify spread in the pelvis or to lymph nodes.

Examination under anaesthesia is essential:

• The clinical extent of the growth is assessed.

• Hysteroscopy and curettage of the uterine cavity are performed and a biopsy taken in all cases, even those that seem the most obvious clinically.

• A rectal examination is important to exclude invasion of the rectum itself. The clinical extent of growth in the parametrium is also more easily felt rectally.

• Cystoscopy excludes involvement of the bladder.

Radiotherapy

This is the first line of attack in advanced stages or in poor-risk patients. It cannot be used if the bladder is invaded because of the risk of fistula formation. In some cases chemotherapy may be given before radiotherapy or surgery to reduce the size of the tumour, so reducing the field needed for radiotherapy.

Radiotherapy is delivered by the use of the cathetron; an empty container is inserted into the uterus and vaginal fornices and clamped into position. Its position is checked and several high-intensity cobalt sources are after-loaded and deliver the irradiation. The apparatus is contained in a sealed unit and radiation delivered by remote control, thus eliminating danger to staff.

Caesium may be used as a preliminary to surgery or combined with external radiotherapy to the lateral pelvic walls. A tube containing 50 mg caesium is put into the uterus and two ovoids or flat boxes containing a further 60 mg are packed into the vagina. Care is taken to give a minimal dose of radiation to the rectum. The caesium is left for 22 hours and three applications are usually given, the second a week after the first and the third 2 weeks after the second. This method has largely been replaced by the cathetron or linear accelerator to give total pelvic irradiation.

Chemotherapy

Increasingly multiagent chemotherapy with *cis*-platinum, vinblastine and bleomycin is used in combination with radiotherapy. In stage 2 disease it may be used to reduce the size of the tumour in order to allow surgery to take place rather than radiotherapy and give an overall better prognosis.

Surgery

Surgical excision is suitable for all stage 1 and some stage 2 cases. Wertheim's radical abdominal hysterectomy is the treatment of choice, removing the uterus, tubes, ovaries, broad ligaments and parametrium, the upper half or two-thirds of the vagina, and the regional lymph glands (Fig. 20.1). Sentinel node marking reduces the need to remove all lymph nodes, improving the morbidity of the operation without affecting survival rates.

In younger women with stage 1 disease who are lymph node negative and wish to retain their fertility, removal of the cervix alone (trachelectomy) can be performed with good results. The internal os of the cervix is commonly rendered incompetent, so an intra-abdominal stitch is placed round the base of the uterus to try to prevent a second trimester loss. Once the woman's family is complete

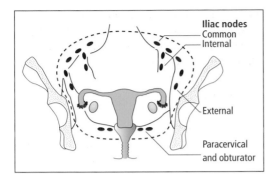

Figure 20.1 The extent of pelvic tissue removed at Wertheim's radical abdominal hysterectomy.

it is wise to perform Wertheim's hysterectomy to prevent recurrence.

Pelvic exenteration

In some advanced cases where carcinoma of the cervix has spread, extensive surgery must be undertaken as the only hope of cure for the patient. It is reserved mainly for patients in good general health with extensive disease involving the bladder or rectum.

Anterior exenteration consists of removing the uterus and adnexae, vagina, bladder and urethra. The ureters are implanted into the colon or into an ileal loop opening on to the abdominal wall.

Posterior exenteration removes the uterus and adnexae, vagina, descending colon and rectum, leaving a colostomy. This is suitable for posterior growths involving the colon or rectum.

In *total exenteration* the two operations are combined and the patient left with an ileal loop and a colostomy.

Results of treatment

These are best assessed by a 5-year follow-up, which in most centres shows a cure rate of up to 80% with stage 1 and about 10% with stage 4 disease.

This range of cure emphasizes the value of early diagnosis and treatment; the tragedy is that so many women worldwide do not receive treatment until the disease is advanced. In the UK most of these will never have had a smear test or failed to have regular checks in later years.

Complications of treatment

Complications may follow treatment with irradiation or surgery. Radiotherapy treatment can flare up infection in the renal tract or exacerbate pelvic abscess. Caesium proctitis may prove troublesome.

The mortality risk with Wertheim's hysterectomy is now only 1% in experienced hands. In addition to any complications of severe abdominal surgery, there is a risk of ureteric fistula which has been reported to be as high as 8% of patients submitted to Wertheim's hysterectomy after irradiation.

Palliation

When nothing can be done to cure the patient of cancer, everyone concentrates on making her last weeks or months as comfortable as possible. Death may occur mercifully from uraemia or haemorrhage, but many women suffer severe and intractable pain in the final stages of the disease.

Analgesics must be used liberally in sufficient amounts to relieve pain. Epidural anaesthesia and/or nerve blocks may be helpful. Chordotomy is sometimes used in intractable pain. If there is severe rectal pain, colostomy may be necessary. Opiates are of great help here and must be retained in the profession's therapeutic armamentarium, prescribing and dispensing being under strict control. Addiction is not a concern in those with advanced pelvic cancer and dosage should be liberal once started.

Malignant tumours of the uterus

Endometrial carcinoma

Aetiology

- Mean age of presentation is 56 years. Four-fifths of the women are menopausal and it is rare under the age of 40.
- Associated with hyperoestrogenic states:
  — obesity
  — diabetes
  — late menopause
  — prolonged use of unopposed oestrogens

— oestrogen-secreting tumours
— long-term tamoxifen usage.
• May be associated with:
— previous pelvic irradiation
— lower parity.

Pathology

• Usually an adenocarcinoma
• More often well differentiated than anaplastic
• May be associated with squamous metaplasia where, if excessive, becomes an adenocanthoma
• May be associated with pyometra or haematometra, secondary to cervical stenosis
• Spreads by invasion through the myometrium and by filling the uterine cavity
• Spreads via cervical lymphatic drainage involving the iliac and para-aortic nodes
• Tumours of upper uterus may spread along the lymphatics in the round ligaments to the deep inguinal nodes
• In advanced cases, the bloodstream spread may carry to the lungs, liver and bones.

Symptoms

• Postmenopausal bleeding: this symptom should be assumed to be caused by carcinoma of the endometrium until proved otherwise
• Blood-stained discharge
• Irregular bleeding.

Signs

• Less commonly, uterine enlargement
• Bleeding through the cervix.

Investigations

Ultrasound to assess dimensions of any tumour and to show endometrial thickness (Fig. 20.2).

Staging

Box 20.2 shows the clinical staging of endometrial cancer.

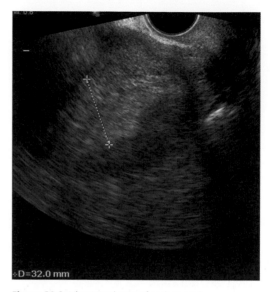

Figure 20.2 Ultrasound scan of endometrial cancer.

Box 20.2 Staging of endometrial cancer

Stage 1   Carcinoma confined to the body of the uterus
Stage 2   Extension to the cervix
Stage 3   Extension outside the uterus but within the true pelvis
Stage 4   Involvement of the:
(a) bladder
(b) rectum
(c) extension outside the true pelvis

Treatment

The treatment of uterine carcinoma is usually surgical:

• The surgical management of well-differentiated carcinoma involves a total abdominal hysterectomy and bilateral salpingo-oophorectomy (TAH/BSO) with pelvic lymphadenectomy. Increasingly the technology of marking and only removing the affected nodes (sentinel node) has reduced the morbidity of radical lymphadenectomy.
• In women with high-grade disease (grade 3 or grade 2 with >2 cm invasion), >50% myometrial invasion or cervical involvement or adverse patho-

logical subtypes (adenosquamous, clear cell or papillary serous carcinoma), a full staging laparotomy
involving omental biopsy, lymph node sampling
and inspection of the upper abdomen is required
in addition to the TAH/BSO.
- Radical hysterectomy is indicated if there is cervical involvement.

Radiotherapy is rarely employed alone unless the
patient is unable to withstand a surgical procedure.
It may be used as adjuvant treatment if adverse factors are identified in the pathology review:
- >50% myometrial invasion
- poorly differentiated high grade disease
- adenosquamous, clear cell or papillary serous
carcinoma
- positive pelvic lymph nodes.
The pelvic lymph node status determines whether
radiotherapy is given to the vault alone or to the
vault and the pelvic side wall.

Hormone therapy: progestogens inhibit the rate
of growth and spread of endometrial carcinoma.

Prognosis

The overall outlook for endometrial cancer is good
because it presents early (Fig. 20.3).

Rarer tumours

Choriocarcinoma

A malignant tumour arising from chorionic tissue
following a hydatidiform mole, abortion or pregnancy; considered in Chapter 7.

Sarcoma

Occurs in:
- childhood as sarcoma botryoides
- postmenopausal women with a fibroid.

It is highly malignant and radioresistant, spreads
via the bloodstream and is diagnosed late. Treatment is a TAH/BSO. Recurrences are treated with
multiagent chemotherapy.

Mixed mesodermal tumours

These arise from mesodermal cells of the ovarian
ducts and may contain primitive muscle cells,

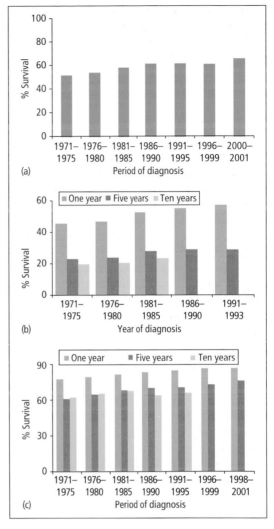

Figure 20.3 Five-year survival rates for (a) cervical, (b) ovarian and (c) corpus uteri cancers in England and Wales.

myxomatous tissue, cartilage and glands. They
present with abnormal bleeding and treatment is
by hysterectomy or occasionally by exenteration.
Vascular spread is common, prognosis poor.

Carcinoma of the ovary

Primary carcinoma of the ovary is now the most
common malignant tumour found in gynaecology
in the UK and an important cause of death in
women, accounting for some 4000 deaths annually

in England and Wales. It is a disease of middle and old age with 90% of cases in women >45 years. It is often diagnosed late because of its lack of symptoms and it commonly metastasizes quickly and widely—hence, a screening test would be helpful (see Chapter 19).

Risk factors relate to ovulatory history and the past activity of the germinal epithelium:

• Increased risk: no pregnancies
• Decreased risk: many pregnancies; use of oral contraceptives.

Ovarian carcinoma may be cystic, arising usually from a benign cyst, or solid. Solid epithelial carcinoma may be papillary, an adenocarcinoma or an undifferentiated carcinoma. Most ovarian cancers are epithelial in origin and many are poorly differentiated by the time of presentation. It may arise in one of the special ovarian tumours such as granulosa cell tumour or dysgerminoma. Although accounting for only 1–2% of tumours, the latter are treatable using modern chemotherapy.

Spread of ovarian carcinoma

The main route of spread of carcinoma of the ovary is transcoelomically via the general peritoneal cavity, to the greater omentum and the peritoneum of the pouch of Douglas in particular. Ascites is frequent. Malignant tumours are often bilateral. Spread via the lymphatics leads to involvement of the para-aortic glands; further spread may involve the supraclavicular glands. Bloodstream spread is unusual; death generally occurs from complications resulting from massive transcoelomic peritoneal secondaries, particularly bowel obstruction. Staging is shown in Box 20.3. Figure 20.4 shows diagrammatically the spread of ovarian tumours.

Metastatic ovarian tumours

The ovary is a frequent site for secondary malignancy because of its rich blood supply. Adenocarcinoma is the most common and the primary site may be the uterus, other ovary, breast, stomach or large bowel. Secondary tumours in the ovary generally reproduce the cell structure of the primary growth.

Box 20.3 Staging classification of ovarian carcinoma

Stage I	Tumour limited to the ovaries
IA	Tumour limited to one ovary
IB	Tumour limited to both ovaries
IC	IA or IB with capsule ruptured
	or
	surface involvement
	or
	malignant cells in ascites/peritoneal washings
Stage II	Tumour involves one or both ovaries with pelvic spread
IIA	To tubes or uterus
IIB	To other pelvic tissues
IIC	IIA or IIB with malignant cells in ascites/peritoneal washings
Stage III	Tumour involvement of abdominal cavity
IIIA	Microscopic peritoneal metastasis beyond pelvis
IIIB	Macroscopic peritoneal metastasis >2 cm diameter
	or
	involvement of retroperitoneal or inguinal nodes
IIIC	Tumour in pelvis with involvement of small bowel
	or
	omentum
Stage IV	Distant metastases
	Liver
	Bowel
	Pleural fluid with malignant cells

Krukenberg's tumour is an uncommon form of secondary carcinoma of the stomach or large bowel. The ovaries are enlarged by solid tumours, usually bilateral, which may reach 20 cm. Histologically they are characterized by the presence of signet ring cells that have undergone mucoid degeneration, so that the nucleus is pushed to one side by a droplet of mucin.

Possibly a small number of Krukenberg's tumours are primary in the ovary; patients have been known to survive for many years after removal of Krukenberg's tumours with no primary tumour found despite extensive investigation. This is not inconsistent with a microscopic slow-growing primary growth somewhere in the gastrointestinal tract that cures itself.

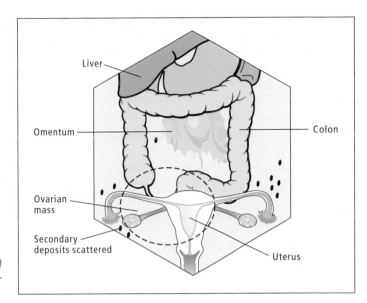

Figure 20.4 Metastatic spread of ovarian cancer: omentum; local; peritoneum; liver.

Investigation of ovarian tumours

Imaging

- Ultrasonography: can reveal the size of the ovarian cyst as well as suspicious features of malignancy, which include solid as well as cystic areas, spread through the capsule of the cyst/ovary, papillary growths within the cyst and abnormal Doppler patterns demonstrating abnormal blood flow.
- CT/MRI of the abdomen and pelvis: more accurately delineates the spread of disease showing peritoneal deposits, omental deposits, para-aortic node involvement and/or liver metastases, ureteric obstruction (rare in ovarian cancer).
- Chest X-ray: shows pleural effusions and/or hilar lymphadenopathy.

Blood tests

- Tumour markers: CA-125, CA-19.9, CEA (carcinoembryonic antigen). If any of these are raised they are used postoperatively to track the success of treatment and the onset of recurrence.
- Liver function tests to detect spread to the liver.
- Urea and electrolytes.
- Full blood count.

The latter two do not help in staging the disease but are important for preoperative assessment.

Treatment of ovarian tumours

The treatment of malignant ovarian tumours is surgical removal as soon as the tumour is diagnosed. If the tumour is apparently malignant, and where ascites is present, laparotomy should always be undertaken. Ascites may be associated with a benign tumour such as a fibroma, and even if there are metastases the prognosis is not hopeless. It may be possible to remove secondary masses in the omentum and, if the primary tumour is removed, secondaries sometimes regress. An ovarian tumour, even if very large, is best removed intact. Tapping the fluid carries a risk of spilling the contents and contaminating the peritoneal cavity.

Carcinoma of the ovary should be treated initially by surgery, which should involve total hysterectomy, bilateral salpingo-oophorectomy and omentectomy, and para-aortic node sampling, although in young women a normal, uninvolved ovary might be left. In advanced cases, as much tumour as possible should be removed at a debulking operation and the greater omentum should be excised. A search should be made for peritoneal metastases, including those on the upper and under surface of the liver. CT or MRI to check that the peritoneal cavity is free from secondary deposits may be carried out 3–6 months after the original operation.

Even in apparently advanced disease the ultimate prognosis appears to be improved by surgical removal of the main tumour masses. The first operation offers the best chance of cure. It should be done by an experienced gynaecological oncologist, preferably working in a specialist centre of gynaecological oncology, who will do the widest excision with the least damage to the ureters, bladder and intestines.

Radiotherapy is not much used in the management of ovarian cancer; the tumours are rarely radiosensitive and radiation would have a deleterious effect on the bone marrow in the lumbar vertebrae.

Chemotherapy with cytotoxic agents gives more hopeful results. Carboplatin has replaced cisplatin because it has fewer side effects on renal function and peripheral nerves. In combination with other agents such as paclitaxel, the platinum compounds give a significant improvement in results.

Prognosis

Like all cancers early diagnosis favours a good prognosis, with many women with stage 1 disease living to die from a different pathology. Unfortunately the general prognosis for ovarian carcinoma is poor because it tends to present so late, <20% surviving for 5 years. Factors that worsen prognosis are:

- advanced stage of disease
- poorly differentiated tumour
- how much tumour remains after surgery.

Carcinoma of the fallopian tube

Primary

- A rare malignancy occurring in older women.
- Papillary carcinoma may be solid or alveolar.
- Sometimes there is a vaginal discharge of an orange–yellow colour.

Treatment is as for ovarian carcinoma.

Secondary

Metastases in the tube most commonly come from cancer of the ovary or uterus.

Malignant disease of the vulva

Intraepithelial neoplasia

In vulval intraepithelial neoplasia (VIN), the malignant cells are limited to the outer layers of the epidermis and there is no spread to the underlying tissues and no metastases. The whole layer is infiltrated with malignant cells.

Clinical features

The patient has irritation or soreness of the vulva. The appearance may be that of vulval dystrophy or there may be a red area with a serpiginous outline. VIN may remain dormant for years or assume the characteristic of invasive carcinoma.

Diagnosis depends on biopsy.

Treatment is by a wide excision with a margin of healthy skin and epithelium.

Squamous carcinoma

Vulval carcinoma is less common than other gynaecological cancers. The squamous form is the most common malignant tumour of the vulva. It occurs mainly in the older age group, with a peak incidence at about 60 years of age. The condition is associated with vulval dystrophy (see Chapter 6).

Pathology

The primary growth is an ulcer with a raised, everted edge and indurated base. Multiple primaries may be found; sometimes the inner sides of both labia minora are involved. The growth may also arise on the clitoris.

Methods of spread

The growth may spread by direct extension and contact to other parts of the vulva, vagina or anus.

Secondary spread is mainly via the lymphatics. Owing to the rich lymphatic drainage of the vulva, the glands that tend to be involved are:

- superficial inguinal group of both sides
- inguinal

- femoral
- iliac
- aortic.

In untreated cases, the glands in the groin may break down to form a fungating ulcerated mass of growth.

Clinical features

Carcinoma of the vulva commonly begins as a small nodule, often unnoticed by the patient at first. It grows in size and becomes ulcerated with discharge and bleeding. It tends to grow on the inner surface of the labia minora in elderly women and may remain unnoticed except for slight discomfort and soreness from the discharge until an advanced stage.

Differential diagnosis

To differentiate malignancy from other causes of a lump in the vulva or of ulceration is the main problem. All lumps or ulcers of the vulva must be fully investigated, including a biopsy.

Treatment

Treatment of carcinoma of the vulva is vulvectomy and dissection of all the superficial and deep inguinal glands, and occasionally the iliac glands. The vulva itself is widely excised with the glands through separate incisions over each groin. Wide excision in advanced growths may have to include removal of the lower part of the urethra, vagina or anal canal depending on site.

In operable cases, a 5-year cure rate of about 70% is achieved. The prognosis depends mainly on involvement of the lymphatic glands.

Radiotherapy

Carcinoma of the vulva is relatively radioresistant whereas the surrounding normal tissues are radiosensitive. Hence, it is not employed usually, but high-voltage treatment may be used for recurrences.

Chemotherapy

This is not a primary treatment for squamous epithelioma or cancer of the vulva, but as with carcinomas of the anus it is being used more often for recurrence.

Basal cell carcinoma

This uncommon tumour presents as an indolent ulcer without invasion of the underlying tissues. Diagnosis is made by biopsy.

The treatment consists of local excision with a margin of normal skin.

Malignant melanoma

Fortunately this highly malignant tumour is rare. It may present as a melanotic nodule or a pedunculated tumour. The best treatment is to perform a vulvectomy and if nodes are involved, an *en bloc* dissection. Cases with diffuse spread of melanoma may be treated by radiotherapy.

Chapter 21

The menopause

The menopause is defined as the cessation of menstruation for more than 1 year. The climacteric is a longer period during which the reproductive organs involute. These time zones overlap each other in time just as they do in youth with the two processes of menarche and puberty.

The mean age of menopause in the UK is 51 with a normal range 45–56 years. Premature menopause (ovarian failure) is defined as the cessation of menses with a raised follicle-stimulating hormone (FSH) level >30 IU/L for >1 year before the age of 40 (see Chapter 3).

Physiology

At the end of reproductive life, the ovaries become less able to produce oocytes due to:
- a lack of primordial follicles, because all have been used/atrophied
- more refractory receptor function in the granulosa and thecal cells.

The falling oestrogen levels result in a large increase in FSH. The endometrium does not proliferate.

The ovarian stroma produces androstenedione, which converts in peripheral fat to estrone,

a weaker oestrogen than estradiol, the steroid on which the woman has depended for much of her reproductive life. Menstruation stops as a result of a lack of cyclical oestrogen and progesterone.

Symptoms

At the menopause 60% of women are relatively asymptomatic, 25% have mild symptoms and 15% have moderate-to-severe symptoms. The two most common symptoms are:
- hot flushes
- dryness of the vagina.

There is often a loss of libido, part of which is hormonal.

Mood swings, nervousness, anxiety, irritability and depression are all measured in this group of women. The decrease of oestrogens may reduce their modulatory role on brain monoamine synthesis.

Symptoms are found more commonly in those who had premenstrual tension or dysmenorrhoea. The symptoms are less frequent in Asian and African–Caribbean women, possibly associated with better maintenance of oestrogen levels by peripheral conversion in these groups.

Loss of collagen leads to uterovaginal prolapse and wrinkling of the skin, again rarer in African–Caribbean women.

Lecture Notes: Obstetrics and Gynaecology, 3rd edition. By Diana Hamilton-Fairley. Published 2009 by Blackwell Publishing. ISBN: 978-1-4051-7801-3.

Hot flushes

These are the feeling of heat over the face and upper part of the body, usually lasting for 30–60 seconds. They are followed by perspiration of this area, which may render the woman wringing wet. These flushes usually last for a year or so and in up to a quarter of women at least 4 years. This is probably due to an increase in the sympathetic nervous system drive mediated through the central neurotransmitters. They come on more at night in bed and can wake a woman up.

Dry vagina

The cervix and vagina are oestrogen dependent. Secretions from the cervix and the surface glands are diminished and the vaginal epithelium becomes thinner, less elastic, with a reduced blood supply; atrophic vaginitis follows. Dryness and, therefore, dyspareunia are common. Extra lubrication may be required or oestrogen cream.

Other genital changes

The breasts become atrophic and the nipples flatten. The uterus becomes smaller. There is less support from the cardinal, uterosacral and uteropubic ligaments so prolapse may occur (see Chapter 22).

Other symptoms

The lower oestrogen levels lead to atrophy of the urethra causing frequency of micturition, dysuria and urgency (urethral syndrome). This is commonly confused with symptoms of urinary tract infection but does not improve with antibiotics. The weakness of the supporting muscles and the cardinal ligaments allows stress incontinence to start at this age.

The pulling back of the posterior wall of the urethra often exposes the sensitive anterior wall, which becomes inflamed. A small polyp or caruncle may occur on the posterior wall.

The reduction of oestrogens leads to an increase in the levels of low-density lipoproteins, cholesterol and triglycerides. This is accompanied by a catch-up rate for women of ischaemic heart disease (IHD).

Mood suppression and memory disturbance have been associated with the menopause.

Long-term symptoms

Most of the above symptoms disappear within a year or two but those on the skeleton stay forever.

The calcium part of the skeleton is reabsorbed, whereas the collagen framework stays the same. This leads to osteoporosis (Fig. 21.1).

Women lose calcium at different rates and so the need for replacement oestrogens differs from one woman to another. Those with established osteo-

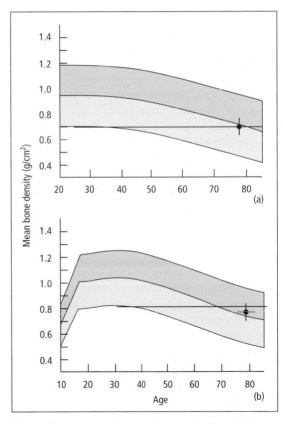

Figure 21.1 Bone density graph for women showing the normal range for (a) hip and (b) lumbar spine against increasing age. The thickened line represents the threshold for increased risk of bone fracture. The filled circle is the result for a 77-year-old woman who is becoming osteoporotic.

porosis should be treated with bisphosphonates. In reproductive life, while oestrogen synthesis is high, women are protected from IHD and coronary occlusion. After the menopause, this does not occur and 10 years later, the rate of IHD is as high in women as in men.

There is no evidence that hormone replacement therapy (HRT) protects women against IHD or stroke; in fact there is trend towards an increase in stroke and an excess of IHD which increases with age.

Postmenopausal therapy

There has been increasing controversy about the use of HRT because of a reported increase in the risk of developing breast cancer, cerebrovascular events, thrombosis and IHD. The consensus view is that, in women who do not have significant symptoms, the risks of taking HRT outweigh the benefits and it is therefore not recommended.

There are circumstances where therapy should be considered:

- Women with significant symptoms—hot flushes, vaginal dryness
- Surgical or irradiation oophorectomy
- Premature menopause.

All treatment modalities contain oestrogen or progesterone, oestrogen and progestogen continuous combined or sequential.

1 For postmenopausal symptoms: short-term oestrogen replacement for women who have symptoms, principally hot flushes and dry vagina for up to 5 years. The aim should be to use the lowest effective dose of oestrogen for the shortest period of time. It is usual to give it in a cyclical fashion of 28 days. This causes remission of symptoms in most women, once the correct dose has been achieved.

If the symptoms return after treatment ceases then the woman can be continued on HRT provided that she understands and accepts the risks of longer-term use.

2 Pelvic irradiation or surgical removal of the ovaries: longer-term replacement therapy is indicated in order to prevent osteoporosis if this occurs before the age of 50. Oestrogen is a potent factor in the maintenance of bone mineralization. Low oestrogen levels lead to a thinning of trabecular bone and eventually osteoporosis. This leads to an increased risk of fractures of the hip and wrist and compression fractures of the vertebrae, resulting in dowager's hump. Some women may require testosterone replacement, specifically to maintain or improve their libido. This may be associated with androgenic side effects and the long-term implications have not been evaluated.

3 Premature menopause: HRT can be used in young women for treating symptoms and preventing osteoporosis.

Progestogens are added in the second half of the cycle in all women who have a uterus to prevent a build-up of endometrium with possible hyperplasia, or atypical hyperplasia and then malignancy.

Owing to the cyclical nature of the treatment, the endometrium that develops during the oestrogen phase is shed after withdrawal and so there appears to be a continuation of menstrual periods (usually light).

Continuous combined treatments are available so that the woman remains amenorrhoeic.

There is no evidence that HRT improves clinical depression or Alzheimer's disease. It may improve minor mood disturbances but the effect is usually short-lived.

Types of HRT

The hormone may be given in a number of ways, as described below.

Orally

This is the most common and the most convenient. Compliance may be patchy and patients may forget, rendering the therapy ineffective.

Transdermal patches and gels

Oestrogen and progestogens are readily absorbed through the skin. There is the advantage of the oestrogen not having to pass through the portal system after absorption, where much would be destroyed. Hence, higher tissue levels of the oestrogens are achieved. The patches need to be changed only every third/seventh day and so compliance is higher. More recently, sprays have been developed.

Implants

Oestrogens can be given in a retard preparation by implantation under local anaesthesia. The pellets can be inserted into the abdominal wall or the thigh under the fascia lata. They last up to 6 months and are easily replaced so compliance is not relevant. Occasionally the oestrogens are given with testosterone to provide some stimulus to the libido, but this increases the risk of IHD.

Repeated use of oestrogen implants can lead to very high levels of oestrogen. As the implant wears off the woman may experience menopausal symptoms even though the serum estradiol levels are still within or above physiological levels. This may lead to women requesting their implants more and more often, leading to dangerous levels of estradiol with an increased risk of thrombosis. Early replacement of implants should therefore be avoided.

Progesterones should be taken by mouth during the second half of each cycle in order to get a withdrawal bleed and prevent build-up of the endometrium in women with a uterus.

This method is most commonly used by women who have had a hysterectomy and do not require progesterone.

Vaginally

Steroids are absorbed through the vaginal epithelium, but a large dose is needed in the vagina to get a reasonable dose inside the body. However, if vaginal dryness or irritative bladder symptoms are the main symptom, this is a good route.

Preparations

1 Orally: Progynova, estradiol or Premarin (estrone); progestogen: norethisterone 1 mg/day for at least 10 days.
2 Subcutaneous implant: 50–100 mg estradiol (±100 mg testosterone).
3 Patches of estradiol 25 or 50 μg with norethisterone acetate 1 mg (12 days).
4 Vaginal application: estriol or estradiol as a cream or pessary high in the vagina twice a week.
5 Non-bleed preparations: these can be either oestrogen with continuous progestogen or non-oestrogenic compounds (tibolone) that mimic oestrogen's effect on menopausal symptoms and bone.

If the uterus has been removed previously, the supplementary progestogen is not required. Unless treatment is stopped for an interval, the doctor and the patient will never know if the treatment is still required.

Side effects of HRT

HRT has minimal side effects. A few women may experience abdominal bloating and breast tenderness, which usually resolves after 2 or 3 months.

Complications of HRT

Malignancy

There is no evidence of any increase in malignancy of the *cervix* or *ovary*.

Neoplasia of the *endometrium* may follow unopposed oestrogen; the risk increases with the duration of use:
- three- to six fold after 5 years of use
- tenfold after 10 years.

Adding cyclical progestogens virtually eliminates this risk.

Breast cancer is stimulated by higher oestrogen levels. Meta-analysis indicates that the relative risk of *breast cancers* is about 1.3 times up to 10 years and exceeds this with longer-term therapy. Continuous combined preparations have been shown to increase the risk of breast cancer twofold after 5 years and threefold after 10 years of use. The increased risk declines back to baseline within 5 years of stopping treatment. Obviously, a woman with a family history of breast cancer should be counselled before starting HRT.

Continued periods

Regular monthly bleeding going on into the 60s is a nuisance. It often reduces in amount but still occurs. In an attempt to prevent this, progestogens may be given in a wider spread but lower dose throughout the cycle.

Tibolone (2.5 mg daily), a gonadomimetic, possesses weak oestrogenic, progestational and androgenic properties. It can be used to treat flushes, and psychological and libido problems, and is not accompanied by regular withdrawal bleeding symptoms, although it is not absolute especially if used by women early in the menopause.

Some women have a weight gain due to water retention when they start the oestrogens, but this settles after a few months. Some women develop depression-like premenstrual tension during the progestogen phase. Changing the dose of added progestogens will help this.

Uterine enlargement

Hyperplasia of the uterus may lead to an increase of bleeding. Any pre-existing fibroids may rarely continue their growth, whereas normally after the menopause their growth stops.

Postmenopausal bleeding

Postmenopausal bleeding is bleeding from the genital tract occurring 6 months or more after the menopause. It is a serious symptom that may indicate the presence of malignant disease in the genital tract. Every woman with postmenopausal bleeding should be assumed to have a carcinoma until a full investigation has proved to the contrary. If she is on HRT the bleeding may be 'breakthrough' where the progestogen is not adequate to prevent the endometrium from bleeding.

The following are chief causes.

The vulva

- Carcinoma
- Urethral caruncle.

Rectal bleeding and haematuria must be excluded.

The vagina

- Carcinoma
- Vaginitis, especially atrophic vaginitis
- Foreign bodies, especially pessaries.

The cervix

- Carcinoma of the ectocervix
- Carcinoma of a cervical canal polyp
- Benign cervical polyp.

The endometrium

- Polyp
- Carcinoma
- Atrophic endometritis
- Sarcoma
- Mixed mesodermal tumours.

The fallopian tube

- Carcinoma.

The ovary

- Feminizing tumours
- Granulosa cell tumour
- Theca cell tumour.

Investigation of postmenopausal bleeding

- Inspection of vulva and urethra
- Cervical smear
- Bimanual vaginal examination
- Transvaginal ultrasound scan
- Hysteroscopy and endometrial biopsy.

Hormone treatment

Withdrawal bleeding may follow administration of oestrogens for menopausal symptoms. This should not be assumed to be the cause of any postmenopausal bleeding until a full investigation including cytology and curettage has excluded more sinister causes.

Chapter 22

Pelvic floor disorders

In most adult women, when standing, the uterus is anteverted, the fundus directed forward and anteflexed, the body of the uterus bent forward on the cervix.

However, vaginal examinations always take place with the woman lying down. Then the body of the uterus often angles back to become axial, ie in line with the long axis of the vagina. Hence, although it is true that in the anatomical position four-fifths of uteri are anteverted and one-fifth retroverted; at vaginal examination, about 40% are anteverted, 40% axial and 20% retroverted.

The structures that maintain the position of the uterus are:
- the cardinal or transverse ligaments
- the uterosacral ligaments.

These are attached to the sides of the supravaginal cervix and lower uterus, leaving the body of the uterus mobile in all directions and capable of growth during pregnancy. The normal uterus is mobile, altering its position when the bladder or rectum becomes distended.

The secondary support of the uterus is the muscular pelvic floor (see Chapter 1).

Lecture Notes: Obstetrics and Gynaecology, 3rd edition. By Diana Hamilton-Fairley. Published 2009 by Blackwell Publishing. ISBN: 978-1-4051-7801-3.

Prolapse

Prolapse is a downward descent of the female pelvic organs as a result of weakness of the structures that normally retain them in position. Both descent and prolapse are relative terms and perceived differently, but are more frequently encountered in women who have borne children and rarely in nulliparous women. Prolapse does not usually become apparent until after the menopause when there is general shrinking and weakening of the supports of the pelvic organs. It is less common in people of African descent.

A prolapse resembles a hernia because there is protrusion of part of the abdominal contents through an aperture in the supporting structures. Protrusion takes place between the two levatores ani and, in more severe cases, through the orifice of the vagina.

Symptoms

Symptoms of genital prolapse are variable and do not bear much relation to the physical signs found on examination but more to the degree of traction on the pelvic ligaments. The symptoms tend to worsen with the day's activities and can be relieved by lying down. The following are the most common complaints:
- A feeling of fullness of the vagina.
- A lump coming down.

- A dragging sensation or bearing down in the back or lower abdomen.
- Vaginal discharge due to an ulcer of the ectocervix usually when the uterus has descended beyond the vaginal introitus. A blood-stained discharge may occur if there is ulceration.
- Difficulty with coitus may be experienced if the cervix protrudes or is greatly elongated.
- Urinary symptoms include:
  — *frequency* of micturition is common and is often daytime only
  — *nocturnal frequency* may be present if there is added cystitis
  — *urgency* of micturition due to weakness of the bladder sphincter mechanism and urge incontinence may occur in some cases
  — there may be *difficulty in emptying* the bladder completely and the woman may find that she has to push the prolapse up with a finger to complete the act of micturition
  — complete *retention of urine* follows urethral overstretch
  — *stress incontinence* when mild is common in women even without prolapse; this is considered later in this chapter.
- Rectal symptoms: many women with prolapse complain of constipation and this may be caused by difficulty in emptying the rectum completely because it bulges into the vagina. Others notice discomfort on sitting on a firm surface; the vaginal wall over the rectocoele can bulge down between the labia. With age, the labia become atrophic and less protective and the prolapsed vagina is exposed to trauma when sitting on hard surfaces.

Physical signs

The woman should first be examined in the dorsal position when she is asked to strain and cough. While she does, the anus may be supported to spare her the embarrassment of an involuntary escape of flatus or faeces. In case of doubt, she may be asked to stand up or walk about for a short time before testing for prolapse again on the bed.

The degree of descent of the cervix is tested with a finger in the vagina. The woman is then asked to adopt Sim's position (Fig. 22.2). She lies on her left

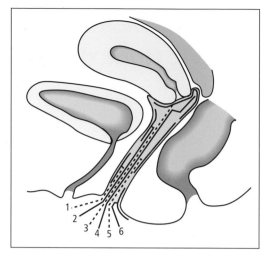

Figure 22.1 Analysis of the areas involved in a prolapse: 1 dislocation of the urethra; 2 cystocoele; 3 descent of cervix and uterus; 4 enterocoele; 5 rectocoele; 6 deficient perineum.

side with her left leg straight and her right leg bent up against her abdomen. Her right arm and shoulder should be turned away from you and her buttocks towards the edge of the couch nearest to the examiner. Sim's speculum is then gently introduced along the posterior wall of the vagina. A cystourethrocoele is usually obvious and the distance from the introitus to the bulge can be measured using a special ruler. The woman is asked to cough and any leakage of urine and/or descent of the cervix noted. As the speculum is withdrawn any posterior vaginal wall prolapse can be noted.

Where there is a complaint of stress incontinence, examination is best made with some urine in the bladder; the urethra and bladder neck may then be supported with two fingers to demonstrate that this manoeuvre controls the incontinence.

Classification

Six components of a genital prolapse (Fig. 22.1) are recognized.

1 *Dislocation of the urethra*: the urethra is displaced downwards and backwards off the pubis. It may be also dilated, becoming an urethrocoele. This arises from damage to or weakness of the triangular ligament (urethrocoele).

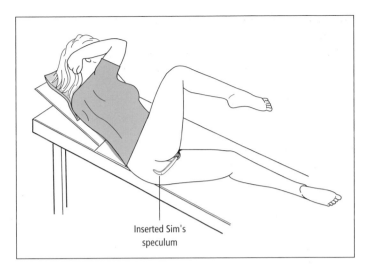

Figure 22.2 The left lateral position or Sim's position.

Inserted Sim's speculum

2 *Cystocoele*: hernia of the bladder trigone following weakness of the vaginal and pubocervical fascia. The bladder base descends and later a bladder pouch is formed which may contain residual urine increasing the risk of a urinary tract infection.

3 *Uterine prolapse*: descent of the uterus and cervix:

— *first degree* with a descent of the uterus, but the cervix remains within the upper vagina

— *second-degree* uterine descent when the cervix reaches down to the vulva on straining, but does not pass through it

— *third degree* or *procidentia* when the cervix and some or the entire uterus are prolapsed outside the vaginal orifice. In practice the fundus of the uterus usually remains within the vagina, but there is an associated inversion of the vagina.

4 *Enterocoele* or pouch of Douglas hernia: a prolapse of the upper part of the posterior vaginal wall. The hernia contains the peritoneum of the pouch of Douglas often with a loop of bowel. Enterocoele may occur together with other types of genital prolapse, especially procidentia. It is also seen in prolapse after a hysterectomy.

5 *Rectocoele*: a prolapse of the lower part of the posterior vaginal wall due to weakness or divarication of the levatores ani; the rectum bulges into the vagina.

6 *The perineal body*: this may be deficient and part of the anal canal may bulge into the vagina. It follows inadequately sutured tears after childbirth or by failure of healing in such tears.

Differential diagnosis

The diagnosis of prolapse is not difficult but it can be hard to decide if it is the cause of the patient's main symptoms. It must be distinguished from:
- vaginal or periurethral cysts
- tumours of the vagina
- a diverticulum of the urethra
- urethral caruncle
- urethral mucosal prolapse.

Symptoms similar to those of prolapse may be caused by:
- varicose veins of the vulva
- haemorrhoids
- rectal prolapse
- cystitis
- vaginitis with congestion of the vagina
- pressure from a large abdominal tumour.

Stress incontinence must be distinguished from other causes of incontinence of urine such as urge incontinence and incontinence resulting from neurological disease.

Prevention

Careful management of labour is important. Episiotomies and tears must be carefully sutured in layers. More important is postnatal pelvic floor and abdominal muscle exercises preferably taught by a physiotherapist. These exercises can be taught antenatally.

Prevention of vault prolapse after hysterectomy is helped by suture of the cardinal and uterosacral ligaments to the vaginal vault.

Treatment

Treatment of prolapse may be conservative or surgical.

Physiotherapy

This can be successful, chiefly in young women after recent childbirth where the vaginal walls and pelvic floor are mainly affected. It is less effective in uterine prolapse. Exercises to strengthen the pelvic floor muscles are carried out under the supervision of a physiotherapist including the voluntary retention of weighted cones in the vagina to strengthen the pelvic muscles. This may be combined with electrotherapy to the pelvic floor muscles. Sets of weighted cones encourage correct pelvic floor contraction by requiring the woman to hold the cone in the vagina for increasing amounts of time.

Conservative treatment

Many types of pessary and support have been devised for prolapse. Their use is only temporary, the better cure being a repair operation. With modern techniques of surgery and anaesthesia, surgery can safely be undertaken in most cases of prolapse.

The indications for pessaries are:
- prolapse during pregnancy
- prolapse immediately after delivery
- when another pregnancy is desired within a short time
- in patients unfit for surgery on medical grounds
- in patients who decline an operation.

Pessary treatment

A plastic ring pessary that fits well surrounds the cervix, pointing slightly forward, and resting between the posterior fornix and the anterior vaginal wall. It supports a vault prolapse by stretching the vaginal wall whereas a cystocoele is directly supported by it. It is less successful in controlling a rectocoele; if the perineum is deficient, the pessary will tend to slip or even fall out.

Pessaries are made in 5 mm sizes from 50 mm to 120 mm.

There are a few cases where a ring pessary fails to control prolapse and surgery cannot be performed. In these cases there are other appliances. The cup-and-stem pessary consists of a sheet of vulcanite or plastic with a stem, to which are attached tapes that are tied to a belt. It is removed at night for cleaning and is thus less likely to cause ulceration. It is a useful long-term pelvic floor support, but rarely used.

Disadvantages
- Ulceration of the vagina and cervix.
- A neglected pessary may become embedded in the vaginal wall and may be removed only with great difficulty.
- A carcinoma of the vagina may develop.

Surgery

The best results from operations for repair of prolapse depend on the degree of descent of the various components of the genital tract together with the judgement and expertise of the surgeon. They should be performed only if there are no urinary symptoms and/or there is no evidence of genuine stress incontinence or significant detrusor instability.

Many surgeons perform *vaginal hysterectomy* when operating for prolapse, an operation of choice when prolapse is combined with menorrhagia or where there are small uterine fibroids. Vaginal hysterectomy is preferred in cases of uterine procidentia.

Anterior colporrhaphy and posterior colpoperineorrhaphy
These operations are designed to restore the support to the vagina from the levator ani and muscles of the perineum. Women with urinary symptoms and vaginal prolapse should all undergo urodynamic investigation before deciding on surgical

treatment. The reasons for doing urodynamics include the following:

• If genuine stress incontinence is demonstrated vaginal surgery is not the treatment of choice.

• If the patient has detrusor instability, vaginal surgery may make it worse and there is an increased risk of postoperative urinary retention and/or infection.

• The first operation for urinary problems gives the best chance of success and it is therefore essential to opt for the operation with the highest cure rate.

New surgical techniques for uterovaginal prolapse have been introduced. These include sacrospinous fixation, where the uterosacral ligaments are fixed to the sacrospinous ligament via the vaginal, laparoscopic or abdominal route, which is being increasingly used with good effect.

Anterior colporrhaphy and posterior colpoperineorrhaphy may be combined with *amputation of the cervix*, and shortening and suture of the cardinal ligaments; this is the Fothergill or Manchester operation (rarely performed).

The following are the reasons for amputating the cervix:

• The supravaginal cervix may be elongated.

• After suture of the cervix, repair of the vaginal vault is more satisfactory.

• The cervix is often unhealthy and infected.

• A possible site for future carcinoma has been removed.

The cervix should not be amputated in young women who may wish to bear children and in cases where there is no vaginal vault prolapse.

Abdominal operations may be combined with prolapse repair. Abdominal hysterectomy may be required for large fibroids and the prolapse may be repaired under the same anaesthetic or later. Removal of a large tumour may itself lead to cure or improvement of prolapse.

Stress incontinence presents surgical challenges. It can occur with or without prolapse.

Preoperative care

Preparation for surgery is most important. The general condition of the patient is assessed and treatment given for conditions such as obesity and chronic cough. Cardiovascular disease and mild diabetes are common in middle-aged women and may need preoperative treatment.

Ulceration of the vagina can follow exposure of the vaginal tissues outside the body in a procidentia or from long wearing of a ring pessary. The risk of ulceration and infection is reduced by regular changing of the pessary (6-monthly) and using regular topical oestrogen cream. Elderly women find the changing of the pessary uncomfortable because the introitus is commonly less elastic and partially stenosed. It is important that the change is performed by a well-trained professional. The pessary can be made more flexible by pre-soaking it in warm water. Regular changes over a long period of time may be unacceptable to some women and it is common for women to ask for surgical intervention after a few years of using a pessary.

Urinary tract infection is common and must be treated. Urge incontinence and detrusor muscle instability should be treated with antispasmodics and surgery postponed until this urogynaecological aspect has been fully investigated and treated.

Postoperative care

Early movements and deep breathing are encouraged and the patient should get out of bed as soon as possible. The use of a lavatory or commode in private helps to overcome difficulties with micturition and defecation. Laxatives are given as required.

The following are postoperative complications in the first 2 weeks:

• *Chest complications* associated with general anaesthesia.

• *Retention of urine* and urinary tract infection: retention usually requires catheterization. If extensive dissection, especially of the perineal tissues, is carried out during the operation, an indwelling Foley catheter should be inserted at the operation. The bladder should be drained continuously for 3–5 days and the catheter then clamped intermittently for a day to reintroduce the sensation of bladder filling. An antibiotic agent should be given during continuous catheterization to prevent urinary infection.

- *Local sepsis* is unusual with the use of antibiotic prophylaxis.
- *Haemorrhage* may be primary, reactionary or secondary. Blood transfusion may be required and in secondary or reactionary haemorrhage, resuturing of the vagina or cervix to arrest bleeding and packing of the vagina may be needed under anaesthesia in the operating theatre.
- *Pelvic vein thrombosis* and *pulmonary embolism* may occur.

There are remote complications.

- *Vaginal discharge* may persist for some weeks. In some cases it is caused by granulation tissue in the scars, which are best treated with silver nitrate sticks. Sutures used in the repair may not be absorbed. They can be nicked and any excess suture material removed at 2 weeks.
- *Urinary complications* include frequency resulting from irritable bladder or chronic infection. Rarely a vesicovaginal or urethrovaginal fistula develops.
- *Dyspareunia* is common and may be caused by leaving the vagina too small; care must be taken not to reduce the vaginal circumference, especially if a posterior repair follows an anterior wall operation. Dyspareunia may also result from disuse of the vagina as a result of fear. Senile atrophy may also be seen in the older age group of those having repair operations.

Future pregnancies after repair

Successful pregnancy can be achieved after prolapse repair, although if the cervix has been amputated there may be an increased tendency to miscarry. Caesarean section is advisable in most cases, especially if there is fibrosis of the remaining cervix, if there has been an extensive vault repair or where surgery has been done for severe stress incontinence.

Vaginal delivery may rarely be allowed.

Urogynaecology

Physiology

The bladder has two main functions in the human.

1 To act as a reservoir for the storage of urine.
2 To empty this reservoir away from the skin of the body at an appropriate time and appropriate place.

Acting as a reservoir, the normal bladder:
- is lined with waterproof transitional epithelium that does not allow diffusion of the urinary electrolytes across its wall
- has a high compliance, accommodating a large volume of urine (300–500 ml) with a rise of intravesical pressure to only 15 cmH$_2$O
- is able to expand suprapubically and extraperitoneally without hindrance or constraint by bone or pelvic viscera
- maintains the pressure in its outflow tract along the urethra at a higher level than intravesical pressure, thus preventing leakage of urine.

The bladder is an efficient expulsive organ:
- The smooth detrusor muscle is richly innervated by the parasympathetic nervous system outflow of sacral roots 2, 3 and 4.
- At the onset of micturition, the pelvic floor striated muscle is voluntarily relaxed, reducing the intraurethral pressure. The background inhibition of the sacral reflex arc is suppressed. Efferent impulses pass to the detrusor muscle causing a rise in intravesical pressure. This then exceeds the intraurethral pressure and leads to the passage of urine down the urethra.

Urinary incontinence

The involuntary loss of urine may be due to:
- true incontinence from a urinary fistula
- genuine stress incontinence
- detrusor instability (overactive bladder syndrome)
- overflow incontinence
- reflex incontinence.

Urinary fistula

A pathological tract may open between a part of the urinary system and the epithelial surface of the vagina or occasionally the skin. These tracts bypass the normal controlling mechanisms causing development of continuous (true) incontinence. They can be congenital or follow major surgery, surgical delivery or disease such as cancer of the cervix.

• Congenital (rare): the ureter draining the upper pole of one kidney opens on the anterior wall of the vagina. It presents in children with continuous urinary loss. This may result in poorly functioning renal polar hydronephrosis or an ectopic hydroureter.

• Caused by surgery: avascular necrosis leads to weakening of the wall of the ureter or bladder and the development of a ureteric or vesicovaginal fistula:

— gynaecological surgery, particularly if there has been anatomical distortion by infection, endometriosis, carcinoma or by preceding small blood vessel damage (endarteritis) caused by irradiation

— obstetric trauma, in association with obstructed labour where the presenting part causes avascular necrosis of the bladder base or sometimes the rectum, causing the development of a vesicovaginal or rectovaginal fistula respectively.

Genuine stress incontinence

An involuntary loss of urine occurs from the urethra, when the transmitted intra-abdominal pressure causes a rise of the intravesical pressure that exceeds the intraurethral pressure in the absence of a detrusor contraction. Approximately 25% of older women have mild problems and 5–10% severe ones.

Symptoms
Involuntary urine loss associated with a sudden, usually unexpected, rise of abdominal pressure such as coughing, sneezing, laughing or lifting.

Physical signs
The coincidental down-swing of the bladder neck leads to urinary leakage from the urethra; often only a few millilitres are passed.

About 50% are associated with prolapse of the vagina.

Detrusor instability (overactive bladders syndrome)

Incidence: 8–10% increasing with age.

Aetiology
Incompletely understood but may be caused by the following:

• An abnormality in the central nervous system when anxiety and stress result in the loss of ability to inhibit the detrusor reflex and, therefore, the development of detrusor contraction

• A recognized neurological defect, such as spinal trauma, demyelinating disorders or epilepsy

• Intense bladder inflammation, particularly in elderly women.

Symptoms
• Urgency of micturition leading to urge incontinence—an inability to hold on

• Frequency of micturition by both day and night

• Often associated with stress incontinence.

Diagnosis
A diary of fluid intake and urinary emptying, including episodes of incontinence, is often helpful in making the diagnosis as frequency and urgency are highlighted. Drinking large volumes affects the symptoms and sound advice on timing and quantities of fluids can improve quality of life significantly. A quality-of-life questionnaire gives a more objective measure of the impact on a person's ability to function normally. The demonstration of detrusor contraction (>15 cmH$_2$O) on cystometry is provoked by bladder filling or straining and the movement or sound of running water.

Overflow incontinence

Loss of urine when the bladder has become filled, usually associated with either:

• obstructive surgery to the bladder neck or

• denervation of the detrusor muscle (usually by extensive pelvic surgery, neurological defects, diabetes).

Symptoms
• The frequent passage of small volumes of urine

• Hesitation of micturition

• A slow stream

• A sensation of incomplete emptying

• Involuntary leakage when bending or getting out of a chair.

Physical signs
• A palpable bladder
• Leakage on elevation of bladder base
• On cystometry, slow urine flow rate
• High residual urine
• Risk of back pressure to upper urinary tract if chronic.

Reflex incontinence

Reflex involuntary voiding is associated with sensory stimulation of the S2–4 segments. This develops when the higher centres are cut off from the sacral reflex arc and thus micturition ceases to be centrally suppressed. It is triggered when there is a significant increase of the afferent impulses to S2, S3 and S4 from either the bladder or the somatic nerves.

Detrusor contractions are often associated with a simultaneous contraction of the pelvic floor (detrusor dyssynergia), causing partial obstruction of urine flow, unlike the relaxation in centrally organized normal micturition.

Urodynamic investigation of incontinence

• Bladder behaviour can be assessed by keeping fluid output charts to measure the frequency of the volumes of urine passed during the day, with a diary of fluid intake.
• Cystometry (with subtracted abdominal pressure) determines the presence or absence of involuntary detrusor contractions thereby differentiating the stable from the unstable bladder and these pressure measurements may be coupled with video-radiological screening (Figs 22.3 and 22.4).

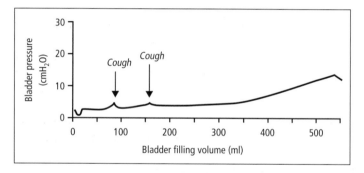

Figure 22.3 Cystometry of a normal bladder filling with rise in intravesical pressure.

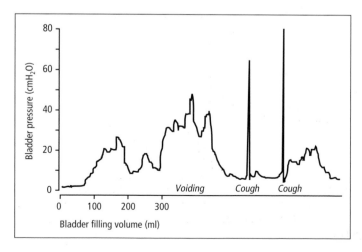

Figure 22.4 Cystometry of filling of an unstable bladder.

- The residual urine can be measured by catheter or pelvic ultrasound.
- Measurement of urinary flow rate with pressure measurements differentiates the obstructed urethra from the poorly functioning detrusor.
- Ultrasound urograms outline defects of the bladder and upper urinary tract and retrograde urography demonstrates ureteric and vesicovaginal fistulas.

Treatment

Stress incontinence

Conservative

- Mild urinary leakage (particularly postnatally): with a good physiotherapist and patient motivation, pelvic floor exercises usually result in improvement.
- Reduction of weight, reduction of excessive physical exertion and the treatment of coughing (smoking cessation) also help.

Surgical

- Sling operation: multiple varieties—using synthetic substances (nylon, Prolene, Teflon, mersilene mesh, tension-free vaginal tapes) or natural tissues (eg round ligament or external oblique aponeurosis). Insertion is usually blind by directed needles through the retropubic space (eg Stamey's procedure). It is commonly done as a day case with the patient returning after 24–48 hours to check the urinary residual with ultrasound.
- Paraurethral injection of collagens to stimulate fibrin formation.
- Vaginal approach: anterior colporrhaphy with bladder neck buttress is a simple operation and permits repair of other prolapses at the same time. Long-term success rate in curing incontinence is approximately 40%.
- Retropubic bladder neck suspension operations: suturing the vaginal wall to the pectineal ligament (Burch procedure) or periosteum over the back of the pubic bone (Marshall–Marchetti–Krantz procedure). These procedures are falling out of use as the sling procedures become more popular.

The unstable bladder (Fig. 22.5)

The symptoms are improved by several means:

- Enthusiastic encouragement, with the help of urinary output volume chart, particularly by incontinence advisers, district nurses and doctors.
- Biofeedback training: this involves training the individual not to respond to the first sensation that their bladder is full, aiming to reach a 4-hour emptying regimen.
- The use of anticholinergic drugs, eg oxybutynin, Pro-Banthine (propantheline bromide), imipramine: these have significant side effects of drowsiness and dry mouth which can make them unsuitable, particularly for women who are working with machinery or driving regularly.
- The use of vaginal oestrogen cream to reduce bladder irritability and the tendency of recurrent urinary infection.

Overflow incontinence

- If obstructed, urethral dilatation or urethrotomy results in improvement.
- If caused by weakened detrusor muscle, continuous drainage with a suprapubic catheter for 2–3 weeks to improve the tone of the detrusor often helps with subsequent bladder training. Occasionally intermittent self-catheterization can be of assistance although infection is common.
- α Agonists—bethanecol.

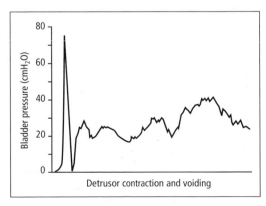

Figure 22.5 Cystometry with detrusor muscle contraction and voiding.

Urinary tract infection

Almost all urinary tract infections develop from the upward spread of the bacteria along the 5 cm of urethra. Infections are associated with:
- the upward passage of organisms during intercourse
- catheterization
- the incomplete emptying of the bladder leading to stagnant urine
- atrophic urethritis from a lack of oestrogens
- poor hygiene after defecation or intercourse.

Symptoms

- Burning dysuria
- Severe urinary frequency
- Urgency of micturition
- Suprapubic discomfort
- Urine odour.

If the infection has spread beyond the bladder to the upper part of the urinary tract then:
- loin pain
- vomiting
- rigors.

Investigations

- Dipstick impregnated with nitrite sensitive amine to screen for bacteria
- Midstream urine culture.

Treatment

- Encouragement of high fluid intake
- Rest in bed if temperature raised
- Rapid use of appropriate antibiotics
- Topical oestrogens in postmenopausal women
- Educational hygiene encouraging postcoital micturition and correct wiping after defecation
- Bladder training with suprapubic catheter if residual urine volumes high.

Urinary frequency

Associated with:
- bladder irritants, eg coffee, cola and fortified wines
- the presence of calculi
- high fluid intake resulting in an increased urinary output
- diabetes mellitus which may present with polydipsia and polyuria
- the use of diuretics
- anxiety, tension and stress, eg outside the examination hall
- development of habits and rituals associated with particular voiding patterns
- insomnia leading to nocturia
- the reduction of any peripheral oedema overnight resulting in increased kidney excretion, bladder filling and nocturia.

Nocturnal enuresis

The involuntary voiding of urine into the bedclothes while asleep.

Aetiology

Not fully known, but the following associations have been noted:
- Deep sleep leading to the loss of suppression of the voiding reflex
- Impairment of the kidneys to concentrate urine while asleep, eg by the persistence of daytime renal excretion pattern
- psychological disturbances such as great unhappiness
- bladder instability in later life.

Treatment

- Frequent waking overnight to ensure regular voiding
- The use of desmopressin and nasal sprays to suppress urine formation while asleep
- Mattress alarms
- Imipramine.

Part 6

Audit of Obstetrics and Gynaecology

Chapter 23

Statistics of reproductive medicine

The population of the world is increasing, although indications are that the boom of the earlier part of the last century is flattening off. In the UK the levels have been fairly steady since the Second World War.

Birth rates are measured in all countries that collect sufficient data. This means that developing countries with poor data sources are not very reliable in measuring birth rates.

The total birth rate is simplest:
• This requires not just knowledge of all the births but also a proper census of the population to derive the denominator (Fig. 23.1). However, it does not relate to the process of birth; no men have babies and few young women or those over 45 do; hence a more sophisticated measure is the general fertility rate.
• The general fertility rate requires a more detailed data analysis of the censuses and is used in western countries. The data for the last years in the UK are shown in Fig. 23.2.

A more readily understandable set of ratios is the completed family size but this can be done only retrospectively (Fig. 23.3).

In the UK the total birth rate is 14 per 1000 and the general fertility rate is 64 per 1000. The completed family size is 1.8, just below replacement level.

There are variations in the monthly birth rate, which is highest from October to March. The rates by days of the week are highest on weekdays (Fig. 23.4a).

As can be seen, the birth rate for babies <2500 g provides a mirror image to the incidence of births and accounts for the higher perinatal mortality rates at the weekend (Fig. 23.4b).

Maternal mortality

Definitions

Deaths of women while pregnant or within 42 days of delivery, miscarriage, termination of pregnancy, from any cause related to or aggravated by the pregnancy or its management but not from accidental or incidental causes. These deaths are further subdivided into direct and indirect causes; *direct* causes are those that result from obstetric complications, whereas *indirect* deaths are those resulting from pre-existing disease or disease that develops during pregnancy secondary to physiological changes of pregnancy.

Major causes of maternal mortality

Maternal mortality has declined dramatically in the last 50 years in the UK (Fig. 23.5), but there are

Lecture Notes: Obstetrics and Gynaecology, 3rd edition. By Diana Hamilton-Fairley. Published 2009 by Blackwell Publishing. ISBN: 978-1-4051-7801-3.

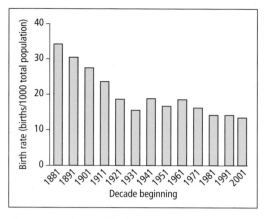

Figure 23.1 The total birth rate in England and Wales (1881–2001) showing numbers of births/1000 total population.

still women who die as a consequence of pregnancy or labour. Globally, 530000 women die each year as a result of complications of pregnancy and labour; only 1% of these deaths occur in the developed world.

According to the 2007 report of the World Health Organization (WHO) on maternal mortality, a woman living in Afghanistan currently has a 1 in 8 lifetime risk of dying during pregnancy or labour. The maternal mortality ratio in Afghanistan is 1800 per 100000 live births. This is higher than the estimated figure of 1000–1500 if women were left entirely without medical assistance.

The figures are similar in Niger (1 in 7) and Sierra Leone (1 in 8), slightly better in Congo, where 2 in 22 women will die of a maternal cause, 1 in 31 in

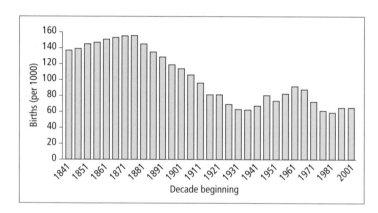

Figure 23.2 The general fertility rate in England and Wales (1841–2001) showing numbers of births/1000 women aged 15–44.

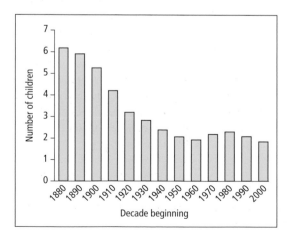

Figure 23.3 Completed family size in England and Wales (1880–2000).

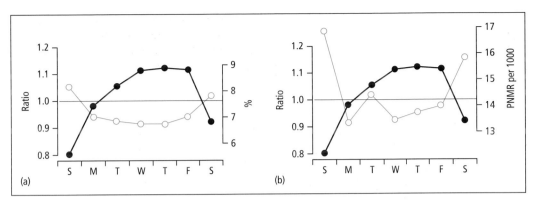

Figure 23.4 Ratio of births by days of the week (for England and Wales) (●—●) against (a) percentage of babies born ≤2500 g (○—○) and (b) perinatal mortality rate per 1000 total births (○—○).

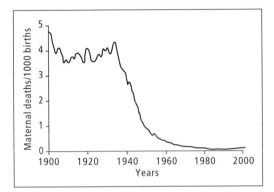

Figure 23.5 Maternal mortality in England and Wales, 1900–1997.

Nepal, 1 in 150 in Morocco and 1 in 840 in Mongolia. In contrast a woman living in Ireland has a risk of only 1 in 47 600, even lower than the UK with a risk of 1 in 8200 (Table 23.1).

The main causes for these deaths in developing countries are haemorrhage, infections, eclampsia, obstructed labour and unsafe abortion. The lack of education and empowerment of women coupled with the unavailability of contraception is a contributory factor to these high lifetime risks of maternal death. Among those women who survive childbirth, there may be significant long-term complications such as fistula, which can have a devastating effect on quality of life.

The UN has made the global reduction of maternal mortality one of its main priorities. At the UN Millennium Summit in 2000, the promotion of gender equality and empowerment of women and the aim to 'reduce by three quarters, between 1990 and 2015, the maternal mortality ratio', were formulated as the third and fifth of eight Millennium Development Goals (Box 23.1).

At the Summit 189 governments committed themselves to supporting these goals. In the UK the Liverpool and London Schools of Tropical Medicine and the Royal College of Obstetricians and Gynaecologists are collaborating to provide education and develop guidelines, promoting safer motherhood in resource-poor countries.

In the UK the major causes are secondary to hypertensive disease of pregnancy, thrombosis and haemorrhage, which are discussed in more detail below. Maternal mortality is expressed as deaths/1000 births or deaths/100000 maternities. In the 3-year period 2002–5 295 women died out of over 2 million births, of which 149 died from obstetric-related causes; the maternal mortality rate (MMR) for direct and indirect deaths was 13.9/100000 maternities. The advances in medical care before pregnancy have led to more women with pre-existing medical conditions becoming pregnant. This has led to indirect maternal deaths making a greater contribution to the MMR. In 2002–5 the MMR for direct deaths was 6.24/100000 compared with 7.7/100000 for indirect deaths. In 1985–87 the rates were 6.1 and 3.8 respectively. However, the combined direct and indirect MMR has hardly changed over the past 15 years.

Table 23.1 Maternal mortality in 2005

Country	Lifetime risk of maternal death of 1 in	Maternal mortality ratio (maternal deaths per 100 000 live births)
Afghanistan	8	1800
Australia	13 300	4
Bangladesh	51	570
Botswana	130	380
Brazil	370	110
Canada	11 000	7
Chad	11	1500
Croatia	10 500	7
Czech Republic	18 100	4
Egypt	230	130
Ghana	45	560
Guatemala	71	290
India	70	450
Ireland	47 600	1
Latvia	8 500	10
Niger	7	1800
Nigeria	18	1100
Nepal	31	830
Romania	3 200	24
Rwanda	16	1300
Sierra Leone	8	2100
Spain	16 400	4
Sudan	53	450
UK	8 500	8
USA	4 800	11
Zimbabwe	43	880

From estimates developed by WHO, Unicef and UNFPA WHO, Geneva (2007) pp. 23–7.

Pregnancy-induced hypertension, pre-eclampsia and eclampsia (MMR 0.85/100 000)

Eclampsia is becoming rarer. When it comes earlier in pregnancy (before 28 weeks) it has a worse effect. Death is from intracranial haemorrhage or renal failure.

To reduce deaths:
- identify high-risk women
- check blood pressure frequently in pregnancy
- admit those with signs of pre-eclampsia (this may be at home for lesser degrees rather than in hospital)
- recognize biochemical and haematological aspects of HELLP (**h**aemolysis, **e**levated **l**iver en-zymes, **l**ow **p**latelets) syndrome (see Chapter 10).

Thromboembolism (MMR 1.94/100 000)

- A third are antenatal and two-thirds after delivery. A third of the latter follow Caesarean section.
- High-risk patients:
  — >35 years
  — obese
  — surgical delivery
  — previous thrombosis.
- Half the deaths are with little warning of previous thrombotic episodes.
- To reduce deaths:
  — prophylactic anticoagulation of high-risk patients
  — avoid risk factors
  — prompt effective treatment on suspicion.

Box 23.1 The Millennium Development Goals

1 Eradicate extreme poverty and hunger
Reduce by half the proportion of people living on less than a dollar a day.
Reduce by half the proportion of people who suffer from hunger.
2 Achieve universal primary education
Ensure that all boys and girls complete a full course of primary schooling.
3 Promote gender equality and empower women
Eliminate gender disparity in primary and secondary education preferably by 2005, and at all levels by 2015.
4 Reduce child mortality
Reduce by two thirds the mortality rate among children under 5.
5 Improve maternal health
Reduce by three-quarters the maternal mortality ratio.
6 Combat HIV/AIDS, malaria and other diseases
Halt and begin to reverse the spread of HIV/AIDS.
Halt and begin to reverse the incidence of malaria and other major diseases.
7 Ensure environmental sustainability
Integrate the principles of sustainable development into country policies and programmes; reverse loss of environmental resources.
Reduce by half the proportion of people without sustainable access to safe drinking water and basic sanitation.
Achieve significant improvement in lives of at least 100 million slum dwellers, by 2020.
8 Develop a global partnership for development
Develop further an open, rule-based, predictable, non-discriminatory trading and financial system.
Address the special needs of the least developed countries, landlocked countries and small island developing states. Deal comprehensively with developing countries' debt.
In cooperation with developing countries, develop and implement strategies for decent and productive work for youth. In cooperation with pharmaceutical companies, provide access to affordable essential drugs in developing countries. In cooperation with the private sector, make available the benefits of new technologies, especially information and communication technologies

Haemorrhage (MMR 0.66/100 000)

Abruptio placentae (placental abruption)
Severe hypovolaemia leads to shock and later renal shutdown. To reduce deaths:

- central venous pressure monitoring
- adequate and quick blood replacement.

Placenta praevia
Repeated and increasing haemorrhage in last trimester of pregnancy. The severe degrees must be treated by caesarean section, which may be a technically difficult operation. To reduce deaths:

- pay more attention to warning bleeds in pregnancy
- have consultant in theatre for caesarean section.

Postpartum haemorrhage (PPH)
Usually from an atonic uterus but can follow cervical trauma. To reduce deaths:

- give oxytocic drug routinely at delivery
- deliver patients at risk in hospital where blood is available (see Chapter 13)
- act promptly using a planned protocol.

Amniotic fluid embolism (MMR 0.8/100 000)

Amniotic fluid entering the circulation causes severe, rapid onset disseminated intravascular coagulation which usually results in a massive post partum haemorrhage. A nationwide reporting system (UKOSS) concentrated on this condition in the last triennium and therefore could be identified as a cause of PPH.

Early pregnancy

Legal abortion (MMR 0.09/100 000)
- Usually after procured and illegal interferences.
- Patients die from haemorrhage, sepsis or renal failure.
To reduce deaths:
- wider use of legal therapeutic abortion
- better contraception.

Ectopic pregnancy (MMR 0.47/100 000)
With reduction of deaths from other forms of haemorrhage this is becoming relatively more important. To reduce deaths:

- admit patients with suspicious symptoms
- act promptly on patients with actual symptoms
- be prepared to laparoscope on suspicion and do not rely on ultrasound and β-hCG (β-human chorionic gonadotrophin) findings alone.

Anaesthesia MMR (0.28/100 000)

Deaths associated with general anaesthesia are reducing greatly in the UK. Inhalation of acid stomach contents in labour under general anaesthetic leads to Mendelson's syndrome. To reduce deaths:
- wider use of regional anaesthetics (eg spinal epidural)
- if general anaesthetic essential, a senior anaesthetist involved and intubation with a cuffed tube.

Other causes

All the other direct causes produce few deaths. Infection (MMR 0.85/100000), once the killer of one in five women in childbirth, is much reduced (although still causing some deaths each year, mostly after caesarean section in labour with prolonged ruptured membranes).

Indirect causes

Pre-existing cardiac disease as a cause is increasing (1.6/100000 in 1991–3 to 2.27/100000 in 2003–5) as more women survive into adulthood with congenital heart disease, although rheumatic fever has dramatically declined as a cause as it is very rare and successfully diagnosed and treated in childhood.

In the triennium 2000–2 suicide was the leading indirect cause of a mother dying. The report recommended that all midwives, health visitors and obstetricians should be trained in detecting early signs of perinatal depression and psychosis with an increase in mental health services for women in pregnancy and around the time of birth. Although the number of inpatient beds for such women has not increased there has been a slight decrease in the number of deaths associated with suicide in 2003–5.

Substandard care

In the UK every maternal death is reported to a central committee—the Confidential Enquiry into Maternal and Child Health (CEMACH), which publishes its confidential findings at 3-yearly intervals. This is not a judicial enquiry and no blame is apportioned to any individual. It is a medical audit where the profession looks closely at its own work and tries to learn from mistakes. The committee tries to assess in each case if an avoidable factor was present: if there was 'some departure from the acceptable standards of satisfactory care'.

In the most recent report, 50% of the deaths directly resulting from pregnancy and delivery were considered to have been avoidable by this definition. It was the patient who made the largest single contribution to this in the antenatal period by either not coming in for care or else ignoring advice given. In labour, the hospital obstetricians and anaesthetists were associated with the highest incidence of substandard care incidents. This was mostly from not paying sufficient heed to warning signs and not having senior-enough doctors in the delivery suite. Shortage of staff and facilities is beginning to be reported in this category. Substandard care from GPs and midwives in these cases was rare.

The following are the most important ways of reducing maternal deaths:
- Improved access to antenatal care
- Improved education in the population of the importance of antenatal care
- More consultant obstetric and anaesthetic involvement on the delivery suite
- Introduction of evidence-based guidelines for all areas of maternity care
- Regular training of all staff including emergency drills for PPH and shoulder dystocia.

Near misses

As maternal deaths are so few, even after national analysis, we cannot draw many statistical conclusions. However, an extended method can be used to increase the database. Here, we look at women who have a firm diagnosis of a given, precisely diagnosed condition and examine the background even though they did not die, eg we could look at those who have lost over 2 litres of blood at a primary PPH. This would be a fairly well-defined group because the loss is so great and we would be able to compare the aetiology and management with that of women who died from PPH. By so doing we would examine about six times as many cases. Similarly, we could look at the reasonably firm diagnosis of pulmonary embolism proven by a scan and, again, examine them as a larger group than those who died from the condition.

The idea of near misses as a method of examination is excellent for an individual hospital or group of hospitals that work as one, but is more difficult to apply regionally or nationally unless the definitions are firmly established.

Risk management

Routine reporting of all incidents that affect the quality of care for the patient are reported to a risk management manager and lead clinician. These may appear minor (past notes unavailable in clinic) or major (delay in obtaining cross-matched blood in a case of major obstetric haemorrhage); however, they can both have a major effect on the standard of patient care and the outcome for the mother and her child. All reports should be a purely factual account and not apportion blame to any individual. The manager and the lead clinician collect all the reports and investigate the problem. This process may highlight a problem in the system of care that needs to be rectified or a need for further staff education, either individually or as a group. Serious adverse incidents are usually investigated locally and then reported to the strategic health authority together with recommendations for preventing such incidents occurring again.

Patient complaints are investigated in a similar way and responses containing the facts of the case, the findings of the investigation and the recommendations are sent to the patient. Patients have the right to request a formal meeting with the hospital after the investigation to express their views and make their own recommendations. Hospitals now employ patient advocates to help patients through this process. The direct communication to the patient reduces the number of cases that proceed to litigation.

Audit is used as a risk management tool. All maternity units in the UK are expected to follow evidence-based multidisciplinary guidelines. These may be developed locally, by the Royal College of Obstetricians and Gynaecologists or the National Institute for Health and Clinical Excellence (NICE). Each unit is expected to audit their care against these guidelines at regular intervals. Each audit should identify areas where the guidelines are not being followed or are inadequate. Recommendations are made to improve the standard of care and the audit repeated to ensure that the changes have improved care. This is called the audit cycle.

Perinatal mortality

The perinatal mortality rate (PMR) is the total of stillbirths and first-week neonatal deaths occurring in every 1000 total births. The definition of stillbirth was changed in 1991 to deaths after 24 completed weeks of gestation from a previous 28 weeks' limit. Hence, a small apparent increase for a short time appears. Figure 23.6 shows the progressive reduction of PMR in 70 years.

In 1997 the PMR was 7.9/1000 total births in England and Wales, and 8/1000 total births in 2005 but it varies across the regions of the country.

Factors influencing PMR

- Low birth weight: babies who weigh <2.5 kg are 300 times more likely to be stillborn (66% of stillbirths) than those who are of normal weight. This is independent of gestational age at delivery.
- Teenage mothers and those >40 have a higher stillbirth rate.
- Obese women (BMI > 30 kg/m²).
- Multiple births: risk of stillbirth is three times greater.
- Place of maternal residence: north-east London has the highest stillbirth rate (7.3/1000) whereas East Anglia has the lowest (3.6/1000), even though they are geographically neighbours.

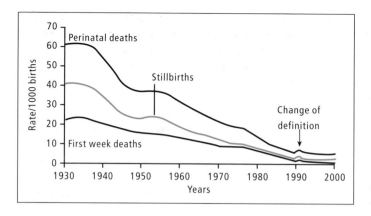

Figure 23.6 Perinatal mortality, still-births and first week neonatal deaths in England and Wales from 1930.

• Social class: the lower social classes have the greatest risk. This is multifactorial, being social, environmental and behavioural. The greater the number of risks (poor housing, poverty, smoking, drug use) the higher the risk.
• Mother's place of birth: women who are recent immigrants have a 30% greater risk of stillbirth than women born in the UK.
• Gender: boys are more likely to be stillborn than girls.
• Method of delivery/perinatal interventions: forceps and breech deliveries are at increased risk. These can be reduced with experienced, well-staffed units and the presence of neonatal intensive care facilities.

Causes of perinatal mortality

Precise causes of perinatal death are often confused by a lack of postmortem information and an insistence on a single or primary cause of death on the certificate:
• Congenital abnormalities: these account for 16% of stillbirths and 22% of neonatal deaths
• Congenital sepsis: systemically acquired infections while *in utero*—1.9%
• Asphyxia, anoxia or birth trauma: 7.5%
• Maternal disorders (diabetes, hypothyroidism): 5.8%
• Maternal obstetric disease: pre-eclampsia 3%
• Rhesus (Rh) haemolytic disease
• Prematurity
• Low birth weight (75% <2500 g)

• Obstetric emergency (placental abruption, cord prolapse, shoulder dystocia).

Classification of causes of perinatal death
• Macerated stillbirths without malformation
• Congenital malformation in either stillbirths or neonatal deaths
• Intrapartum perinatal deaths secondary to asphyxia or trauma or both
• Neonatal deaths as a result of immaturity
• Other specific causes, eg Rh haemolytic disease.

Confidential Enquiry into Maternal and Child Health

The Confidential Enquiry into Stillbirths and Deaths in Infancy (CESDI) is now merged with the maternal deaths into the CEMACH. The Department of Health, in conjunction with the Royal Colleges, set up a CESDI group in each of the NHS regions. These assess, in a confidential way, all deaths from week 20 of pregnancy through childbirth to the end of the first year of life. Although the groupings are disparate, we can derive a subset analysis of perinatal deaths leaving out those aged <24 weeks (large numbers are terminations of pregnancy), and those after the first week of life when the perinatal period finishes; among these the major causes of death include sudden infant death syndrome.

Each group has research midwives who determine more details of each death reported by examining the hospital notes. The central committee then makes recommendations and finds whether there is any degree of substandard care. Recommendations follow from these groups and it is hoped that they can make as great an impact on perinatal deaths as the Confidential Enquiries into Maternal Deaths have made on mothers' care.

Management of perinatal death

When pregnancy ends with the loss of a fetus or a neonate, particular care and support are needed for the couple involved. This is a difficult situation for the parents and relatives, and for the medical and nursing staff. Grief reactions commonly involve the following phases (Fig. 23.7):

1 Initial denial of what has occurred
2 Attempt to apportion blame to themselves
3 Attempt to apportion blame to the doctors and midwives
4 Eventual acceptance of their loss which may take several months.

Problems associated with intrauterine death

- Intrauterine infection
- Difficult induction of labour
- Psychological and possibly psychiatric sequelae
- Disseminated intravascular coagulopathy (DIC) if fetus retained for some weeks—this is a theoretical risk and rarely encountered.

Management of labour

- Confirm the diagnosis of intrauterine death by real-time ultrasound.
- Give the parents time to come to terms with their loss.
- Plan induction of labour at a time that is suitable for the parents, but ensuring that they have a midwife to look after them throughout the period of induction and labour. They are often given mifepristone first to prime the cervix and return 48 hours later to start a prostaglandin induction.
- Arrange facilities for the partner to stay throughout the procedure.

Investigations

- Hb (including HbA1c)
- Cross-match and save serum
- Kleihauer's test
- Clotting studies

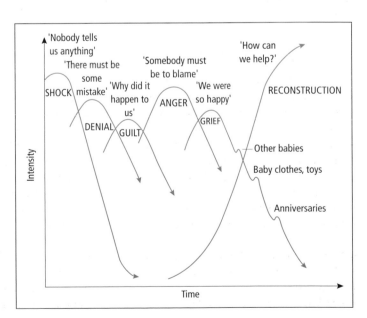

Figure 23.7 Emotional response to bad news. (From Newell S, Darling J (2007) *Lecture Notes on Paediatrics*, 8th edn. Blackwell Publishing, Oxford.)

- Lupus anticoagulant and anticardiolipin antibodies (for systemic lupus erythematosus/antiphospholipid syndrome)
- Fasting blood sugar and HbA1c (for diabetes)
- Liver function tests.

From the baby:

- Karyotype: skin sample, placental biopsy or amniocentesis if the baby looks abnormal
- Surface swabs particularly in the presence of prolonged rupture of membranes
- *Post mortem*: this is essential if the parents are to be given as full an explanation as possible of why their baby died. The consent form for the postmortem examination is very detailed and requires training before taking the consent.

Management

- Induce labour with prostaglandin pessaries given every 3 hours.
- Do not rupture the membranes until the woman is in labour and the cervix is >4 cm dilated if at all
- Keep an accurate fluid balance chart.
- Give liberal analgesia. If the woman wishes to have an epidural ensure that her blood clotting values are normal.
- Discuss whether the couple wish to see the baby after delivery. Parents should be encouraged but not pressed to view their babies.

The babies should be photographed, clothed and looking as natural as possible. These photographs should be filed in case parents wish to see them much later—sometimes they ask a year or so later.

Postnatal care

The woman should be looked after by midwifery staff known to her in the antenatal period. The length of hospital stay is not determined by medical events but more by what the couple want. She may go home as soon as she wishes but should not have the feeling of being sent away. Her GP and community midwife must be informed by one of the medical staff of the loss by telephone.

- Arrange for the mother to be seen by a specialist midwife who is skilled in counselling patients who have lost their babies.
- Ask if she wishes her baby to be baptized and buried; if so, arrange the procedure with the hospital chaplain or other religious leader according to the parent's request.
- Consent for postmortem examination should be obtained from the parents.
- The following procedures should be undertaken:
  — heart blood should be sent for karyotyping and viral studies
  — two Polaroid photographs of the baby should be taken. One should be a general photograph and the other should be a close-up of the baby's face. In addition, foot- and hand-prints and a lock of hair are retained
  — X-ray the baby
  — if available, MRI of baby.
- The consultant should interview the parents before discharge from hospital and explain as far as possible the circumstances surrounding the death.
- The couple are met 4–6 weeks later with all the postmortem evidence to hand.
- The couple should be put in touch with a society, eg Stillbirth, Abortion and Neonatal Death Society (SANDS), or people who have experienced a similar problem.
- Lactation should be suppressed by means of a firm supporting brassiere. Bromocriptine or cabergoline should be offered.
- Women who had to have a hysterectomy or have one surviving twin may need professional psychotherapeutic help.

Self-assessment questions

Chapter 1

1.1

From the list of words/phrases below fill in the blanks:

The uterine artery is a branch of the (1) _____ artery. The uterus is a hollow, muscle-walled organ in direct communication with the (2) _____ and the vagina. Inferior to the uterine artery lies the (3) _____ The ligaments that support the uterus include the (4) _____ and the (5) _____.

(a) external iliac
(b) transverse cervical
(c) pudendal
(d) ureter
(e) pectineal
(f) bladder
(g) fallopian tubes
(h) internal iliac
(i) ovaries
(j) uterosacral

1.2

Which of the following statements are true?
(a) The granulosa cells secrete androstenedione.
(b) The granulosa cells become luteal cells after the release of the oocyte.
(c) Luteal cells secrete progesterone alone.
(d) The ovary contains around 50 000 oocytes at menarche.
(e) The primordial oocytes are found in the cortex of the ovary.

1.3

Which of the following statements are true of the menstrual cycle?
(a) The LH surge causes the oocyte to undergo meiosis reducing the chromosome number in the oocyte to 23.
(b) Estradiol causes the endometrial glands to secrete glycogen.
(c) The endometrium is shed because the spiral arterioles lose their elasticity and start to bleed.
(d) The luteal phase lasts for a fixed duration of 12–14 days.
(e) In the proliferative phase of the cycle the endometrial glands become tortuous.

1.4

Which of the following statements are true?
(a) Estradiol exerts a negative feedback on FSH.
(b) The secretion of FSH and LH is under the control of the thalamus.
(c) FSH catalyses the conversion of testosterone to estradiol.
(d) Testosterone is essential for the production of estradiol.
(e) Progesterone concentrations reach their peak at the time of ovulation.

1.5

Using the words and phrases below label the diagram provided on page 322.
(a) Uterine fundus
(b) Uterine corpus
(c) Endometrium
(d) Isthmus of fallopian tube
(e) Ampulla of fallopian tube
(f) Infundibulopelvic ligament
(g) Internal os of cervix

Lecture Notes: Obstetrics and Gynaecology, 3rd edition. By Diana Hamilton-Fairley. Published 2009 by Blackwell Publishing. ISBN: 978-1-4051-7801-3.

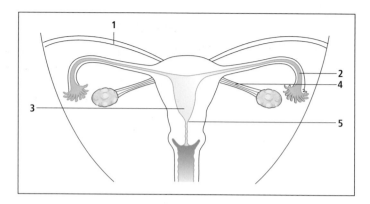

(h) External os of cervix
(i) Fimbriae of fallopian tube
(j) Round ligament

Chapter 2

2.1

Ask a female friend to role-play a patient and practise taking a history using the following role-plays. The instructions for the candidate are that you should take a history from the role-player in 10 minutes. At the end, the candidate may be expected to give a two-sentence summary of the case. The role-player needs to make up a name for herself and fill in some personal details. The scoring scheme may be purely for communication skills or may include marks for information given.

2.2

You are a 22-year-old woman who has come to see the doctor because of painful periods. You have had them since you started your periods at the age of 12. They are becoming worse. The pain is crampy and radiates down the front of your legs. You take Nurofen regularly but it only helps a little bit. The pain starts the day before your period and continues for 3 days. Your periods are regular, bleeding for 5 days in every 26–29 days. You have never been pregnant and are not in a relationship at present. You had a smear last year, which was normal. (All other details are up to the imagination of your role-player!)

2.3

You are a 27-year-old woman who has been trying for a baby for 18 months. You had a child at the age of 22 by a different partner and an ectopic pregnancy 2 years ago. You have never had an infection but, now you come to think about it, you were supposed to take a course of tablets 3 years ago after one of your boyfriends had been to a clinic, but you never bothered. You have been with your current partner, aged 32, for the last 2 years and are planning to get married next year. Your periods are regular and you have no other health problems. Your baby (a boy) was born at term vaginally with no problems. (All other details are up to the imagination of your role-player!)

2.4

You are a 32-year-old woman who is seeing your GP about future contraception. You have had three children and don't really want any more. During your first pregnancy you developed high blood pressure and the baby was delivered at 36 weeks by caesarean section. Your other two children were born naturally. Your mother has diabetes, which was diagnosed in her 50s. Your father is alive and well but has high blood pressure. You do not like taking the pill because you keep forgetting it and it gives you headaches. You are concerned that the other hormonal preparations will make you put on weight, which is a problem for your job as an air hostess. You have never had any other illnesses. You smoke 30 cigarettes a day and drink socially. (All other details are up to the imagination of your role-player!)

Chapter 3

Read the following five clinical scenarios carefully and answer the questions that follow.

Scenario 1

A 16-year-old presents with a history of primary amenorrhoea. She is 1.45 m tall and weighs 53 kg (BMI 25.2). On physical examination her breasts are Tanner stage 2; she has a normal vulva and vagina. Her mother reports that she struggles at school and is being teased because she is so short.

Scenario 2

A 16-year-old girl presents with a history of primary amenorrhoea. She is 1.64 m tall and weighs 47 kg (BMI 17.5). Her breast development is Tanner stage 3 and she has scanty pubic hair; she has a normal vulva and vagina. She represents Greater London in marathon running and is otherwise well.

Scenario 3

A 17-year-old girl presents with a history of secondary amenorrhoea. She is 1.64 m tall and weighs 56 kg (BMI 21). She started her periods at the age of 14 and they were irregular and light until 1 year ago when they stopped. On physical examination she has acne on her face and back which she finds distressing. Her legs and arms are hairy and she has hair on her abdomen in an inverted triangle. Her vulva and vagina are normal. Her mother has type 2 diabetes. She is otherwise well.

Scenario 4

A woman of 24 presents to the clinic with secondary amenorrhoea. Her periods started at the age of 12 and were regular until 2 years ago when they became irregular and light. She has noticed a discharge from her breasts and suffers from severe headaches. On physical examination she has a white discharge from her breasts and is otherwise normal.

Scenario 5

A 15-year-old girl presents to the clinic with primary amenorrhoea. She complains of intermittent abdominal pain and has noticed that her school skirt is becoming tighter. Her weight and height are normal for her age. On examination her breasts are Tanner stage 4 and pubic hair stage 5. Her vulva looks swollen at the introitus and she has a palpable abdominal mass that is tender.

3.1

From the list below choose the single most likely diagnosis for each of the clinical scenarios above.
(a) Androgen insensitivity syndrome
(b) Cryptomenorrhoea
(c) Pregnancy
(d) Polycystic ovary syndrome
(e) Asherman's syndrome
(f) Turner's syndrome
(g) Congenital adrenal hyperplasia
(h) Hyperprolactinaemia
(i) Constitutional delay of puberty
(j) Anorexia/exercise-related amenorrhoea

3.2

From the lists below select the most useful first-line investigations to establish the diagnosis for each clinical scenario.
(a) Ultrasound scan
(b) Ultrasound scan, LH, FSH and testosterone
(c) Ultrasound scan, LH, FSH, prolactin
(d) Chromosome analysis
(e) Pregnancy test
(f) LH, FSH, estradiol
(g) Ultrasound scan, LH, FSH, testosterone, adrenal androgen profile
(h) Thyroid function tests

3.3

From the list below select the most appropriate first-line treatment for each condition.
(a) Weight gain
(b) Removal of gonads/ovaries

(c) Incision of vaginal septum
(d) Referral to the antenatal clinic
(e) Bromocriptine
(f) Progestogerone therapy every 3 months
(g) Creation of a vagina
(h) Oestrogen replacement therapy
(i) Prednisolone
(j) Weight loss

Chapter 4

4.1

Which of the following statements are true?
(a) On semen analysis more than 10% normal forms is considered normal.
(b) The most common cause of anovulatory subfertility is hyperprolactinaemia.
(c) Women with premature ovarian failure (POF) can be successfully treated with follicle-stimulating hormone (FSH).
(d) Male subfertility due to oligospermia can be successfully treated with intracytoplasmic sperm injection (ICSI).
(e) The risk of multiple pregnancy in ovulation induction is around 30%.
(f) The most common cause of anovulatory subfertility is polycystic ovary syndrome.
(g) Progesterone levels should be tested in the mid-follicular phase.
(h) A sperm count of 10 million/ml would be considered normal.
(i) Tubal patency can be checked using ultrasound.
(j) Progesterone levels should be tested in the mid-luteal phase.

4.2

Which of the following are associated with causing tubal damage leading to tubal subfertility?
(a) *Trichomonas vaginalis*
(b) Gonorrhoea
(c) Previous ectopic pregnancy
(d) Use of the oral contraceptive pill
(e) *Chlamydia*

4.3

Match the diagnosis (a–e) to the first-line treatment (1–10) that could be offered to give the best chance of a successful pregnancy.
(a) Bilateral tubal blockage
(b) Polycystic ovary syndrome
(c) Hyperprolactinaemia
(d) Oligospermia due to Klinefelter syndrome
(e) Turner's syndrome

(1) Egg donation
(2) Bromocriptine
(3) FSH
(4) Weight gain
(5) In vitro fertilization
(6) Weight loss
(7) Intracytoplasmic sperm injection
(8) Clomifene
(9) Tubal surgery
(10) Donor insemination

Chapter 5

5.1 OSCE role-play question (10 minutes)

Candidate's instructions: a 14-year-old girl comes to your practice requesting contraception. You are the GP who is going to counsel her. She has no medical illnesses and her weight is normal.

Role-player's instructions: you are a 14-year-old girl who is fully developed. Your periods started when you were 11. You have been going out with a 16-year-old boy in your school for the last 3 months. Your relationship has developed to the point that you are thinking about having sex with him. Your parents do not know about the relationship and you do not want to tell them. You get on reasonably well with your father but he is never at home because he is a long distance lorry driver. You constantly fight with your mother who does not understand you at all and would be horrified that you had a boyfriend. She disapproves of your friends and will not let you go out late at weekends. You tend to defy her and take the consequences in the morning. You know that she would be furious if you got pregnant so you want to be sensible and take precautions so this can't happen. Your friend has told you to go to the GP and get the pill. She has reassured you that she or he cannot tell your parents without your permission. You haven't told your boyfriend because you do not want him to know that you are ready for sex; you just want to be protected in case. You have no medical problems, you smoke three cigarettes a day and are of normal weight. You have never taken any illegal substances. The rest is up to the imagination of the role-player.

5.2 OSCE role-play question (10 minutes)

Candidate's instructions: a woman of 35 comes to your clinic requesting sterilization. She is fit and well and of normal weight. You are the doctor who will counsel her.

Role-player's instructions: you are a woman of 35. You have three children and do not want any more. You have been married for 12 years and your children are 10, 7 and 3 years old, all fit and well. You and your husband have discussed this and have decided that you should have the operation. You have been on the pill for the last 3 years but you know that you should stop taking it because you smoke 40 cigarettes a day. Your periods were regular but quite heavy before you had your youngest daughter. You have no other medical problems and all the children were normal deliveries at term. You do not want to use barrier methods because they are messy and unreliable. You are not keen on a coil because you have heard that they cause heavy periods and infection. You are worried about putting on weight after the operation and have heard that the mini-pill and the injections are also bad for your weight. All other details are up to the role-player.

5.3

Which of the following statements are true about the combined oral contraceptive pill (COCP)?
(a) COCP should be started on the seventh day of a woman's period.
(b) If the woman misses the first two pills in her packet she should use additional protection for at least 2 weeks.

(c) COCP should be taken at the same time of day to ensure protection from unwanted pregnancy.
(d) A past medical history of thrombosis is an absolute contraindication for prescribing the COCP.
(e) Women on antiepileptic medication should be prescribed a pill with a low oestrogen content.

5.4

Which of the following are absolute contraindications to the use of an intrauterine contraceptive device.
(a) Past history of pelvic inflammatory disease
(b) Past history of sickle cell disease
(c) Past history of termination of pregnancy
(d) Past history of an abnormal cervical smear
(e) Past history of heart valve replacement

5.5

Which of the following are recognized methods of emergency contraception.
(a) High-dose oestrogen given in two doses 12 hours apart
(b) High-dose oestrogen and progestogen given in two doses 12 hours apart
(c) High-dose progestogen given in two doses 12 hours apart
(d) Endometrial curettage
(e) Insertion of an intrauterine device (IUD) within 5 days of unprotected intercourse

Chapter 6

6.1

Which of the following statements are true of sexually transmitted infections (STIs)?
(a) Gonorrhoea in women is best diagnosed by cultures of material from the posterior vaginal fornix.
(b) Syphilis is adequately treated in penicillin-allergic pregnant women by erythromycin.
(c) Contact tracing partners of women with first attack genital herpes is helpful.

(d) Bacterial vaginosis should be diagnosed by culture of a high vaginal swab (HVS) for *Gardnerella vaginalis*.

(e) *Chlamydia trachomatis* is routinely diagnosed by nucleic acid amplification tests performed on endocervical swabs.

6.2

Which of the following statements are true about HIV infection?

(a) It is caused by a DNA virus that binds to the CD4 receptor.

(b) Seroconversion commonly presents with a glandular fever-like illness.

(c) In the UK, all patients with a CD4 count below $200 \times 10^6/l$ should be encouraged to start anti-HIV drugs.

(d) Antiretroviral resistance testing can show resistance patterns to both current and previous anti-HIV drugs.

(e) Tenofovir is a nucleotide reverse transcription inhibitor.

6.3

Ask a friend to role-play a patient and practise taking a sexual history using the following role-play. The instructions for the candidate are that you should take the history from the role-player in 8 minutes. At the end, the candidate may be expected to give a 4-minute summary of the case and outline appropriate investigations for this woman. The role-player needs to make up a name for herself and fill in some personal details. The scoring system will award marks for communication skills, history-taking and appropriate investigations (maximum 12 marks).

Role-player's instructions: you are a 35-year-old married woman with two healthy children, aged 5 and 7. You have come to the doctor because of vulval itching. You last had sexual intercourse (unprotected, only divulge if asked) with your husband 3 nights ago and have been together for over 10 years. Recently, your husband went to Thailand on a business trip. Two weeks previously, while he was away, you had sex with a male friend and the condom broke (only divulge this if asked). Your last smear test was normal 1 year ago and you have never had an STI before. You are very worried.

6.4

Which of the following statements about vaginal discharge are true?

(a) Female vulvovaginal candidiasis has a thick creamy discharge and presents with vulval itching.

(b) Twenty per cent of women with symptomatic gonorrhoea complain of a vaginal discharge.

(c) A pH of >4.5 is associated with the presence of bacterial vaginosis.

(d) The release of a fishy odour on addition of alkali to the vaginal discharge is typical of *Trichomonas vaginalis*.

(e) If a woman presents with trichomoniaisis contact tracing should be carried out.

6.5

Which of the following are true?

(a) Examination of patients with psychosexual problems is rarely rewarding.

(b) Ejaculation is under parasympathetic control.

(c) Psychosexual problems are best managed by seeing both partners together.

(d) Vaginismus occurs only with penile entry into the vagina.

(e) Anorgasmia is more common in men than women.

Chapter 7

7.1

Fill in the blanks in the following sentences from the list below.

In pregnancy the maternal cardiac output increases principally because of a greater (1) _____. Haemoglobin concentrations decrease because of an increased (2) _____ despite an increased (3) _____. The uterus grows by (4) _____ with a blood flow at term of (5) _____ ml/kg per min.

(a) 100–150

(b) red cell volume

(c) stroke volume

(d) 200–250

(e) hypertrophy

(f) plasma volume

(g) pulse rate

(h) red cell mass

(i) mitosis

(j) mean haemoglobin concentration

7.2

Which of the following statements are true?

(a) Fetal haemoglobin shifts the oxygen dissociation curve to the right of that for haemoglobin A.

(b) At birth, changes in the neonatal circulation enable the entire circulating volume to enter the pulmonary tree.

(c) In fetal life oxygenated blood from the umbilical arteries flows directly to the left side of the heart.

(d) During fetal life the lungs are filled with amniotic fluid.

(e) Exposure to teratogens is more likely to cause congenital abnormalities in the first trimester of pregnancy.

7.3

The functions of the placenta include which of the following?

(a) Transfer of oxygen from the mother to the fetus

(b) Transfer of urea from the mother to the fetus

(c) Prevention of premature labour

(d) Transfer of nutrients from the fetus to the mother

(e) Regulation of fetal metabolism of insulin and glucose

7.4

The smallest diameters of the fetal skull include which of the following?

(a) Mentovertical

(b) Submentobregmatic

(c) Suboccipitobregmatic

(d) Biparietal

(e) Occiptofrontal

Chapter 8

8.1

A woman presents with her second miscarriage. Which of the following pieces of information should she be given in respect of miscarriage?

(a) It is unlikely that she has done/taken anything to cause the miscarriage.

(b) She has a 75% chance of miscarrying again.

(c) She may try again for a pregnancy after one normal period.

(d) She has a 25% chance of miscarrying again.

(e) Most miscarriages are due to an abnormality in the baby.

8.2i

A 27-year-old woman attends A&E with acute left-sided lower abdominal pain. She has vomited once. Her last period was 3 days ago and seemed light to normal. On examination her pulse is 115/min, blood pressure 106/64, temp 37.1°C. Her abdomen is tender with rebound particularly in the left iliac fossa. What is the most likely diagnosis?

(a) Acute appendicitis

(b) Ruptured ectopic pregnancy

(c) Unruptured ectopic pregnancy

(d) Pelvic inflammatory disease

(e) Ruptured ovarian cyst

8.2ii

Her urinary pregnancy test is positive. What immediate treatment should you arrange for her

(a) Fluid resuscitation

(b) Blood transfusion

(c) Left salpingectomy

(d) Admit and await results of serum hCG

(e) Ultrasound scan

8.2iii

Following her treatment what advice would you give her?

(a) You would recommend the IUCD as her best form of contraception.

(b) She should wait 1 month before trying for pregnancy again.

(c) She has an 80% chance of a successful pregnancy next time.

(d) She should attend for an ultrasound scan at 6 weeks when she conceives again.

(e) She should have an ultrasound in 6 weeks' time to check that the uterus is empty.

8.3

Which of the following statements are true of a hydatidiform mole?

(a) May be associated with early onset pre-eclampsia.

(b) Is more common in the UK than in the Far East.

(c) Should be treated with methotrexate.

(d) Should be followed up for a minimum of 1 year in a specialist centre.

(e) Is associated with a higher than average hCG concentration.

8.4

Which of the following is true of choriocarcinoma?

(a) There is early spread to bones.

(b) Cisplatin is the chemotherapeutic agent of choice.

(c) Hysterectomy is indicated only if there is severe bleeding.

(d) After hydatidiform mole the risk of choriocarcinoma is 40%.

(e) After hydatidiform mole the risk of choriocarcinoma is 4%.

Chapter 9

9.1

Mrs Walker is 36 weeks' pregnant in her first pregnancy. Please examine her and give your conclusions to the examiner. (Mannequins are available to practise on, although ideally you should perform the examination on a woman in the antenatal clinic, having asked her permission to do so first. Remember that you should always have a female chaperone with you whenever you examine a woman.) As you examine the woman run through the examination and present to a clinician or fellow student who will score against the checklist in Answers to self-assessment questions, p. 344.

9.2

Which of the following investigations are performed at the first antenatal visit in the UK?

(a) Toxoplasmosis

(b) Rubella

(c) Cytomegalovirus (CMV)

(d) Syphilis

(e) Hepatitis A

9.3

Which of the following are used as indicators of fetal well-being beyond 24 weeks of pregnancy?

(a) Liquor volume

(b) Fetal lie

(c) Fetal movements

(d) Uterine artery Doppler ultrasonography

(e) Umbilical artery Doppler ultrasonography

9.4

A woman presents at 12 weeks of pregnancy. She has had two live births at term, delivered a live baby at 21 weeks who died within a few minutes of birth, one pregnancy loss at 8 weeks and an intrauterine death at 25 weeks. Which one of the following correctly expresses her gravidity and parity?

(a) Gravida 6 Para 4 + 1

(b) Gravida 6 Para 3 + 2

(c) Gravida 5 Para 33 + 2

(d) Gravida 5 Para 4 + 1

(e) Gravida 6 Para 5 + 0

9.5

Causes for intrauterine growth restriction (asymmetrical small for gestational age) include:

(a) Essential hypertension
(b) Maternal obesity
(c) Smoking tobacco
(d) Abnormal placental implantation
(e) Rubella

Chapter 10

10.1

Which of the following statements are true?
(a) Pre-eclampsia is defined as a rise in the diastolic blood pressure after 20 weeks of pregnancy by >15 mm/Hg from the booking blood pressure without proteinuria.
(b) Women with pre-eclampsia are at increased risk of developing gestational diabetes.
(c) Pre-eclampsia is defined as a rise in the diastolic blood pressure after 20 weeks of pregnancy by >15mm/Hg from the booking blood pressure with proteinuria.
(d) The most dangerous risk of pre-eclampsia for the mother is cerebral oedema leading to fitting.
(e) The most dangerous risk of pre-eclampsia for the mother is developing HELLP syndrome.

10.2

A woman of 38 presents at 36 weeks in her first pregnancy with a headache. The symphysiofundal height is 35 cm, cephalic presentation with the head 4/5 palpable per abdomen. Her blood pressure is 174/112, pulse 82 beats/min, temperature 36.7°C. The CTG is reassuring. Her reflexes are brisk bilaterally with 4 beats of clonus in each ankle. Which of the following is the most appropriate treatment?
(a) Magnesium sulphate infusion followed by delivery of the baby.
(b) Magnesium sulphate infusion with hydralazine followed by delivery of the baby.
(c) Immediate delivery of the baby.
(d) Phenytoin infusion with hydralazine followed by delivery of the baby.
(e) Diazepam with hydralazine followed by delivery of the baby.

10.3

Anti-D should be given to all women who are Rh negative in which of the following scenarios?
(a) Threatened miscarriage
(b) Following the birth of a baby whose blood group is A negative
(c) Following the birth of a baby whose blood group is A positive
(d) Ectopic pregnancy
(e) Medical termination of pregnancy

10.4

A woman of 28 presents at 34 weeks of pregnancy with constant abdominal pain and a small amount of bleeding. Her symphysiofundal height is 37 cm; her uterus is tender and firm. The CTG shows unprovoked decelerations. Her pulse is 108 beats/min and her blood pressure 100/60 mmHg. What is the most likely diagnosis?
(a) Placenta praevia
(b) Cervical cancer
(c) Von Willebrand's disease
(d) Placental abruption
(e) Cervical polyp

10.5

Polyhydramnios is associated with which of the following?
(a) Gestational diabetes
(b) Fetal renal agenesis
(c) Pre-eclamptic toxaemia
(d) Obstetric cholestasis
(e) Tracheo-oesophageal fistula

10.6i

A woman presents with vaginal bleeding and abdominal pain at 38 weeks of pregnancy. She has a pulse of 120 beats/min with a blood pressure of 86/54. The most important diagnosis to exclude is:
(a) Major placenta praevia
(b) Placental abruption
(c) The onset of labour

(d) Carcinoma of the cervix

(e) Intrauterine fetal death

10.6ii

Which of the following should you do as a matter of urgency

(a) Listen to the fetal heart and start a CTG.

(b) Perform an ultrasound scan to check the placental site and the presence of the fetal heart.

(c) Insert two large-bore cannulas and take blood for full blood count and group and save.

(d) Insert two large-bore cannulas and send blood for full blood count; cross-match 4 units and coagulation screen.

(e) Ring the anaesthetist, haematologist and consultant obstetrician to ask them to attend.

Chapter 11

11.1

Which of the following statements are true?

(a) Women with gestational diabetes commonly present with ketoacidosis.

(b) Women with a first-degree relative suffering from type 1 diabetes are at increased risk of developing gestational diabetes.

(c) Women with pre-existing type 1 diabetes are at increased risk of developing pre-eclamptic toxaemia.

(d) Gestational diabetes is most commonly controlled by diet alone.

(e) Gestational diabetes usually requires insulin therapy.

11.2

Gestational diabetes is associated with an increased risk for the fetus of:

(a) Unexplained stillbirth beyond 40 weeks of pregnancy

(b) Hypoglycaemia following birth

(c) Shoulder dystocia

(d) Congenital abnormality

(e) Neonatal jaundice

11.3

Common causes of anaemia in pregnancy include:

(a) Vitamin B_6 deficiency

(b) Vitamin K deficiency

(c) Folate deficiency

(d) Vitamin B_{12} deficiency

(e) Iron deficiency

11.4

Which of the following statements are true?

(a) Women with β-haemolytic streptococci are at increased risk of going into premature labour.

(b) Babies born to women with β-haemolytic streptococci are at increased risk of hypoglycaemia.

(c) β-Haemolytic streptococci are a vaginal commensal in up to 20% of women.

(d) Women with β-haemolytic streptococci should be treated with penicillin during labour.

(e) Women with β-haemolytic streptococci should be treated with penicillin antenatally to prevent infection in the neonate.

Chapter 12

12.1

Put the following sentences into the correct sequence/order to describe the passage of the fetus through the birth canal.

(a) The fetal head engages in a transverse position.

(b) The fetal head extends round the symphysis pubis.

(c) The fetal head flexes as it descends into the birth canal.

(d) The fetal head restitutes to a transverse position.

(e) The fetal head most commonly rotates through 90° so that the occiput becomes anterior as it reaches the levator ani.

12.2

During normal labour which of the following are recommended to monitor the well-being of the mother and fetus?

(a) The mother's pulse rate should be recorded every 30 minutes in the active phase of labour.

(b) In the first stage of labour the descent of the baby's head should be measured by its distance above or below the ischial spines.

(c) The fetal heart should be checked every 30 minutes in the first stage of labour with a Sonicaid.

(d) The mother's urine output should be measured hourly.

(e) The fetal heart rate should be checked after every contraction in the second stage.

12.3

Which of the following are indications for commencing continuous electronic fetal monitoring (EFM)?

(a) A woman at term in spontaneous labour who ruptures her membranes and has meconium-stained liquor.

(b) A woman at term in spontaneous labour who ruptures her membranes and has clear liquor.

(c) A woman at term in spontaneous labour who has had a deceleration detected using a Pinard Stethoscope every 30 minutes.

(d) A woman who ruptured her membranes 6 hours ago, has clear liquor and is in spontaneous labour.

(e) A woman at term in spontaneous labour who has had a previous caesarean section.

12.4

In normal labour which of the following statements are true?

(a) Uterine contractions are generated in the lower segment of the uterus.

(b) The rate of cervical dilatation in a first labour should be >0.5 cm/h.

(c) The latent phase should not exceed 8 hours in a first labour.

(d) The second stage of labour should not exceed 2 hours in duration in a woman with an epidural.

(e) An episiotomy should be performed in most women.

Chapter 13

13.1

A woman in her first pregnancy is admitted in spontaneous labour at 39 weeks. On examination the presentation is cephalic, 2/5 palpable. The cervix is 1 cm long and firm, 1 cm dilated posterior to the head and the head is 2 cm above the spines. Which of the following statements are true?

(a) She is in the active phase of the first stage of labour.

(b) Her Bishop's score is <4.

(c) She is in the latent phase of the first phase of labour.

(d) Her Bishop's score is >4.

(e) She should be encouraged to mobilize and re-examined in 4 hours.

13.2

Which of the following presenting positions can be delivered spontaneously vaginally?

(a) Face presentation

(b) Brow presentation

(c) Occipitotransverse

(d) Occipitoposterior

(e) Vertex presentation

13.3

Which of the following statements are true?

(a) Breech presentation is more common in pre-term babies.

(b) Most women with a breech presentation should be offered external cephalic version at 37–38 weeks.

(c) Breech presentation is more common at term than at 34 weeks.

(d) Breech presentation is associated with a higher perinatal mortality regardless of the mode of delivery.

(e) Caesarean section should be offered to all women with twins where the presentation is cephalic in the first twin and breech in the second twin.

13.4

List the five conditions that should be met before undertaking an surgical vaginal delivery for a cephalic presentation.

13.5

Which of the following are true about primary postpartum haemorrhage (PPH)?
(a) It is defined as a loss of blood of >500 ml.
(b) It is more common following a spontaneous vaginal delivery.
(c) The most common cause is uterine atony.
(d) It can be prevented by giving Syntometrine with the birth of the anterior shoulder.
(e) It is more common in women with pre-eclampsia.

13.6

Which of the following features of a cardiotocograph (CTG) would be considered non-reassuring in labour?
(a) Baseline variability of 5–15 beats/min
(b) Early decelerations in the second stage of labour
(c) Late decelerations in the first stage of labour
(d) A fetal heart rate of 170 beats/min
(e) Accelerations

Chapter 14

14.1

A woman on the postnatal ward bursts into tears when you go and see her 48 hours after the birth of her baby. Which of the following might indicate that she is at high risk of developing postnatal depression?
(a) She does not show any interest in her infant who is crying insistently.
(b) She is bottle-feeding the baby.
(c) She is unable to sleep.
(d) Her mother had severe postnatal depression.
(e) Her partner has recently left her and was not present at the birth of the baby.

14.2

A woman presents 10 days after a normal vaginal delivery with a raised temperature of 38.4°C. Match the additional information given in 1–5 to the five most likely of the diagnoses (a)–(j)
1 She has passed several clots and is in pain. Her uterus is 16 weeks size and tender.
2 She complains of pain on passing urine. Her left loin is tender.
3 She complains of right breast tenderness and has a fluctuant mass in the upper quadrant.
4 She complains of a productive cough with chest pain particularly on inspiration.
5 Her left leg is swollen and tender with erythema particularly over the inner aspect of her calf where she has varicose veins.
(a) Breast engorgement
(b) Salpingitis
(c) Pyelonephritis
(d) Bronchitis
(e) Deep vein thrombosis
(f) Retained products of conception
(g) Pulmonary embolism
(h) Thrombophlebitis
(i) Cystitis
(j) Breast abscess

14.3

Which of the following would be appropriate management/treatment of the conditions in 1–5 of Question 14.2.
(a) Increased fluid intake and antibiotics
(b) Broad-spectrum antibiotics with physiotherapy
(c) Heparin i.v. followed by 6 months of anticoagulation
(d) Oral flucloxacillin with good breast support
(e) Broad-spectrum antibiotics i.v. alone
(f) Flucloxacillin i.v. with support stockings
(g) Heparin i.v. followed by 3 months of anticoagulation
(h) Broad-spectrum antibiotics and surgical incision and drainage
(i) Broad-spectrum antibiotics i.v. with evacuation of retained products
(j) Oral broad-spectrum antibiotics alone

Chapter 15

15.1

List the five elements of the Apgar score.

15.2

A baby is born in the following condition at 1 minute. She is pink with a heart rate of 120 beats/min. She is not moving or crying and has taken a few irregular gasps. Her limbs are flaccid but she is moving her facial muscles. What is her Apgar score?

(a) 9
(b) 8
(c) 7
(d) 6
(e) 5

15.3 OSCE question

Candidate's instructions: during an antenatal visit at 32 weeks, Jane Wooller says that she is unsure whether she wants to breast-feed her baby and wishes to discuss this with you. You are expected to discuss the advantages and disadvantages of breast-feeding versus bottle-feeding.

Role-player's instructions: you are Mrs Jane Wooller, a 34-year-old woman in her first pregnancy. You are now 32 weeks. The midwife discussed breast-feeding with you at the booking visit but you didn't take much in because it seemed so far away then as an issue. You have been to two antenatal classes where breast-feeding has been discussed among the mothers to be. You thought that you would definitely breast-feed but found that during the discussion you felt rather revolted by the idea, particularly feeding in public. You are a very private person who, before pregnancy, took a great pride in your appearance and figure, and you want to get back to your original clothes size as soon as possible after the birth. Breast-feeding sounds rather invasive of your privacy and you do not relish leaking breast milk onto your clothes. However, you do want to do the best for your baby. The rest is up to the role-player's imagination.

15.4

Which of the following babies are at increased risk of developing significant neonatal jaundice?

(a) Group A negative baby born to a group A positive mother
(b) Group A negative baby born to a group A negative mother
(c) Group A positive baby born to a group A negative mother
(d) Group A positive baby born to a group B positive mother
(e) Group A positive baby born to a group A positive mother

Chapter 16

16.1 OSCE question

Candidate's instructions: a 37-year-old woman, Elizabeth Parker, has come to see you in your GP surgery. She has only recently moved to your area. She is complaining of heavy periods. Please take a history. You have 7 minutes.

Role-player's instructions: you are Mrs Elizabeth Parker, a 37 year old. Over the last 2 years your periods have become increasingly heavy. They are regular every 28 days and last for 7–10 days. They used to last only 5 days. You have noticed that the first 4 days are particularly heavy with clots the size of 50p pieces. On the first day you can bleed so heavily that you have to change every 30 minutes to 1 hour. At night you wear two pads, a tampon and an incontinence pad, and still have to change in the middle of the night. You have painful periods but this has not changed. You have three children and you were sterilized when you were 35. Before this you had been on the combined oral contraceptive pill. You smoke 25 cigarettes a day so you had stopped the pill. Your last smear test was 2 years ago and was normal. You are otherwise fit and well. All other details are up to the role-player.

16.2

From the list below select the three most relevant investigations for Mrs Parker.

(a) Endometrial biopsy
(b) Transvaginal ultrasound scan
(c) Hormone profile
(d) High vaginal swab
(e) Cervical smear
(f) Hysteroscopy
(g) Full blood count
(h) Thyroid function tests

16.3

The investigations are all normal. What is the most appropriate first line treatment?
(a) Mirena IUS
(b) Norethisterone from day 15 to day 26 of the cycle
(c) Antifibrinolytic therapy during the menses
(d) Paracetamol during menses
(e) Endometrial ablation

16.4

A woman is admitted for a total abdominal hysterectomy. Which of the following are routine prophylactic measures for all women undergoing this procedure?
(a) Co-amoxiclav 1.2 g i.v. intraoperatively
(b) Subcutaneous low-molecular-weight (LMW) heparin intraoperatively
(c) Flowtron boots intraoperatively
(d) TED stockings
(e) Phenoxymethylpenicillin 1 g i.v. intraoperatively

16.5

When consenting a woman for a total abdominal hysterectomy, which of the following should be included on the consent form as possible complications?
(a) Infection
(b) Haemorrhage
(c) Removal of the ovaries
(d) Damage to the ureters
(e) Damage to the bladder

Chapter 17

17.1 OSCE question

Candidate's instructions: Rosemary Beckett, a woman of 32, is referred to the gynaecology clinic by her GP. She gives a 2 year history of increasingly severe period pains. You are expected to take a history and outline your initial management of Mrs Beckett.

Role-player's instructions: you are Rosemary Beckett, a 32-year-old primary school teacher. You have been married for 3 years. You have never been pregnant and use condoms for contraception. You tried the pill in your early 20s but found that it made you feel depressed. Your periods are regular but have been becoming increasingly painful over the last 2 years. The pain starts as a low constant ache in your back radiating to the front. It starts 3–4 days before your period, is worst on the first 2 days of your period and then subsides. Sex is uncomfortable in some positions, particularly before your period. The pain can be acute and is deep inside, especially when your husband is particularly vigorous. He is sympathetic but you feel that it is beginning to affect your relationship because your libido is less than when you first married. You and your husband are planning to have a baby within the next 2 years and are worried that the pain may prevent pregnancy. You have no past medical or surgical history of relevance, no allergies and take Nurofen for the pain, but no regular medication. All other details are up to the role-player.

17.2

Submucous fibroids are commonly associated with which of the following?
(a) Constant lower abdominal pain
(b) Menorrhagia
(c) Vomiting
(d) Secondary dysmenorrhoea
(e) Ectopic pregnancy

17.3

A 24-year-old woman presents with unilateral abdominal pain, vomiting, abdominal rebound

and guarding. She is apyrexial and her LMP was 1 week ago. Which of the following is the most likely diagnosis?
(a) Pelvic inflammatory disease
(b) Bleeding into a corpus luteal cyst
(c) Ruptured corpus luteal cyst
(d) Torted dermoid cyst
(e) Ruptured mucinous cystadenoma

17.4

Which of the following is true of benign ovarian cysts?
(a) May undergo degeneration
(b) May rupture causing acute abdominal pain
(c) May contain well-differentiated tissues
(d) May contain altered blood
(e) May secrete testosterone

17.5

A 19-year-old woman presents with right iliac fossa pain. The pain came on gradually and was associated with nausea and vomiting. She has not opened her bowels for 36 hours. On examination she has a temperature of 37.6°C. Abdominal examination reveals tenderness in the right iliac fossa (RIF) with guarding and rebound. Vaginal examination reveals mild tenderness on the right with no cervical excitation. What is the most likely diagnosis?
(a) Appendicitis
(b) Pyelonephritis
(c) Torted right ovarian cyst
(d) Small bowel obstruction
(e) Ruptured right ovarian cyst

Chapter 18

18.1

What are the four stages of breast cancer screening?

18.2

List the risk factors for breast cancer.

18.3

Which of the following agents are used in adjuvant therapy?

(a) Gosvelin
(b) Anastrozole
(c) Cisplatin
(d) Provera
(e) Methotrexate

18.4

List the three main areas that should be treated in a case of primary breast cancer.

Chapter 19

19.1

OSCE question: at the next station you are expected to take a cervical smear from the pelvic floor model provided. (Some universities may use gynaecologically trained assistants—women who have volunteered to assist in the training of medical students and doctors in performing vaginal examinations.) Find a pelvic floor model and practise doing a vaginal examination and taking a cervical smear as if in an examination.

19.2

Which of the following statements are true?
(a) Cervical screening should be offered to all women from age 25 to age 64.
(b) Cervical screening gives an accurate diagnosis of the degree of cervical intraepithelial neoplasia.
(c) Women with an abnormal cervical smear graded moderate dyskaryosis should be referred for colposcopy.
(d) Women with an abnormal cervical smear graded moderate dyskaryosis should have a repeat smear performed 6 months later.
(e) Cervical smears taken during pregnancy are more likely to give a false-negative result.

19.3

A woman of 35 is referred to colposcopy with a smear result of severe dyskaryosis. Place the following description of the examination in the correct order.

(a) A biopsy is taken of an unstained area.

(b) A note is made of the areas that turn white and how rapidly they do so.

(c) The area is excised using loop diathermy under local anaesthetic.

(d) Acetic acid 4% is painted onto the cervix.

(e) Iodine solution is painted onto the cervix and the unstained areas noted.

19.4

List the six main reasons why the UK cervical screening programme is not 100% effective.

19.5

List the five measures that have been put in place to try to improve the effectiveness of screening in the UK.

Chapter 20

20.1

Which of the following statements are true?

(a) Carcinoma of the cervix is the most common gynaecological malignancy.

(b) More women die of ovarian cancer than any other gynaecological malignancy.

(c) Cervical cancer most commonly presents with postmenopausal bleeding.

(d) Endometrial cancer most commonly presents with postmenopausal bleeding.

(e) Ovarian cancer most commonly presents with postcoital bleeding.

20.2

A woman of 48 presents with postcoital bleeding; her last smear was 8 years ago and was normal. She is otherwise well. On examination she has an ulcerated lesion on her cervix that bleeds on contact. The vulva, vagina and uterus all feel normal. Which of the following should be undertaken to investigate the cause of her postcoital bleeding?

(a) CT scan of abdomen and pelvis

(b) Liver function tests

(c) Biopsy of her cervix

(d) Chest X-ray

(e) Hysteroscopy and curettage

20.3

A woman of 63 presents with a hard fixed abdominal mass noticed by her GP when she complained that her clothes were becoming tighter. Her menopause was 12 years ago and she has had no vaginal bleeding. She has no other abnormalities on examination. What is the most likely provisional diagnosis?

(a) Stage 3 carcinoma of the ovary

(b) Stage 3 carcinoma of the cervix

(c) Stage 1 carcinoma of the ovary

(d) Stage 3 carcinoma of the uterus

(e) Stage 4 carcinoma of the ovary

20.4

Which of the following are useful preoperative staging investigations for the woman in Question 20.3?

(a) Hysteroscopy and curettage

(b) CT scan of abdomen and pelvis

(c) Serum tumour markers

(d) Chest X-ray

(e) Urea and electrolytes

20.5

A woman of 63 presents with an offensive discharge from her vagina. She admits that her vulva has been very itchy and sore for several years. Over the last few months she has noticed occasional blood stains on her pants and a lump on her left labia. Her GP has treated her with antibiotics to no effect. Which of the following are the most appropriate investigations for this woman?

(a) Examination and biopsy of her vulva

(b) High vaginal swab

(c) Abdominal palpation particularly in both groins

(d) Cervical smear

(e) Hysteroscopy and curettage

Chapter 21

21.1 OSCE question

Candidate's instructions: you are the junior doctor seeing a Mrs Hilda Black, a 48 year old, for her preoperative assessment. She is about to be admitted for a total abdominal hysterectomy and bilateral oophorectomy for menorrhagia that has not responded to medical therapy. She wishes to discuss her options for hormone replacement therapy (HRT). You are expected to answer her questions.

Role-player's instructions: you are Mrs Hilda Black, a 48-year-old housewife. You have had very heavy, painful periods for the last 5 years. You have tried all forms of medical therapy with minimal improvement and have finally decided to have a hysterectomy. The consultant has discussed removal of your ovaries and, as your grandmother died of ovarian cancer, you have decided to have them removed as well. The consultant gave you some leaflets on HRT but they have left you rather confused. You have come to the hospital for your preoperative check-up and have a list of questions you wish to ask the doctor about your options for HRT.

1 What sort of HRT will I need to take?
2 How long should I take it for?
3 What are the side effects?
4 How will I take it?
5 What are the benefits of taking HRT?
6 What are the possible long-term risks of HRT?
Try not to allow the candidate to take a history from you and move on to the questions.

21.2

A woman of 53 presents with vaginal bleeding. Her menopause was 4 years ago and she has been on oral cyclical HRT since then. She is very happy with her HRT but has noticed that she has been bleeding between her packets. The bleeding lasts for a few days and can be quite heavy. Which of the following diagnoses are possible causes of her bleeding?
(a) Endometrial polyp
(b) Subserosal fibroid
(c) Atrophic vaginitis
(d) Ovarian cancer
(e) Cervical cancer

21.3

List the investigations that should be undertaken in this woman with reasons.

Chapter 22

22.1

A woman of 52 is referred to the gynaecology outpatients by her GP. She is complaining of urinary incontinence. You are expected to take a history from her.

Role-player's instructions: you are Mrs Sarah Ball, a 52-year-old primary school teacher. Over the last 5 years you have been increasingly troubled by suddenly leaking small amounts of urine when you cough, run or do any form of exercise. You used to go to aerobic classes but have given them up. You are also finding it difficult at school—several of the children have commented on a smell of urine in the classroom and you feel very embarrassed. You empty your bladder between each class but still notice some leaking as you move round the classroom. You wear a panty-liner all the time, which you find irritating. You have to get up to the toilet twice every night. The amount that you pass is normal; occasionally you have to go again 5–10 minutes after emptying your bladder. You have noticed some backache and a feeling of something coming down. You have had three children all born vaginally—the first baby was delivered by forceps and you had a lot of stitches. Your last period was 3 years ago. Your last smear was 2 years ago and smears have always been normal. You are not taking HRT because your mother died of breast cancer. You smoked 20 cigarettes a day until 4 years ago. Your weight has gradually increased since you stopped smoking. You are otherwise fit and well.

22.2

Describe how you would examine and manage this patient.

22.3

List five principal complications of vaginal repair operations (colporrhaphies).

22.4

Define genuine stress incontinence.

22.5

Which of the following are common symptoms of detrusor instability?
(a) Urgency
(b) Slow urinary stream
(c) Incomplete emptying
(d) Nocturia
(e) Frequency

Chapter 23

23.1

Give the definitions for the following:
1   Total birth rate

2   General fertility rate
3   Maternal mortality
4   Maternal mortality rate
5   Perinatal mortality rate

23.2

Give the three most common direct causes of maternal mortality.

23.3

Give three measures that can be undertaken to improve standards of care.

23.4

Give three maternal factors that affect the perinatal mortality rate.

23.5

Following the death of a baby what investigations should be performed?

Answers to self-assessment

Chapter 1

1.1 (1) h, (2) g, (3) d, (4) b or j, (5) b or j

The uterine artery is a branch of the (1), (h) *internal iliac* artery. The uterus is a hollow, muscle-walled organ in direct communication with the (2), (g) *fallopian tubes* and the vagina. Inferior to the uterine artery lies the (3), (d) *ureter*. The ligaments that support the uterus include the (4), (j) *uterosacral* and (5), (b) *transverse cervical*.

1.2 b, e

See pp. 4, 9, 12. The granulosa cells secrete estradiol. Once the oocyte has been released they become luteal cells and secrete estradiol and progesterone. At menarche there are around 500 000 oocytes in the ovary.

1.3 a, d, e

See pp. 1–13. At the time of the luteinizing hormone (LH) surge the oocyte undergoes meiosis but with an unequal distribution of the cellular cytoplasm, forming an oocyte ready for fertilization and the first polar body with 23 chromosomes in each. Glycogen is secreted in the luteal (secretory) phase of the cycle from the effects of progesterone on the endometrial glands. The endometrium is shed because the spiral arterioles go into spasm, causing hypoxia and death of the endometrium. The follicular phase (from day 1 of the cycle to ovulation) can be very variable (compare polycystic ovaries), whereas the luteal phase is of a fixed duration.

1.4 a, c, d

Estradiol exerts a negative feedback on follicle-stimulating hormone (FSH) (ie when estradiol levels are low FSH levels rise). FSH and LH are controlled by the *hypo*thalamus, which secretes gonadotrophin-releasing hormone (GnRH). Testosterone is the major precursor of estradiol and is secreted by the theca cells under the influence of LH; the testosterone passes to the granulosa cells and is converted to estradiol, catalysed by FSH. Progesterone starts to be secreted only at the time of ovulation and reaches its peak 7 days after ovulation in a non-conception cycle.

1.5 See figure below.

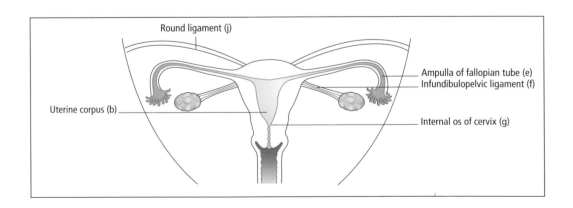

Round ligament (j)

Ampulla of fallopian tube (e)
Infundibulopelvic ligament (f)

Uterine corpus (b)

Internal os of cervix (g)

Chapter 2

Marking scheme

The marking schemes vary from medical school to medical school. Some mix marks for communication and details of the history together into one question. Some may group aspects of the question together and allow examiners to give a mark of 0, 1 or 2 depending on how well the candidate does in each section. The scheme outlined below gives a list of the things that may give you a mark (shown in parentheses) or that may be included in a group and is therefore only a guide to possible marks. It is wise to ask your medical school how their marking scheme is structured. You can then devise your own marking sheets and use the cases for practice.

Communication

- Introduces themselves (1)
- Eye contact (1)
- Picks up on verbal clues. Patients often do not remember all the relevant details of their history immediately but may say something that implies that you have an opportunity to ask another question to help them remember or feel comfortable answering the question, eg the first patient may not be in a relationship because of dyspareunia and she may give a clue when answering the question about whether or not she has a boyfriend; the second patient may not remember the episode of being asked to take some tablets, or may know that she had had an infection causing her ectopic pregnancy, but feels a bit stupid for not having followed medical advice. (1)
- Picks up on non-verbal clues. Non-verbal clues include patients not looking at you, wriggling on their chair, not answering the question. You should notice this and re-ask the question in a different way or challenge the patient gently if she is looking very diffident or refusing to answer the question. (1)
- Use of non-medical language (1)
- Listens (1)
- Allows questions (1)
- Structured history. This is marks for a logical order to the history which leads to a full assessment of the patient's problem. Do not get bogged down in irrelevant detail such as a long surgical history or detailed system questions because you will run out of time. Learn the list of headings and go through them quickly, ignoring negative answers and going into further detail for a positive answer. (1/2)
- Accurate summary (1)

History-taking

- Identifies main complaint (1)
- Explores main complaint appropriately (1)
- Ascertains all details of main complaint (1)
- Last menstrual period (LMP)/menstrual history (1)
- Past gynaecological/sexual health history (1)
- Past obstetric history (1)
- Past medical and surgical history (1)
- Family history (1)
- Social history (1)
- Medication/allergies (1)
- Summary (1)

The first three of these may be grouped together to give a score of 0–2.

In some medical schools the role-player may give marks for communication—did you trust this doctor, would you see him or her again, did you understand what they told you?—are questions that may be asked. Role-players have been shown to be very accurate in picking out the students who will do well and those who will not.

Chapter 3

The relevant information for each scenario is given below:

1 Turner's syndrome is associated with short stature in 100% of cases. Her ovaries are dysgenetic so they do not ovulate, giving her a low oestrogen with a high LH and FSH. She should receive oestrogen replacement in the form of the pill or HRT. Egg donation is her only means of becoming pregnant.

2 This young girl has a low body mass index (BMI) and does a lot of exercise. Both of these predispose young women to hypogonadotrophic hypogonadism. They have a low oestrogen and low LH and FSH. The most appropriate treatment is weight gain and a reduction in exercise (unlikely to be accepted in a talented athlete, but they can still gain weight). Treatment for fertility should not be started until weight gain has been achieved.

3 This young girl has the stigmata of polycystic ovary syndrome—secondary oligoamenorrhoea, acne and hirsutism. Her family history of type 2 diabetes makes her more likely to be insulin resistant, leading to anovulation and hirsutism. Her LH may be raised, and her FSH and estradiol will be normal whereas her testosterone will be raised. First-line treatment should be the pill with a non-androgenic progestogen (cyproterone acetate, desorgestrel, gestone). To achieve fertility clomiphene is the first line of treatment.

4 Galactorrhoea is diagnostic of hyperprolactinaemia. Her LH, FSH and estradiol will be low and her prolactin raised. First-line treatment is with a dopamine agonist. This is usually all that is required to restore menses and fertility.

5 This is a classic presentation of cryptomenorrhoea—imperforate hymen. All her hormone profile will be normal. First line of treatment is surgery—a cruciate incision in the hymen. Menses will continue normally and fertility will be unaffected.

Answers

3.1 (1) f, (2) j, (3) d, (4) h, (5) b
3.2 (1) d, (2) f, (3) b, (4) c, (5) a
3.3 (1) h, (2) a, (3) f, (4) e, (5) c

Chapter 4

4.1 a, d, f, i, j
Women with premature ovarian failure (POF) do not respond to FSH; their only recourse to achieve pregnancy is through egg donation. The risk of multiple pregnancy is 10%. A sperm count of >20 million/ml with >50% motility and >10% normal forms is considered normal.

4.2 b, c, e
4.3 (a) 5, (b) 8, (c) 2, (d) 10, (e) 1
Tubal surgery is less successful than in vitro fertilization (IVF) in achieving an intrauterine pregnancy in women with tubal damage. The first-line treatment for ovulation induction in women with polycystic ovary syndrome (PCOS) is clomiphene. FSH is successful for women with hypogonadotrophic hypogonadism. Klinefelter syndrome men should not be offered intracytoplasmic sperm injection (ICSI) because of the high risk of triploidy in the offspring.

Chapter 5

5.1 Marking scheme as for communication in Chapter 2 and:

- History of menarche and cycle length (1)
- Nature of relationship with boyfriend including his age (1)
- Implications of starting sex at this age (1)
- Relationships within the family (1)
- Telling her that she is below the legal age for sex (1)
- Trying to persuade her to tell her parents (1)
- Agreeing that this consultation is confidential (1)
- Discussing the pros and cons of the oral contraceptive pill (1)
- Explaining how to take the pill and the 7-day rule (1)
- Bringing the consultation to a close (1)

Following the Gillick case doctors are able to prescribe contraception for under-age girls and are bound to keep it confidential from her parents if the girl so wishes. This does not, however, remove the responsibility of the doctor to act in the best interests of the girl. She should be encouraged to tell her parents/guardian. She should be aware of the risks of entering into a sexual relationship—increased risk of PID, finding it unsatisfactory/painful, need for cervical smears and of pregnancy even if on the pill. When you have agreed to give her the pill it is important to give her the advice on how to take it (see p. 50).

5.2 Marking scheme:
- Establishes age and size of family (1)
  - Establishes stability of relationship (1)
  - Discusses male sterilization (1)
  - Discusses alternative methods
    including Mirena (1)
  - Agrees to sterilization (1)
  - Explains operation/day case (1)
  - Explains failure rate (1:300) (1)
  - Explains that sterilization is
    irreversible and permanent (1)
  - Explains need for mini-laparotomy
    if necessary (unlikely) (1)
  - Reassures about weight gain and
    periods (1)

Vasectomy (male sterilization) should always be discussed as there are fewer risks of the operation compared to laparoscopy. The stability of the relationship is very important although difficult to assess because divorce followed by a new partnership is a common reason for women to request reversal of sterilization. Couples sometimes feel that removing the threat of further pregnancies will solve their relationship difficulties; this is seldom the case. There is no evidence that contraceptive pills in any form increase weight gain but it is a commonly held belief among women.

5.3 b, d

The combined oral contraceptive pill (COCP) should be started on the first day of a period. By missing the first two pills in a packet the pill-free interval has been lengthened beyond 7 days, significantly increasing the risk that ovulation will occur. The COCP does not need to be taken at the same time each day, although the progestogen-only pill does because the mechanism for pregnancy prevention is not by suppression of ovulation. Antiepileptic medication interferes with the metabolism of the COCP so a higher dose of oestrogen is required to suppress ovulation (50 mg vs 35 mg).

5.4 a, e

Intrauterine contraceptive devices (IUCDs) do not increase the risk of a sickle cell crisis but a careful sexual history should be taken. An IUCD does not increase the risk of cervical cancer.

5.5 b, c, e

Oestrogen alone does not reduce the risk of implantation. High-dose progestogen alone is now the recommended form of oral emergency contraception. Oral emergency contraception is effective only up to 72 hours after unprotected intercourse whereas an IUCD can be used up to 5 days after intercourse. Endometrial curettage does not prevent implantation.

Chapter 6

6.1 e

Gonorrhoea is best diagnosed by endocervical culture on specialized media. High diagnostic yields occur if multiple sites are cultured, ie endocervix, urethra and anorectum. Erythromycin is used to treat penicillin-allergic pregnant women but has poor transplacental distribution. In addition, it is not as reliable as penicillin or doxycycline in the treatment of syphilis. Therefore, it is recommended that the mother be re-treated with doxycycline after breast-feeding has stopped. Consideration should be given to treating the baby with procaine penicillin at birth. First attack genital herpes can occur months or years after initial infection with the herpes virus, so contact tracing has limited value. Bacterial vaginosis is best diagnosed by Gram stain of high vaginal swab (HVS) material and culture for *Gardnerella vaginalis* is no longer recommended. Endocervical specimens should be used to test for *Chlamydia trachomatis* and this is usually done by nucleic acid amplification tests.

6.2 c, e

Human immunodeficiency virus (HIV) is a retrovirus and contains RNA and the reverse transcriptase enzyme that allows a DNA copy of the single RNA strand to be made. HIV uses the CD4 receptor to enter cells. Most seroconversions are asymptomatic. Patients with CD4 counts between 200 and 350 × 10^6/l will also be encouraged to start anti-HIV drugs if they have severe HIV-related symptoms, had an opportunistic infection or a rapidly falling CD4 count in the presence of a high viral load. Antiretroviral resistance testing may give false reassurance about susceptibility to anti-HIV drugs used in the past as resistant virus may be archived in the body and re-emerge under selective pressure should the drug be introduced. Tenofovir belongs to a new class of nucleotide reverse transcriptase inhibitors.

6.3 Marking scheme:

- Communication:
  - ○ Introduces themselves (1)
  - ○ Eye contact (1)
  - ○ Pick up anxiety over sexually transmitted infection (STI) (1)
- History-taking:
  - ○ Asked about extramarital partners (1)
  - ○ Asked about condoms (1)
  - ○ Took a drug history (1)
  - ○ Asked about nature of discharge (1)
  - ○ Asked about past STIs (1)
- Investigations
  - ○ Offered full STI screen* (2)
  - ○ Offered HIV test (1)
  - ○ Discussed 3-month window period for HIV (1)

6.4 a, c, e

Fifty per cent of women with gonorrhoea present with vaginal discharge. The release of a fishy odour on addition of alkali is typical of bacterial vaginosis not trichomonas infection, although the acid conditions of the vagina provide an ideal culture medium for *Trichomonas*.

6.5 a, c

Ejaculation is under sympathetic control mediated by adrenoreceptors. Psychosexual problems usually involve conflicts, often between couples. Psychosexual medicine works best when both members of the couple participate in the therapeutic intervention and understand the rationale. Vaginismus can be observed during the clinical examination on insertion of a speculum or fingers during a bimanual examination. Anorgasmia occurs more commonly in women than men and has both psychological and physical causes.

Chapter 7

7.1 (1) c, (2) f, (3) h, (4) e, (5) a

In pregnancy the maternal cardiac output increases principally because of a greater (1), (c) *stroke*

---

* Half a mark for each of chlamydial infection, trichomoniasis, gonorrhoea and syphilis.

volume. Haemoglobin concentrations decrease because of an increased (2), (f) *plasma volume* despite an increased (3), (h) *red cell mass*. The uterus grows by (4), (e) *hypertrophy* with a blood flow at term of (5), (a) *100–150 ml/kg per min*.

If you got any of these wrong please reread the text, pp. 91–3.

7.2 b, e

Fetal haemoglobin has a higher oxygen affinity than haemoglobin A and shifts the dissociation curve to the left as it becomes saturated with oxygen at lower oxygen concentrations. In fetal life oxygenated blood flows in the umbilical vein and deoxygenated blood in the umbilical arteries. In fetal life the lungs are filled with fluid, produced by the pneumocytes, that has a different chemical composition to amniotic fluid. This is confusing because the lungs do not develop properly in the absence of amniotic fluid (anhydramnios), presumably because growth factors in amniotic fluid are absorbed from the fetal mouth and gut as the fetus drinks the amniotic fluid, although we do not have direct evidence for this. Fetal organogenesis is complete by 12 weeks of gestation, although growth and maturation of all tissues continue throughout pregnancy. Exposure to infections in the second trimester (eg rubella, toxoplasmosis, cytomegalovirus [CMV], listeriosis) can lead to learning difficulties, blindness, deafness, etc., because of failure of maturation rather than congenital abnormality.

7.3 a, c, e

The placenta acts as a filter so that nutrients, oxygen and hormones pass from the mother to the fetus whereas waste products pass from the fetus to the mother. Human placental lactogen regulates the metabolism of insulin and glucose. Progesterone from the placenta relaxes the uterine muscle, helping to maintain the pregnancy.

7.4 b, c, d

- b = face presentation
- c = vertex presentation
- d = dimension used in ultrasound and is one of the diameters of a vertex presentation

All of these have an average diameter of 10 cm. The largest diameter is the mentovertical with an average diameter of 13 cm.

Chapter 8

8.1 a, c, d, e

After two miscarriages the chances of a successful pregnancy next time are 75%. Most miscarriages are the result of chromosomal abnormalities in the baby that are not inherited and occur by chance. In giving this piece of information many parents assume that there is something wrong with them, so it is important to present this with sensitivity and emphasize that it is a chance occurrence in most miscarriages. Women should also be advised to take folic acid to reduce the risk of neural tube defects.

8.2i b

The pain is on the wrong side for an appendix particularly as her temperature is normal. She is tachycardic and has a lower than average diastolic blood pressure, so you should be concerned that she has an ectopic pregnancy and treat accordingly, or until excluded. A ruptured ovarian cyst can present in this way but it is very rare and seldom associated with vomiting.

8.2.ii c

Rapid transfer to theatre to stop the bleeding is the most effective treatment for a ruptured ectopic pregnancy.

8.2.iii d

It is essential that women present early in subsequent pregnancies if they have had an ectopic to locate the implantation site as early as possible and so minimize the risk of a further rupture.

8.3 a, d, e

Hydatidiform mole is more common in the Far East than in the UK. It is associated with hyperemesis and early onset pre-eclamptic toxaemia (PET). Because of the risk of developing choriocarcinoma, regular follow-up with serial human chorionic gonadotrophin (hCG) estimations is essential. Surgical evacuation is the treatment of choice with chemotherapy used for those with persistently raised hCG concentrations.

8.4 c, e

Choriocarcinoma spreads to the lungs. Forty per cent of cases of choriocarcinoma follow a hydatidiform mole whereas the risk of developing choriocarcinoma after a hydatidiform mole is 4%.

Chapter 9

9.1 Checklist (see p. 118).
- Introduction and verbal consent to examine.
- Check with woman for areas of tenderness.
- Inspection: the abdomen is distended compatible with pregnancy. Check for scars, rashes, linea nigra (pigmented midline), anaemia, fetal movements.
- Palpation: measure symphysiofundal height (SFH), lie, presentation, engagement, fetal movements, liquor volume.
- Auscultation of fetal heart with a Pinard or Doppler ultrasonography.
- Some stations also require that you take the blood pressure and check the urine. It is common in exams for albumin or glucose to be added to the urine to catch out the unwary student.

9.2 b, d

Toxoplasmosis and CMV are not routinely screened in the UK, although in regions with a high prevalence they may be. Syphilis is easily treated with penicillin and prevents transmission to the fetus. For rubella, although immunization cannot be given in pregnancy, knowing the immunity status allows the non-immune woman to avoid contact with children or adults with rubella and to be immunized in the postnatal period. Hepatitis B is screened but not hepatitis A, because the latter usually resolves with no risk of transmission to the baby whereas the former may affect the baby postnatally and immunization can be offered at birth to the neonate.

9.3 a, c, e

A reduced liquor volume has been shown to be one of the most sensitive indicators for fetal distress. Polyhydramnios may be associated with gestational diabetes or fetal abnormality, eg tracheooesophageal fistula. Fetal movements are a good indicator of well-being. Umbilical artery Doppler ultrasonography is reassuring if the pressure index and flow are normal. Uterine artery Doppler ultrasonography is used as an identifier of a woman at increased risk of developing PET if notches are present at 20 and 24 weeks. An abnormal fetal lie may be associated with congenital abnormalities but is not a predictor of fetal distress.

9.4 b

This woman is in her sixth pregnancy so she is Gravida 6. She has had three babies born after 24 weeks of pregnancy although one died—Para 3. She has had two pregnancy losses <24 weeks—Para 3 + 2. Even though the 21-week-gestation baby was born alive it is still classified as a miscarriage because the gestation is less than the legal definition of viability—24 completed weeks of pregnancy.

9.5 a, c, d

Obesity usually causes excessive growth of the fetus (macrosomia). Rubella is usually associated with symmetrical SGA (small for gestational age) because the main effects are on the developing brain of the fetus not on the placenta.

Chapter 10

10.1 c, d

Raised blood pressure without proteinuria is called pregnancy-induced hypertension and is rarely associated with increased risks for the mother or fetus. Women with gestational diabetes are at increased risk of developing PET rather than the other way around. An eclamptic fit secondary to cerebral oedema can be fatal to both the mother and the baby whereas HELLP syndrome is usually more insidious in onset and resolves spontaneously after delivery of the baby.

10.2 b

This woman is at high risk of developing eclampsia and requires immediate treatment for her blood pressure and cerebral irritation (fulminating pre-eclampsia). Magnesium sulphate has been shown to be the most effective prophylactic treatment for pre-eclampsia. It does have an effect on hypertension but is quite slow acting. This woman's blood pressure is at a level that predisposes her to cerebral haemorrhage. Hydralazine given in bolus doses every 15 minutes until the diastolic blood pressure is between 90 and 100 mmHg acts more rapidly. Once the blood pressure is controlled, the baby should be delivered by whichever method is most appropriate.

10.3 a, c, d, e

All pregnant women should have their blood group checked regardless of gestation or site of the pregnancy. Anti-D should be given when there is any bleeding in pregnancy. The most common cause of rhesus isoimmunization is now the failure to give anti-D after a miscarriage, therapeutic abortion or ectopic pregnancy.

10.4 d

Placenta praevia, cervical cancer and cervical polyp/ectropion can present with an antepartum haemorrhage but are usually painless. Von Willebrand's disease predisposes a woman to bleeding but the diagnosis is usually known before pregnancy. Placental abruption can be concealed so the uterus may be large for dates as a result of haemorrhage behind the placenta. The uterus is classically tender and hard (woody). The maternal tachycardia suggests haemorrhage. Young women can maintain their blood pressure despite a large loss of blood, so it is easy to underestimate the degree of haemorrhage.

10.5 a, e

Renal agenesis is associated with anhydramnios because the fetus does not excrete any urine. PET is associated with oligohydramnios particularly if there is intrauterine growth restriction. Obstetric cholestasis does not alter the liquor volume. In a fetus with tracheo-oesophageal fistula, the fetus is unable to ingest the amniotic fluid and so liquor volume increases.

10.6i b

Placenta praevia and carcinoma of the cervix do not present with pain. This patient is showing signs of hypovolaemic shock which is unheard of in normal spontaneous labour. The baby may well be dead but the important diagnosis to exclude is an abruption.

10.6ii d

In an abruption the amount of visible loss is often less than the true amount. Resuscitation of the mother takes precedence over all else so it is the most important. Once the cannulas are in, non-cross-matched blood can be given and/or colloids until the cross-matched blood arrives. Informing senior staff and getting help are very important because it takes a whole team to save these women.

The welfare of the baby comes second to that of the mother so finding the fetal heart by CTG (cardiotocography) or ultrasound can occur once the mother's condition is more stable or she is ready for delivery.

Chapter 11

11.1 c, d

Ketoacidosis is never seen in gestational diabetes and is very rare even in women with type 1 diabetes. Women with a first-degree relative with type 2 diabetes (non-insulin dependent/late onset) are at increased risk of developing gestational diabetes. It is most commonly controlled by diet alone. All women with diabetes, whether pre-existing or gestational, are at increased risk of developing PET.

11.2 a, b, c, e

Congenital abnormalities are rare in gestational diabetes but three times more common in poorly controlled pre-existing diabetes.

11.3 c, e

Iron and folate deficiencies are the two most important common causes of anaemia in pregnancy. Supplements should be given, particularly if the diet is not balanced (eg strict vegetarians).

11.4 a, c, d

β-Haemolytic streptococci are a vaginal commensal that cannot be eradicated with penicillin because they will return, so there is no point in treating it before labour. The main risk to the neonate is of pneumonia and/or septicaemia, which is associated with a high perinatal mortality. Treatment of the mother with penicillin during labour reduces the risk to the baby.

Chapter 12

12.1 c, a, e, b, d

See pp. 177–91. If possible find a doll and a model pelvis and rehearse the stages of rotation and delivery of the fetal head.

12.2 c, e

See p. 179.

12.3 a, c, e

Meconium may be a sign of fetal hypoxia and so all fetuses should be electronically monitored. Electronic fetal heart rate monitoring (EFM) is indicated if a deceleration is heard on intermittent monitoring. An alteration in the fetal heart rate is often the first sign of impending scar dehiscence in labour after a caesarean section. Spontaneous rupture of membranes with clear liquor is not an indication for EFM, provided that the onset of labour is spontaneous.

12.4 b, c, d

Uterine contractions are generated in the fundus of the uterus and pass down the uterus to the lower segment. In a woman using epidural anaesthesia who is fully dilated the normal practice is to allow the head to descend for 1 hour and for the woman to push for 1 hour. If the baby is not delivered she should be assessed by an obstetrician and decision made with regard to delivery. Women with an epidural should be continuously electronically monitored.

Chapter 13

13.1 b, c, e

The WHO definition of the active phase of labour is when the cervix is 4 cm or more dilated. To revise Bishop's score, see p. 184. In early labour women should be encouraged to mobilize because this encourages the fetal head to descend and put pressure on the cervix, helping it to dilate.

13.2 a, d, e

Brow presentation cannot deliver spontaneously because the presenting diameter is the largest (13 cm). Occipitotransverse diameter is also large and the baby requires rotation to occipitoanterior (vertex position) before delivery. Occipitoposterior positions can deliver spontaneously although they commonly require intervention with forceps.

13.3 a, b, d

Most babies who are breech before 34 weeks turn to become cephalic so that the incidence at term is 3% compared with 10% in preterm babies. The more preterm the infant, the higher the likelihood of a breech presentation. Offering external cephalic version (ECV) before 37 weeks is often a waste of time: first the baby may spontaneously turn to cephalic and second the baby is more likely to revert to breech if turned before 37 weeks but highly unlikely to do so beyond 37 weeks. Breech presentation is associated with an increased prevalence of congenital abnormalities, and at term the perinatal morbidity and mortality are higher even if the baby is delivered by caesarean section. There is no evidence that the outcome for the second twin is improved by elective caesarean section if the first twin is cephalic, because the first twin will have dilated up the vaginal passage and the second twin is usually smaller than the first twin.

13.4

1 Adequate analgesia
2 Head <1/5 palpable per abdomen
3 Empty bladder
4 Full dilatation
5 Head at spines or below

13.5 a, c, d

Syntometrine is a combination of Syntocinon and ergometrine, both effective uterotonics that reduce the incidence of postpartum haemorrhage (PPH) significantly. Neither spontaneous vaginal delivery nor pre-eclampsia (in the absence of HELLP syndrome) increases the risk of PPH.

13.6 c, d, see p. 189.

Chapter 14

14.1 c, d, e

Bottle-feeding does not predispose a woman to develop postnatal depression (PND) unless she wanted to breast-feed and is unable to—this would be rare at only 48 hours after birth. Sleeplessness, a strong family history and a recent life event all predispose a woman to PND. Rejection of the infant is more likely to be an early sign of postnatal psychosis.

14.2 (1) f, (2) c, (3) j, (4) d, (5) h

A high temperature in a woman passing clots is most likely to indicate retained products of conception with endometritis. Salpingitis is usually a late sequela. The left loin tenderness would indicate pyelonephritis rather than cystitis. The fluctuant mass in her breast makes the diagnosis one of breast abscess rather than simple engorgement. Pulmonary emboli rarely present with a temperature >38°C or a productive cough, although pleuritic pain is common. Deep vein thrombosis usually gives a low-grade pyrexia or none at all, with deep pain in the muscle of the calf rather than tenderness and erythema.

14.3 (1) i, (2) a, (3) h, (4) b, (5) f

Flucloxacillin is a broad-spectrum antibiotic that is particularly effective against *Staphylococcus aureus* and is used for any infection near the skin. A breast abscess is unlikely to settle without surgical incision and drainage. All urinary tract infections require increased fluid intake and antibiotics. Bronchitis with a temperature as high as this may go on to develop into pneumonia, and so physiotherapy is very helpful to clear the infected tissue from the lungs. Retained products of conception are a focus for infection and should be removed after 24 hours of broad-spectrum antibiotics to reduce the risk of uterine perforation and bleeding.

Chapter 15

15.1

1 Heart rate
2 Respiratory effort
3 Muscle tone
4 Reflex irritability
5 Colour

15.2 d

- Heart rate >100 = 2
- Respiratory effort, irregular = 1
- Muscle tone, flaccid = 0
- Reflex irritability, grimace = 1
- Colour, pink = 2

15.3 Marking scheme:

Breast-feeding

For (5 marks)

- Breast milk is designed for babies
- Contains right balance of nutrients
- Contains immunoglobulins
- Reduces infections in the baby particularly gastrointestinal upset
- Cheap and always available on demand
- No bottles to make up or heat up
- No sterilizing kit needed

Against (5 marks)

- Engorged breasts
- Cracked nipples
- May not be enough milk

- May leak but can get pads
- Exposed in public but more acceptable now; with special bras and clothes can be very discreet
- Have to take baby with you
- Only one that can feed the baby

15.4 c, d

If the baby is rhesus negative and the mother positive fetal blood cells cannot sensitize the mother. If the baby is positive and the mother negative, the fetal cells can sensitize the mother who makes anti-D antibodies, which then cross the placenta and haemolyse the fetal red blood cells causing jaundice. At birth the antibodies persist in the baby's circulation and, combined with the normal breakdown of blood cells, can lead to significant jaundice. A baby of blood group A born to a mother with blood group B may suffer from an ABO incompatibility because the antigens and antibodies on the surface of the baby's red blood cells are different from those of the mother. They commonly become severely jaundiced in the first 24 hours of life. It is rare if the mother is blood group O.

Chapter 16

16.1 Marking scheme:
- Introduction and getting basic details (1)
- Menstrual history (0–4)
  - Previous cycle
  - Change in nature of period
  - Protection used
  - Impact on life
- Past contraceptive history (1)
- Last smear test (1)
- Past obstetric history (1)
- Social history (1)
- Medication and allergies (1)

16.2 b, e, g

Hysteroscopy and endometrial biopsy are not routine in women under the age of 40 because endometrial cancer is rare in this age group. They are indicated if the ultrasound scan is abnormal (see p. 234). Cervical pathology is common and may not be visible to the naked eye so a smear is always indicated even if it has been done quite recently. A full blood count is a reasonably objective measure of

blood loss because a Hb of <11 g/dl with a microcytic picture indicates anaemia secondary to menstrual blood loss. Thyroid function tests are rarely informative in an asymptomatic woman. It is rare for women to become menopausal below the age of 40 (3%) so a hormone profile is likely to be normal. PCOS usually presents much earlier

16.3 c

First line treatment with non-hormonal medication has been shown to be the most effective first-line therapy with the fewest side effects. Antifibrinolytics, antiprostaglandins and fenamates are the most effective. Paracetamol is ineffective. Norethisterone is effective only if taken continuously. Mirena IUS is a second- or third-line therapy whereas endometrial ablation is indicated only if all other treatments have failed.

16.4 a, c, d

Phenoxymethylpenicillin does not affect anaerobic organisms and so is not suitable for infection prophylaxis in gynaecology. Subcutaneous heparin is reserved for women at high risk of thrombosis. TED stockings and Flowtron boots are recommended internationally for all women undergoing pelvic surgery.

16.5 All are correct

Although damage to the bladder and ureters is a rare complication it is serious, so women should be warned. The ovaries may need removal if they are very adherent to the uterus or abnormal. Infection and haemorrhage are a risk for all operations however small.

Chapter 17

17.1 Marking scheme:
  History
- Nature of pain: (0–2)
  - Site, onset, cyclicity, radiation
- Dyspareunia: (0–2)
  - Nature, deep, relationship, sensitivity
- Menstrual history: (0–2)
  - Regular, normal flow, contraception, desire for fertility,
- Logical sequence: (0–2)
  - Past medical, surgical, gynaecological and obstetric history, SH, FH, medication, allergies

- Management: (0–2)
  - Endometriosis, pelvic examination, ultrasonography, laparoscopy

17.2 b, d

Submucous fibroids protrude into the uterine cavity and are lined by endometrium. The increased surface area and the increased vascularity of the fibroid commonly lead to menorrhagia. The uterus recognizes the fibroid as being abnormal and tries to extrude it through the cervix, commonly causing severe secondary dysmenorrhoea. Constant lower abdominal pain is usually associated with fibroid degeneration. Vomiting and ectopic pregnancy are rare associations.

17.3 d

Pelvic inflammatory disease (PID) presents with a pyrexia of >38°C, bilateral pain and no vomiting. Bleeding into or rupture of a cyst can cause localized peritonism but rarely vomiting. A torted ovarian cyst is commonly associated with vomiting.

17.4 b, c, d, e

Fibroids degenerate whereas ovarian cysts can rupture causing acute abdominal pain. Dermoid cysts contain well-differentiated tissues such as teeth, hair, sebaceous glands, renal, neural and other tissues. Endometriomas or luteal cysts that have bled internally contain altered blood (chocolate cysts). Ovarian cysts can secrete androgens (Sertoli–Leydig cell tumours/androblastomas) or oestrogen (granulosa cell tumours).

17.5 a

This is a classic presentation of appendicitis. Pyelonephritis usually presents with loin pain, a swinging pyrexia of >38°C, vomiting, frequency and dysuria. A torted ovarian cyst is not usually associated with pyrexia or absence of bowel movements. Bowel obstruction presents with generalized abdominal pain and apyrexia and a ruptured ovarian cyst rarely causes gastrointestinal symptoms.

Chapter 18

18.1

1 Mammography for all women aged 50–65
2 Clinical examination
3 Ultrasound/MRI
4 Needle cytology

18.2

1 *Genetic*: mutations in either of the two recognized breast cancer genes (*BRCA*-1 and *BRCA*-2) Cowden's syndrome and ataxia telangiectasia.

2 *Hormonal factors*: early menarche, late menopause, no full-term pregnancies, full-term pregnancy occurring after the age of 40. HRT of all types but particularly continuous combined HRT (see Chapter 21).

3 *Environmental factors*:
- Radiation.
- Alcohol increases the risk of breast cancer in a dose-dependent manner.
- Diet has a large effect on breast cancer risk. Diets rich in fresh fruit and vegetables are associated with a much lower risk of breast cancer (50% reduction).

18.3 a, b, e

Cisplatin is commonly used in ovarian cancer but is not effective for breast cancer. Provera is used in endometrial cancer. Other adjuvant therapies include tamoxifen, cyclophosphamide, 5-fluorouracil and epirubicin.

18.4

1 Breast itself (breast primary)
2 Axillary lymph nodes
3 Micrometastases

Chapter 19

19.1 Marking scheme (potential 15 marks)
- Introduces him- or herself (1)
- Fills in the form correctly:* (0–3)
  - Name and address of woman
  - Date of birth
  - Hospital/NHS number (if known)
  - GP's name and address
  - Clinical details
  - Last menstrual period
  - Hormone treatment/IUCD
- Fills in slide correctly: (0–3)
  - Name of woman
  - Date of birth

* Not always expected under exam conditions but vital in clinic.

○ Date of test

○ Hospital/NHS number (if known)

- Explains procedure and obtains consent   (0–2)
- Assembles and inserts speculum correctly   (1)
- Uses Aylesbury spatula (not blunt ended):   (0–2)
  ○ Rotates spatula through 360°
- Removes speculum correctly   (1)
- Wipes both sides of spatula onto slide   (1)
- Fixes slide with fixative   (1)

It is difficult to remember that a model should be spoken to as if she were a real woman. Most OSCE questions award marks for the communication part of the vaginal examination. It is therefore vital that the student practises this acting technique with a model and a critical observer before the examination.

19.2 a, c

All women with a single cervical smear showing mild/moderate/severe dyskaryosis should be referred to colposcopy. Colposcopy with a cervical biopsy is essential for an accurate diagnosis of the degree of cervical intraepithelial neoplasia (CIN). The correlation between the degree of dyskaryosis and CIN is not strong and so cervical screening does not give an accurate diagnosis. The guideline for the referral of mild dyskaryosis has recently been updated. The previous practice of repeating the smear after 6 months and referring to colposcopy if the smear is abnormal again has been changed such that all these women should be referred for colposcopy. Additionally if a woman has three abnormal smears in the preceding 5 years which may not have been consecutive, she should be referred for colposcopy if she has not already been seen. In pregnancy the cervical smear is more likely to give a false-positive result than a negative result.

19.3 d, b, e, a, c

It is important that 4% acetic acid be painted onto the cervix before staining with iodine because the density of the white staining and the rapidity of change give an idea of the degree of abnormality whereas iodine shows only the area of abnormality. A biopsy should be taken before undertaking treatment to give an accurate histological diagnosis. The loop diathermy can distort the histology result due to heat artefact.

19.4

1 Not all women attend for cervical screening.

2 There will be false negatives (inadequate sampling/misinterpretation of the slide by a cytopathologist/glandular abnormality).

3 The infrequency of screening may miss a rapidly progressive case.

4 Treatment may be incorrectly given.

5 Treatment may not be adequate (full excision may not be achieved/reported on histology).

6 Recurrences may occur even if treatment was initially effective.

19.5

1 GPs keep a computerized register of all patients by age and sex.

2 The computer generates automatic letters of recall every 3 years for all women between the ages of 20 and 64.

3 Results are sent to the woman and her GP regardless of where the test was taken.

4 GPs are rewarded financially for achieving a >85% uptake of the programme.

5 Smear tests are offered in a variety of community and hospital-based clinics.

Chapter 20

20.1 b, d

Ovarian cancer is now the most common gynaecological malignancy (breast cancer is not classified as a gynaecological malignancy) and carries the poorest prognosis because most cases present with stage 3. Cervical carcinoma most commonly presents with postcoital bleeding whereas endometrial cancer presents with postmenopausal bleeding. Ovarian cancer remains asymptomatic until late in the disease when women usually present with a pelvic mass and/or ascites.

20.2 a, c, d

This woman has carcinoma of the cervix until proved otherwise. Staging for cervical carcinoma includes:

- Examination under anaesthetic (including rectovaginal examination to assess the size of the tumour, parametrial spread, extension into the rectovagina; septum).

- Cystoscopy and sigmoidoscopy to assess bladder and bowel involvement.
- Biopsy of the suspicious area.
- Chest X-ray.
- IVU.

CT or MRI may be offered if available to give further information on tumour size nodal involvement but does not alter the FIGO staging, which is determined by the above investigations.

20.3 a

Carcinoma of the uterus and cervix nearly always present with vaginal bleeding. Stage 1 cancer of the ovary usually presents with a mobile mass which is rarely palpable per abdomen because ovarian cancer often spreads beyond the ovary at diameters <10 cm. Stage 4 ovarian cancer can be diagnosed clinically only if there are palpable supraclavicular glands, a pleural effusion or a palpable liver edge—all of these are rare. The most common stage of ovarian carcinoma at presentation is stage 3.

20.4 b, c, d

A hysteroscopy and curettage is not helpful in ovarian carcinoma but essential in the staging and diagnosis of uterine and cervical carcinoma. Although urea and electrolytes are essential preoperative tests they are not useful in the staging of ovarian cancer. Imaging of the chest, abdomen and pelvis should confirm the stage of the disease before surgery, giving the surgeon and the patient useful information about the nature of the proposed surgery and its likely success. Together with the medical oncologists a plan for postoperative chemotherapy can be drawn up and the patient made fully aware of what is in store before major surgery.

20.5 a, c

This woman has vulval carcinoma until proven otherwise. A careful examination of her vulva will reveal an ulcerated area that is probably secondarily infected. A swab and a biopsy should be taken from the ulcerated area. A high vaginal swab, cervical smear and hysteroscopy are unlikely to be informative. Abdominal palpation is indicated to detect enlarged inguinal nodes.

Chapter 21

21.1 Marking scheme:

1 Oestrogen only	(1)
2 Ideally till the age of 55 or a minimum of 2 years	(1)
3 Minimal side effects, transient breast tenderness and abdominal bloating	(1)
4 Can take orally, transdermally or by implant every 6 months	(1)
5 Main benefit is long-term reduction in risk of osteoporosis	(1)
6 Long-term increased risk of breast cancer particularly after 5 years	(1)

General ability to discuss with the patient, ability to give accurate information, reassures the patient, appreciates her concerns and helps her make a decision (0–4)

21.2 a, e

Endometrial polyps are a common cause of postmenopausal vaginal bleeding. Atrophic vaginitis may spontaneously bleed but this is more common after sexual intercourse. It is also rare in women who are on HRT because they do not get vaginal dryness. Subserosal fibroids usually become inactive following the menopause even in women on HRT. Ovarian cancer virtually never presents with vaginal bleeding whilst cervical cancer often does.

21.3

- Inspection of vulva and vagina to check for vulval ulceration. Urethral caruncle, atrophic vaginitis (unlikely in this woman).
- Speculum examination of the cervix; to exclude cervical polyp, ectropion or frank carcinoma.
- Cervical smear: to detect carcinoma *in situ* or cervical dysplasia.
- Bimanual vaginal examination: to exclude uterine enlargement.
- Transvaginal ultrasound scan: to check for endometrial abnormalities including polyps.
- Endometrial biopsy: to ensure that the histology of the endometrium is normal.
- Hysteroscopy and biopsy if transvaginal scan is abnormal or equivocal.

Chapter 22

22.1 Marking scheme:
- Introduction, name and age of patient (1)
- Identifying main complaint accurately (1)
- History taking
- Leaking when coughing/exercising
- Nocturia
- Symptoms of prolapse
- Disruption to life } (0–4)
- Past obstetric history
- Past gynaecological history
- Family history
- Social history } (0–4)

22.2
- Abdominal palpation to check for masses.
- Vaginal examination: dorsal initially to check for descent and the size of the uterus and presence of any pelvic masses.
- Place her in Sim's position. Ask her to cough. Note presence or absence of cystourethrocoele and uterine descent. Note any urinary leaking.
- Management: her symptoms are suggestive of genuine stress incontinence. She requires urodynamic assessment with video cystourethrography before deciding on treatment. While awaiting this she should be referred to the physiotherapists for pelvic floor exercises, including voluntary retention of vaginal cones. If urodynamics confirm a diagnosis of GSI (genuine stress incontinence) a retropubic or vaginal sling operation will give her the best chance of cure rather than a vaginal colporraphy.

22.3 Any five of the following:
1 Urinary tract infection
2 Local infection
3 Primary or secondary haemorrhage
4 Urinary retention
5 Dyspareunia/vaginal stenosis
6 Venous thrombosis
7 Vaginal discharge
8 Chest infection
9 Fistula formation.

22.4 An involuntary loss of urine from the urethra when the transmitted intra-abdominal pressure causes a rise in the intravesical pressure, which exceeds the intraurethral pressure in the absence of a detrusor contraction.

22.5 a, d, e

Incomplete emptying and a slow urinary stream are more often associated with overflow incontinence. Frequency and urgency are the most common symptoms of detrusor instability but are not specific enough to establish the diagnosis without urodynamic investigation.

Chapter 23

23.1
1 Total birth rate = births per year 1000 midyear population.
2 General fertility rate = births per year 1000 women aged 15–45.
3 Maternal mortality: deaths of women while pregnant or within 42 days of delivery, miscarriage, termination of pregnancy, from any cause related to or aggravated by the pregnancy or its management but not from accidental or incidental causes.
4 Maternal mortality rate = no. of maternal deaths/1000 births or 100000 maternities.
5 Perinatal mortality rate = total of stillbirths deaths in the first 7 days of life >24 weeks of gestation/1000 births.

23.2 Hypertensive disease of pregnancy, thromboembolism, haemorrhage.

23.3 Introduction of evidence-based guidelines, incident reporting and investigation, regular audit.

23.4 Place of residence, past nutrition and diseases, education, social class, age and parity.

23.5 Full blood count, fasting blood sugar and HbA1c, Kleihauer's test, clotting studies, lupus anticoagulant and anticardiolipin antibodies, Liver function tests, postmortem examination, fetal karyotyping, X-ray or MRI of the baby if postmortem examination declined.

Appendix

Additional reading

Newell S & Darling J (2007) *Lecture Notes on Paediatrics*, 7th edn. Oxford: Blackwell Publishing.

Confidential Enquiry into Maternal Deaths—Saving Mothers Lives 2003–5. (ISBN 978-0-95335368-2)

Confidential enquiry into stillbirth and death in infancy (CESDI) 2000–2

Healthcare Commission (2008) Towards better births: a review of maternity services in England

Websites and relevant published guidelines

NICE guidelines: www.nice.org.uk

- Caesarean section
- Osteoporosis
- Assessment and treatment of fertility
- Electronic fetal monitoring
- Induction of labour
- Anti-D immunoglobulin for Rh prophylaxis
- Confidential enquiry into maternal and child health
- Intrapartum care
- Antenatal care
- Postnatal care

RCOG guidelines 1999–2002: www.rcog.org/guidelines

- Male and female sterilization
- Antenatal corticosteroids
- Gestational trophoblastic disease
- Alcohol consumption in pregnancy
- Amniocentesis
- Anti-D immunoglobulin for Rh prophylaxis
- Breast cancer (pregnancy after)
- Breech presentation (management)
- Chickenpox in pregnancy
- Early pregnancy loss: management
- Eclampsia (management)
- Endometriosis (investigation and management)
- Genital herpes in pregnancy
- HRT and venous thromboembolism
- Instrumental vaginal delivery
- Pelvimetry: clinical indications
- Perineal repair
- Peritoneal closure
- Placenta praevia: diagnosis and management
- Recurrent miscarriage: management
- Small for gestational age fetus: investigation and management
- Third- and fourth-degree perineal tears following vaginal delivery: management
- Thromboembolic disease in pregnancy and the puerperium
- Tocolytic drugs for women in preterm labour
- Tubal pregnancies

Index

Page numbers in *italics* represent figures, those in **bold** represent tables